FAQs in
DIABETES, ENDOCRINOLOGY AND METABOLISM

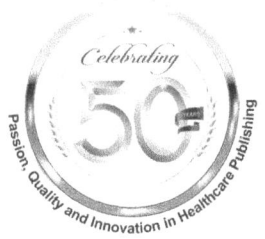

FAQs in
DIABETES, ENDOCRINOLOGY AND METABOLISM

M Saifuddin
MBBS (DMC) FCPS (Medicine) MD (Endocrinology)
FACE (USA) FACP (USA) FRSM (UK)
Training in Advance Endocrinology
(Singapore, MAYO Clinic USA)
Fellowship Training
(Harvard Medical School, Massachusetts General Hospital)
Assistant Professor
Department of Endocrinology
Dhaka Medical College
Dhaka, Bangladesh

Foreword

Md Faruque Pathan

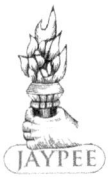

JAYPEE BROTHERS MEDICAL PUBLISHERS
The Health Sciences Publisher
New Delhi | London | Panama

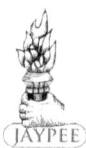 **Jaypee Brothers Medical Publishers (P) Ltd.**

Headquarters
Jaypee Brothers Medical Publishers (P) Ltd
4838/24, Ansari Road, Daryaganj
New Delhi 110 002, India
Phone: +91-11-43574357
Fax: +91-11-43574314
Email: jaypee@jaypeebrothers.com

Overseas Offices

J.P. Medical Ltd
83 Victoria Street, London
SW1H 0HW (UK)
Phone: +44 20 3170 8910
Fax: +44 (0)20 3008 6180
Email: info@jpmedpub.com

Jaypee-Highlights Medical Publishers Inc
City of Knowledge, Bld. 235, 2nd Floor
Clayton, Panama City, Panama
Phone: +1 507-301-0496
Fax: +1 507-301-0499
Email: cservice@jphmedical.com

Jaypee Brothers Medical Publishers (P) Ltd
Bhotahity, Kathmandu, Nepal
Phone: +977-9741283608
Email: kathmandu@jaypeebrothers.com

Website: www.jaypeebrothers.com
Website: www.jaypeedigital.com

© 2019, Jaypee Brothers Medical Publishers

The views and opinions expressed in this book are solely those of the original contributor(s)/author(s) and do not necessarily represent those of editor(s) of the book.

All rights reserved. No part of this publication may be reproduced, stored or transmitted in any form or by any means, electronic, mechanical, photocopying, recording or otherwise, without the prior permission in writing of the publishers.

All brand names and product names used in this book are trade names, service marks, trademarks or registered trademarks of their respective owners. The publisher is not associated with any product or vendor mentioned in this book.

Medical knowledge and practice change constantly. This book is designed to provide accurate, authoritative information about the subject matter in question. However, readers are advised to check the most current information available on procedures included and check information from the manufacturer of each product to be administered, to verify the recommended dose, formula, method and duration of administration, adverse effects and contraindications. It is the responsibility of the practitioner to take all appropriate safety precautions. Neither the publisher nor the author(s)/editor(s) assume any liability for any injury and/or damage to persons or property arising from or related to use of material in this book.

This book is sold on the understanding that the publisher is not engaged in providing professional medical services. If such advice or services are required, the services of a competent medical professional should be sought.

Every effort has been made where necessary to contact holders of copyright to obtain permission to reproduce copyright material. If any have been inadvertently overlooked, the publisher will be pleased to make the necessary arrangements at the first opportunity. The **CD/DVD-ROM** (if any) provided in the sealed envelope with this book is complimentary and free of cost. **Not meant for sale.**

Inquiries for bulk sales may be solicited at: jaypee@jaypeebrothers.com

FAQs in Diabetes, Endocrinology and Metabolism

First Edition: **2019**

ISBN: 978-93-5270-617-4

Dedicated to

My father for endless love
My mother for continuous care
Momotaj Begum for love and care
Zaima Saif and Zahin Saif for innocent love.

Foreword

It is a great pleasure and honor for me to write the foreword for *FAQs in Diabetes, Endocrinology and Metabolism* by M Saifuddin. This book is written in very easy and simple manner in questions and answers format. The author is one of the renowned Endocrinologist of Bangladesh and very young and dedicated to the field of Endocrinology. Students of undergraduate and postgraduate level will be very beneficial with the book. Sometimes, it is not very easy to describe a topic in a simple way, but the author did it very successfully.

Lastly, thanks to the author to let me to write the foreword of the book. May Almighty bless him.

Md Faruque Pathan
Professor and Head
Department of Endocrinology
BIRDEM General Hospital and Ibrahim Medical College
Dhaka, Bangladesh

Preface

With blessings of the Almighty, it become possible to bring out the first edition of *FAQs in Diabetes, Endocrinology and Metabolism*. When I was a postgraduate student of Endocrinology, I always feel for a book that have all the information necessary to pass in the examination and written in very easy and simple manner in questions and answers form. That feelings step me forward to write this book. For a physician like me it is very difficult to write a medical book, as we are very busy all over days with a morning at Government Medical College and evening at private practice. It takes around five long years to complete the script. The book is in questions and answers format, very easy and comfortable to read.

I have collected written, objective structured practical examination (OSPE) and other format Endocrinology questions from different undergraduate and postgraduate institutes and try to solve every question in the book. I have updated the contents of the book as per all the latest guidelines by various endocrine organizations all over the world, especially American Association of Clinical Endocrinologists (AACE) guidelines, American Diabetes Association (ADA), European Association for the Study of Diabetes (EASD), American Thyroid Association (ATA) guideline, also other organizations of the world. I must acknowledge to all the authors of the guidelines, position statements, also acknowledge to all the authors and publishers of reference books mentioned in the Bibliography. I hope this will be usable for students, as they will get easy and comfortable arrangement of all the endocrine questions.

M Saifuddin

Acknowledgments

I must acknowledge my teachers, colleague doctors and students who helped endlessly to write down the book.

- Professor Md Faruque Pathan, Professor (Endocrinology), BIRDEM
- Professor Zafar A Latif, Professor (Endocrinology), BIRDEM
- Professor Hajera Mahtab, BIRDEM
- Professor AK Azad Khan, BIRDEM
- Dr Shahjada Selim, Assistant Professor (Endocrinology), BSMMU
- Professor SM Ashrafuzzaman, Professor (Endocrinology), BIRDEM
- Professor Hossain Shahid Ferdous, Professor (Endocrinology), Popular Medical College
- Professor Tofail Ahmed, Professor (Endocrinology), BIRDEM
- Dr Mohammod Feroz Amin, Associate Professor (Endocrinology), BIRDEM
- Professor M Fariduddin, Professor (Endocrinology), BSMMU
- Professor MA Hasanat, Professor (Endocrinology), BSMMU
- Professor Md Abdul Mannan, Professor (Endocrinology), Anwer Khan Modern Medical College
- Professor MA Jalil Ansari, Professor (Endocrinology), Dhaka Medical College
- Professor Laique Ahmed Khan, Retired Professor (Endocrinology), Rangpur Medical College
- Professor Abdus Saleque Mollah, Retired Professor (Endocrinology), Chittagong Medical College
- Professor Md Nazrul Islam Siddiqui, Professor (Endocrinology), Mymensingh Medical College
- Muhammad Hafizur Rahman, Professor (Endocrinology), Dhaka Medical College
- Dr Indrajit Prasad, Associate Professor (Endocrinology), Dhaka Medical College
- Dr Ajit Kumar Paul, Associate Professor (Endocrinology), Mainamati Medical College
- Professor Nizamul Karim Khan, Retired Professor (Endocrinology), Mymensingh Medical College
- Dr Mir Mosarraf Hossain, Associate Professor (Endocrinology), Sir Salimullah Medical College
- Dr AHM Aktaruzzaman, Associate Professor (Endocrinology), NITOR
- Dr Samir Kumar Talukder, Associate Professor (Endocrinology), Rangpur Medical College
- Dr Md Shah Emran, Assistant Professor (Endocrinology), Sylhet Medical College
- Dr Farhana Aktar, Assistant Professor (Endocrinology), Chittagong Medical College
- Dr Tanjina Hossain, Assistant Professor (Endocrinology), Green Life Medical College
- Dr Abul Bashar Mohammad Kamrul Hasan, Endocrinologist, Mymensingh Medical College

- Dr Imtiaj Mahbub, Assistant Professor (Endocrinology), Rajshahi Medical College
- Dr Debasish Kumar Ghosh, Assistant Professor (Endocrinology), Khulna Medical College
- Dr Faria Afsana, Assistant Professor (Endocrinology), BIRDEM
- Dr Sultana Marufa Shefin, Assistant Professor (Endocrinology), BIRDEM
- Dr Md Qamrul Hassan, Assistant Professor (Endocrinology), Rangpur Medical College
- Dr Taaniyah Haq, Assistant Professor (Endocrinology), BSMMU
- Dr Abul Kalam Mohammad Aminul Islam, Assistant Professor (Endocrinology), Colonel Malek Medical College, Manikganj
- Dr Md Anwar Hossain, Assistant Professor (Endocrinology), Shahid Syed Nazrul Islam Medical College, Kishoreganj
- Dr Rushda Sarmin Binte Rouf, Endocrinologist, BIRDEM
- Dr Yasmin Aktar Khan, Consultant Endocrinologist, Bangladesh Medical College
- Drs Kazi Ali Hassan, Noor-E-Nazneen and Shah Alam
- Drs Md Shahinur Rahman, Mohammad Abdul Hannan (Tareq) and Mohammad Ripon
- Drs Sharmin Jahan, Ahsanul Haq Amin and Marufa Mustari
- Drs Nazmul Kabir Qureshi, Md Abu-jar Gaffar and Mohammad Rafiq Uddin
- Drs Mohammad Atiqur Rahman, Mashfiqul Hasan and ATM Jabed Hasan
- Drs Mohammed Mahboob Iftekhar and Ahmed Salam Mir.

I am also grateful to Shri Jitendar P Vij (Group Chairman), Mr Ankit Vij (Managing Director) and Ms Chetna Malhotra Vohra (Associate Director—Content Strategy) of M/s Jaypee Brothers Medical Publishers (P) Ltd, New Delhi, India, for continuous inspiration to write this book. Last but not the least, gratitude to my wife and kids for endless love and care all the time.

Contents

Section 1 DIABETES

1. Definition, Diagnosis, and Classification of Diabetes Mellitus — 3
2. Pathogenesis of Diabetes Mellitus — 13
3. Fibrocalculous Pancreatic Diabetes — 20
4. Exercise in Diabetes Mellitus — 25
5. Oral Antidiabetic Drugs — 30
6. Insulin — 39
7. Hypoglycemia — 51
8. Diabetic Ketoacidosis and Hyperosmolar Nonketotic Coma — 57
9. Diabetic Retinopathy — 64
10. Diabetic Nephropathy — 69
11. Diabetic Neuropathy — 80
12. Diabetic Foot — 86
13. Dyslipidemia in Diabetes Mellitus — 92
14. Preconceptional Care in Diabetic Patients — 99
15. Gestational Diabetes Mellitus — 101
16. Diabetes Mellitus and Surgery — 105
17. Diabetes Mellitus and Ramadan — 108
18. Sick-day Management of Diabetic Patients — 112
19. Skin Manifestation of Diabetes Mellitus — 114
20. Prevention of Diabetes Mellitus — 116

Section 2 ENDOCRINOLOGY

A. Pituitary and Hypothalamic Disorders

21. Hypopituitarism — 121
22. Pituitary Adenoma — 126
23. Acromegaly — 133
24. Prolactinoma — 141
25. Diabetes Insipidus — 148
26. Short Stature — 152

B. Thyroid Disorders

27. Thyrotoxicosis — 159
28. Hypothyroidism — 177
29. Thyroid Nodules — 188
30. Thyroid Neoplasm — 192

C. Bone and Mineral Disorders

31. Hypercalcemia — 198
32. Hypocalcemia — 205
33. Osteoporosis — 211

D. Adrenal Disorders

34. Incidental Adrenal Mass — 221
35. Cushing Syndrome — 223
36. Adrenocortical Insufficiency — 236
37. Judicious Use of Glucocorticoid — 246
38. Endocrine Hypertension — 250
39. Pheochromocytoma — 256
40. Congenital Adrenal Hyperplasia — 266

E. Reproductive Endocrinology

41. Puberty	271
42. Male Hypogonadism	279
43. Male Infertility	289
44. Gynecomastia	298
45. Erectile Dysfunction	301
46. Hirsutism	307
47. Polycystic Ovarian Syndrome	309
48. Female Infertility	314
49. Amenorrhea	324
50. Menopause	330
51. Precocious Puberty	335
52. Miscellaneous Endocrine Disorders	337

Section 3 METABOLISM

53. Spontaneous Hypoglycemia	343
54. Homocystinuria	346
55. Phenylketonuria	347
56. Obesity	348
57. Alkaptonuria	351
58. Glycogen Storage Disease	352
59. Lysosomal Storage Disease	353
60. Galactosemia	354
61. Wilson Disease	355
62. Hemochromatosis	356

63. Acute Intermittent Porphyria — 357

64. Renal Tubular Acidosis — 359

65. Hypomagnesemia — 361

66. Nonalcoholic Fatty Liver Disease — 362

67. Gout — 364

Bibliography — *367*

Index — *369*

SECTION 1

DIABETES

1. Definition, Diagnosis, and Classification of Diabetes Mellitus
2. Pathogenesis of Diabetes Mellitus
3. Fibrocalculous Pancreatic Diabetes
4. Exercise in Diabetes Mellitus
5. Oral Antidiabetic Drugs
6. Insulin
7. Hypoglycemia
8. Diabetic Ketoacidosis and Hyperosmolar Nonketotic Coma
9. Diabetic Retinopathy
10. Diabetic Nephropathy
11. Diabetic Neuropathy
12. Diabetic Foot
13. Dyslipidemia in Diabetes Mellitus
14. Preconceptional Care in Diabetic Patients
15. Gestational Diabetes Mellitus
16. Diabetes Mellitus and Surgery
17. Diabetes Mellitus and Ramadan
18. Sick-day Management of Diabetic Patients
19. Skin Manifestation of Diabetes Mellitus
20. Prevention of Diabetes Mellitus

CHAPTER 1

Definition, Diagnosis, and Classification of Diabetes Mellitus

Q. Define diabetes mellitus (DM).

Ans. Diabetes mellitus (DM) is a metabolic disorder characterized by chronic/persistent hyperglycemia together with disturbances of carbohydrate, protein, and fat metabolism resulting from defects of insulin secretion, insulin action, or both associated with long-term damage, dysfunction, and failure of different organs, for example, eyes, kidneys, nerves, and blood vessels.

Q. Classify diabetes mellitus etiologically.

Ans.

- **Type 1 diabetes:** β-cell destruction usually leading to absolute insulin deficiency
  - Autoimmune
  - Idiopathic
- **Type 2 diabetes:** Range from predominantly insulin resistance with relative insulin deficiency to predominantly secretory defect with insulin resistance
- **Other specific types:**
  - **Genetic defects of β-cell function:**
    - Chromosome 20, hepatocyte nuclear factor (HNF)-4α maturity onset diabetes of the young 1 (MODY 1)
    - Chromosome 7, glucokinase (MODY 2)
    - Chromosome 12, HNF-1α (MODY 3)
    - Chromosome 13, insulin promoter factor-1 (MODY 4)
    - Chromosome 17, HNF-1β (MODY 5)
    - Mitochondrial DNA mutation
  - **Genetic defects of insulin action:**
    - Type A insulin resistance
    - Lipoatrophic diabetes
  - **Disease of exocrine pancreas:**
    - Fibrocalculous pancreatic disease
    - Chronic or recurrent pancreatitis
    - Hemochromatosis
    - Trauma/pancreatectomy

- Neoplasia
- Cystic fibrosis
– **Endocrinopathies:**
  - Cushing syndrome
  - Acromegaly
  - Thyrotoxicosis
  - Glucagonoma
  - Pheochromocytoma
– **Drug or chemical induced:**
  - Glucocorticoids
  - Thiazide diuretics
  - Phenytoin
  - Pentamidine
  - Diazoxide
  - Nicotinic acid
  - Thyroid hormones
– **Infections:**
  - Congenital rubella
  - Cytomegalovirus (CMV)
  - Mumps
  - Coxsackie B
– **Other genetic syndromes associated with diabetes:**
  - Down syndrome
  - Turner syndrome
  - Klinefelter syndrome
  - Friedreich ataxia
  - Myotonic dystrophy
  - Wolfram syndrome/DIDMOAD (DI, DM, OA, nerve deafness)
  - Prader-Willi syndrome
  - Laurence-Moon-Bardet-Biedl syndrome
- **Gestational DM.**

Q. Mention precaution about interpretation of measured glucose.

Ans.
- Blood glucose in mmol/L × 18 = mg/dL
- Red blood cells (RBCs) continue to metabolize/glycolysis glucose after blood collection, thus ↓ in glucose level. Avoided by rapid centrifugation, plasma separated, and frozen until estimation
- Whole blood glucose concentration is 12%–15% lower than plasma concentration
- Venous glucose is similar to arterial and capillary level when fasting
- After meal, venous glucose concentration is 10% lower than arterial concentration
- If patient has IV line, blood should be drawn from opposite arm to prevent mixing with infusion.

Chapter 1: Definition, Diagnosis, and Classification of Diabetes Mellitus

Q. Mention criteria for diagnosis of DM.

Ans. According to American Diabetic Association:
- Fasting plasma glucose (FPG) ≥7 mmol/L. Fasting is defined as no calorie intake for ≥8 h

  Or
- Two-hour plasma glucose ≥11.1 mmol/L during oral glucose tolerance test (OGTT) as described by WHO using a glucose load containing equivalent of 75 g anhydrous glucose dissolved in water

  Or
- HbA_1C ≥6.5. The test should be performed in a laboratory using a method that is NGSP (National Glycohemoglobin Standardization Program) certified and standardized to DCCT (Diabetes Control and Complication Trial) assay

  Or
- In patient with classic symptoms of hyperglycemia or hyperglycemic crisis, random blood sugar ≥11.1 mmol/L.

(In absence of unequivocal hyperglycemia, result should be confirmed by repeat testing).

Q. Discuss about oral glucose tolerance test (OGTT).

Ans. OGTT is most reliable method to determine glucose tolerance status.
- **Procedure:**
  - Unrestricted carbohydrate diet containing ≥150 g carbohydrate daily for at least previous 3 days
  - The test should begin in the morning after 8–14 h of overnight fast
  - FPG measured
  - An oral glucose load of 75 g for adult or 1.75 g/kg body weight up to maximum 75 g for children is given in 250–300 mL water. The drink must be completed within 5 min
  - A second sample is collected at 120th minute after glucose drink
  - If glucose is not estimated immediately, blood sample may be preserved with sodium fluoride (6 mg/mL whole blood, it inhibit glucose metabolism by RBC). Blood should be centrifuged and plasma separated and frozen until estimation
  - Smoking, tea, or physical stress is not allowed and person should remain seated during the test
- **Importance of OGTT:**
  - OGTT is only means to identify people with impaired glucose tolerance (IGT)
  - FPG alone fails to diagnose approximately 30% of DM
  - OGTT is needed to confirm or exclude any abnormality of glucose tolerance in asymptomatic person
  - A person of normal fasting glucose or impaired fasting glucose (IFG) if subjected to OGTT may be found as diabetic or IGT
  - OGTT should be done in individuals with FPG 5.6–6.9 mmol/L, RBS 7.8–11 mmol/L, or HbA_1C 5.7%–6.4%

- **Interpretation:** Venous plasma glucose in mmol/L

	Fasting	2-h after glucose load
Diabetic	≥7 or	≥11.1
IGT	<7 and	7.8–11
IFG	5.6–6.9 and	<7.8

Q. Discuss about prediabetes/intermediate hyperglycemia.

Ans. Person at increased risk of diabetes.
- **Categories of prediabetes:**
  - IFG: FPG 5.6–6.9 mmol/L
    OR
  - IGT: 2-h plasma glucose 7.8–11.0 mmol/L during OGTT
    OR
  - HbA_1C 5.7%–6.4%
- **Importance:**
  - High risk in future to develop DM
  - Risk factor for cardiovascular disease (CVD)
  - Associated with obesity (especially abdominal or visceral obesity), dyslipidemia with high triglyceride (TG), low HDL cholesterol, and hypertension (HTN)
- **Management:**
  - Monitored annually with OGTT, HbA_1C
  - Other cardiovascular risk factors should be identified and treated accordingly
  - Metformin should be considered for prevention of type 2 DM in person with prediabetes, especially those with BMI ≥35 kg/m², age <60 years, women with prior gestational diabetes mellitus (GDM), or those with rising HbA_1C despite lifestyle intervention.

Q. What is stress diabetes?

Ans. In some people, abnormal blood glucose result is observed under conditions which impose burden on pancreatic β cell, for example, during infection, MI, or other severe stress. This stress hyperglycemia usually disappears after acute illness resolved. OGTT should be done after recovery from acute illness.

Q. Mention criteria for testing for diabetes or prediabetes in asymptomatic adults.

Ans.
- Testing should be considered in overweight or obese (BMI ≥25 or ≥23 kg/m² in Asian) adults who have one or more of the following risk factors:
  - IFG, IGT, or HbA_1C ≥5.7% on previous testing
  - First degree relative with diabetes
  - Women with prior GDM
  - History of CVD
  - Hypertension (≥140/90 mm Hg or on therapy for hypertension)
  - HDL cholesterol level <35 mg/dL and/or triglyceride level >250 mg/dL

- Women with polycystic ovarian syndrome (PCOS)
- Physical inactivity
- Other clinical conditions associated with insulin resistance (e.g. severe obesity, acanthosis nigricans)
- For all patients, testing should begin at age 45 years
- If results are normal, testing should be repeated at 3-year intervals with consideration of more frequent testing depending on initial results (e.g. those with prediabetes should be tested yearly) and risk status.

Q. **Mention criteria for testing for type 2 diabetes or prediabetes in asymptomatic children ($\leq$18 years).**

Ans.
- Overweight (BMI >85th percentile for age and sex, weight for height >85th percentile, or weight >120% of ideal for height) plus any two of the following risk factors:
  - Family history of type 2 diabetes in first or second degree relative
  - Signs of insulin resistance or conditions associated with insulin resistance (acanthosis nigricans, hypertension, dyslipidemia, PCOS, or small for gestational age birth weight)
  - Maternal history of diabetes or GDM during the child's gestation
- Age of initiation: Age 10 years or at onset of puberty, if puberty occurs at a younger age
- Frequency: Every 3 years.

Q. **What are the goals of treatment of DM?**

Ans.

1. **In adults:**
   - Plasma glucose:
     - Fasting/preprandial: 4.4–7.2 mmol/L
     - 2-h postmeal/peak postprandial: <10 mmol/L
     - In hospitalized patients: 7.8–10 mmol/L in critically ill and noncritically ill patients
     - Blood glucose and HbA_1C goals for children and adolescents with type 1 diabetes: Goals should be individualized and lower goals may be reasonable based on risk–benefit assessment

Before meals (mmol/L)	Bedtime/overnight (mmol/L)	HbA_1C
5.0–7.2	5.0–8.3	<7.5%. A lower goal (<7%) is reasonable if it can be achieved without excessive hypoglycemia

   - HbA_1C: <7%
     - More stringent goal (HbA_1C <6.5%) in selected patients if this can be achieved without significant hypoglycemia includes those with short duration of diabetes,

type 2 diabetes treated with lifestyle or metformin only, long-life expectancy or no significant CVD
- Less stringent goal (HbA$_1$C <8%) in selected patients includes elderly (above 55 years, blood glucose target may be relaxed adding 1.1 mmol/L for each decade), history of severe or recurrent hypoglycemia, hypoglycemic unawareness, advanced microvascular or macrovascular complications, extensive comorbid conditions, limited life expectancy, or long standing diabetes in whom the goal is difficult to achieve with multiple glucose lowering agents, including insulin
- Fasting lipid profile:
  - Total cholesterol: <200 mg/dL
  - LDL cholesterol: <100 or <70 mg/dL with H/o CVD or 30% reduction regardless of baseline LDL
  - HDL cholesterol: >40 (M), >50 mg/dL (F)
  - TG: <150 mg/dL
- BMI: <25 kg/m^2 (for Asian recent recommendation <23 kg/m^2)
- Waist circumference: <90 cm (M), <80 cm (F)
- BP:
  - Less than 140/90 mm Hg
  - Less than 130/80 mm Hg if high risk of CVD, albuminuria, or CKD (estimated glomerular filtration rate (eGFR) <60 mL/min/1.73 m^2)
  - GDM: 120–160/80–105 mm Hg
- Target of diabetic education: teaching, training, and empowerment of patient to take part in treatment plan
- Stop smoking and tobacco intake in any form
- Avoid alcohol.

Q. Discuss about glycated hemoglobin.

Ans.

- Hemoglobin react spontaneously with glucose to form glycated derivatives in a non-enzymatic manner, the extent of which is determined by concentration of glucose in blood
- β chain of hemoglobin A$_0$ react with glucose to form HbA$_1$C (Amadori product)
- Other compounds results from similar reactions of α and β chains of Hb and these can be measured as total glycated Hb
- The test should be performed in a laboratory using a method that is NGSP certified and standardized to DCCT assay.
- **Use:**
  - HbA$_1$C serves as a retrospective indicator of average glucose concentration over previous 6–8 weeks. 50% of variance of HbA$_1$C is determined by average blood glucose concentration over last 30 days, 25% by concentration over last 30–60 days, and remaining 25% by concentration over last 60–120 days. 1% rise of HbA$_1$C corresponds to average increase of 2 mmol/L of blood glucose

- HbA₁C has strong predictive value for diabetes complications
- HbA₁C can be used for diagnosis of DM that has greater convenience (fasting not required), greater preanalytical stability, and less day-to-day variation during stress and illness
- HbA₁C also serves as a check of accuracy of patient's glucometer

- **Limitation:**
  - Greater cost, limited availability of HbA₁C testing in certain regions of developing world, and imperfect correlation between HbA₁C and average glucose in certain individuals
  - HbA₁C does not provide a measure of glycemic variability or hypoglycemia
  - Condition that affect erythrocyte turnover (e.g. hemolysis and Hb variant) can affect HbA₁C. Some conditions that affect measurement of HbA₁C are:
    - IDA ↓
    - Pregnancy ↓
    - Hemoglobinopathies
    - Hemodialysis
    - Erythropoietin therapy
    - Recent blood loss or transfusion
    - Polycythemia

- **Recommendation:**
  - Perform HbA₁C test at least two times a year in patients who are meeting treatment goals and who have stable glycemic control
  - Perform HbA₁C test quarterly in patients whose therapy has changed or who are not meeting glycemic goals

- **Relation of HbA₁C with estimated average glucose(eAG):**

HbA₁C (%)	eAG (mmol/L)
5	5.4
6	7.0
7	8.6
8	10.2
9	11.8
10	13.4
11	14.9
12	16.5

Q. What is fructosamine?

Ans. Albumin contains free amino groups which can react nonenzymatically with glucose to from fructosamine.

- **Advantage:** Fructosamine reflect glucose level over previous 1–3 weeks, remain useful in a number of circumstances, for example, in pregnancy or preconception period where motivation to improve control is high and changes can be evaluated at shorter intervals
- **Disadvantages:**
  - Markedly affect by excessive turnover or excretion of albumin, for example, renal disease
  - Not standardized in the same way as HbA_1C
  - Linkage of fructosamine to average glucose and prognostic significance is not clear as for HbA_1C.

Q. What is brittle diabetes?

Ans. Diabetic individuals whose life is constantly being disrupted by episodes of hypo- or hyperglycemia whatever the cause despite the best attempts of the physician and healthcare team.
- **Etiology:**
  - Erratic eating pattern, for example, in children/eating disorder
  - Irregular lifestyle
  - Unrecognized other endocrine disorder that alter glucose metabolism. For example, Addison disease, Cushing syndrome, or pheochromocytoma
  - Psychological/behavioral disorder or personality disorder
  - Substance misuse or dependence
  - Errors in oral antidiabetics (OAD) or insulin dose/schedule/administration
  - Poorly designed insulin regimen
  - Lipodystrophy at injection sites causing variable insulin absorption
  - Gastroparesis due to autonomic neuropathy
  - Factitious/malingering (need for increased attention)
  - Insulin resistance: at cellular receptor or postreceptor level
- **Evaluation:**
  - Insulin challenge test: Short acting regular insulin 0.1-U/kg administered SC and IV
  - Normal response: ↓ blood glucose level >95 (SC) and >62 mg/dL (IV)
  - If normal response: assess eating pattern, lifestyle, compliance with prescribed regimen, gastric motility, psychological evaluation of patient
  - If abnormal response: Abnormalities of insulin absorption, intracompartmental transfer, receptor or postreceptor function
- **Management:**
  - Patient education regarding OAD/insulin dose, insulin injection technique, dose adjustment
  - Regular meal in correct time, amount, and composition
  - Healthy lifestyle with regular exercise.

Q. Mention components of comprehensive diabetes medical evaluation.

Ans.

1. **History:**
   - Age and characteristics of onset of diabetes [e.g. diabetic ketoacidosis (DKA), asymptomatic laboratory finding]
   - Eating patterns, nutritional status, weight history, sleep behaviors, and physical activity habits
   - Personal history:
     - Presence of common comorbidities and dental disease
     - History of smoking, alcohol, and substance use
     - History of HTN, dyslipidemia
     - Screen for depression, anxiety, and disordered eating
     - Screen for diabetes distress using validated and appropriate measures
     - Screen for psychosocial problems and other barriers to diabetes self-management such as limited financial, logistical, and support resources
   - Treatment history:
     - Review of previous treatment regimen and response to therapy (HbA_1C records)
     - Diabetic education, self-management
     - Current treatment of diabetes including medications, medication adherence, meal plan, results of glucose monitoring, and patient's use of data
   - History of diabetes-related complication:
     - Hypoglycemia episodes
       - Frequency and cause of severe (require assistance for treatment) and mild (self-treated) episodes
       - Time of day when "hypos" are experienced
       - Nature and intensity of symptoms
       - Ability to identify onset (awareness)
     - DKA: Frequency, severity, and cause
     - Microvascular complications: Retinopathy, nephropathy, and neuropathy (sensory including history of foot lesions, autonomic including sexual dysfunction and gastroparesis)
     - Macrovascular complications: IHD, CVD, PAD
   - For women with childbearing capacity, review contraception and preconception planning.

2. **Examination:**
   - Height, weight, BMI, waist circumference
   - Pulse, BP including orthostatic measurement when indicated
   - Head and neck: Thyroid, carotid pulse
   - Eyes: Xanthelasma, cataract, visual acuity (distant and near vision), fundoscopy
   - Oral cavity: Mucosal candidiasis, teeth and gum

- Examination of hand: Cheiroarthropathy, Dupuytren contracture, Carpal Tunnel syndrome
- Axilla: Acanthosis nigricans
- Skin: Diabetic dermopathy/shin spots, granuloma annulare, scleroderma, fungal infection, insulin injection site
- Examination of lower limb:
  - Inspection:
    - Callus of weight bearing area
    - Clawing of toes
    - Loss of planter arch
    - Localized infection, ulcer
    - Fungal infection between toes and nails
  - Circulation: Peripheral pulses, skin temperature, capillary refill
  - Sensation:
    - Light touch: 10 g monofilament
    - Vibration: 128 Hz tuning fork over big toe/malleoli
    - Vibration perception threshold: Biothesiometry
    - Pain: Pin prick/pressure over Achilles tendon
    - Proprioception: Joint position of big toe
  - Reflex: Ankle jerk.

3. **Investigations:**
   - Glucose profile (FBS, 2-h ABF, 2-h AL, 2-h AD)
   - HbA_1C (if not done within past 3 months)
   - Urine R/M/E, spot urine albumin to creatinine ratio (ACR)
   - Serum creatinine and eGFR
   - Fasting lipid profile
   - LFTs
   - Plain X-ray abdomen in patient <30-year age to exclude pancreatic calcification
   - TSH in type 1 DM.

4. **Referrals:**
   - Eye care professional for annual dilated eye examination
   - Dentist for comprehensive dental examination
   - Registered dietitian for MNT
   - Family planning for women of reproductive age
   - Mental health professional, if indicated.

CHAPTER 2

Pathogenesis of Diabetes Mellitus

Q. Discuss pathogenesis of type 1 diabetes mellitus (T1DM).

Ans.

- T1DM is an autoimmune disease involving both cellular and humoral immune pathways leading to selective destruction of insulin secreting β cells of pancreatic islets
- Hyperglycemia with classical symptoms of diabetes occurs only when 70%–90% of β cells have been destroyed
- Some residual β-cell function may be seen (as demonstrated by C peptide study) initially, and transient period of remission can occur producing "honeymoon" phase of the disease.

1. **Genetic factors:**
   - The concordance rate of T1DM among monozygotic twins ranges from 30% to 50% up to 70% compared to only 10%–19% among dizygotic twins
   - More than 85% T1DM occur in individual with no previous first degree family history
   - Human leukocyte antigen (HLA) region within the major histocompatibility complex on short arm of chromosome 6 harbors the main foci involved in genetic susceptibility of T1DM
   - HLA haplotypes DR3-DQ2 and DR4-DQ8 associated with increased susceptibility to T1DM.

2. **Environmental factors:**
   - **Maternal factors:** Gestational infection, higher maternal age, higher birth order, ABO blood group incompatibility
   - **Viral infections:** Mumps, rubella, enterovirus/coxsackie B virus, rota virus, Cytomegalovirus (CMV), Epstein–Barr virus (EBV), etc.
   - **Hygiene hypothesis:** Reduced exposure to microorganism in early childhood limits maturation of immune system and ↑ susceptibility to autoimmune disease
   - **Dietary factors:** Bovine milk (bovine serum albumin), short breastfeeding, various nitrosamines found in smoked meats, cereals, vitamin D deficiency
   - **Factors related to insulin sensitivity or resistance:** Puberty, high energy food, weight gain

- **Psychological stress:** Stress during pregnancy, child-parent separation, difficult adaptation
- **Toxic substances:** Alloxan, streptozocin, vacor.

3. **Pathology:**
   - **Insulitis:** Infiltration of islets with mononuclear cells containing activated macrophages, CD4 and CD8 T lymphocytes, NK cells, B lymphocytes
   - Initial patchiness of the lesion until a very late stage
   - β-cell specificity of the destructive process with glucagon and other hormone-secreting cells in the islets remaining intact.

4. **Autoantibodies in T1DM:**
   - **Glutamic acid decarboxylase (GAD 65) autoantibodies:** Found in 70%–80% of children with new onset T1DM, also 1% of general population. Currently considered as good marker for both prediction and follow up of β-cell dysfunction among individuals at risk
   - **Islet antigen 2 autoantibodies (IA-2Ab):** Found in 60%–70% of children with new onset T1DM. Frequency decreases with increased age of onset
   - **Insulin autoantibodies:** Highly specific as autoantigens of β cell (insulin and its precursor proinsulin) are expressed only in β cells
   - **Zinc transporter and autoantibodies (ZnT8Ab):** Second novel β-cell specific autoantigen in addition to insulin, found in 60%–80% of children with new onset T1DM.

Q. Mention other disorders with type 1 phenotype.

Ans.
- Maturity onset diabetes of the young (MODY) and other forms of monogenic diabetes caused by mutations of mitochondria, amylin or pathways implicated in pancreatic β-cell function
- Latent autoimmune diabetes of adults (LADA)
- Fulminant type 1 diabetes presenting with diabetic ketoacidosis after viral infections
- Another form which revert to clinical course resembling type 2 diabetes after initial ketotic presentation.

Q. What is monogenic diabetes syndrome?

Ans. Monogenic diabetes results from inheritance of mutation or mutations in a single gene.
- **Neonatal diabetes:** Diabetes diagnosed within first 6 months of life
- **MODY:** This subgroup of monogenic diabetes is a result of partial defect in glucose-induced insulin release and accounts for up to 5% of diabetes
- **Criteria:**
  - Onset before the age of 25 years
  - Strong family history of diabetes. DM in 3 generation on vertical transmission (autosomal dominant)

- Nonketotic
- Typical features of type 2 DM (T2DM) absent (nonobese, lack associated insulin resistance)
- No HLA or islet cell autoantibodies association
- Mild fasting hyperglycemia (5.5–8.5 mmol/L) and may initially achieve good glycemic control with diet and tablets/without insulin for 5 years but ultimately insulin treatment is required.

- **Subtypes of MODY:**

Functional defect	Main type	Gene mutated
β-cell glucose sensing	MODY 2	Glucokinase
β-cell transcriptional regulation	MODY 1 MODY 3 MODY 5	HNF-4α HNF-1α HNF-1β

Other types: MODY 4, MODY 6, MODY 7, MODY 8, MODY 9

- **Importance of diagnosing MODY:** These children may be incorrectly diagnosed as type 1 or T2DM leading to nonoptimal treatment regimen and delays in diagnosing other family members.

Q. Discuss LADA/type one and a half diabetes.

Ans.

- LADA is a slowly progressive form of autoimmune disease causing diabetes and is characterized by presence of serum autoantibodies to pancreatic antigens
- Approximately 10% of patients with T2DM having LADA
- Apart from high clinical suspicion, HLA studies may distinguish LADA from classic T1DM
- **Importance of diagnosing LADA:** Early use of insulin instead of sulfonylurea may prevent or reduce the rate of deterioration of β-cell function.

Q. Discuss etiopathological current concept of T2DM.

Ans.

- T2DM is a heterogeneous disorder caused by combination of genetic and environmental factors which adversely affect β-cell function and tissue insulin sensitivity.
- The pathogenesis can be described under two broad headings:
  - Abnormalities of insulin secretion and β-cell defect
  - Insulin resistance
- The impact of two components varies from person to person and in same person from time to time. A few patients may exhibit severe impairment of insulin release and normal sensitivity. Another small group of patients demonstrate exaggerated insulin release, mostly in early phase of the disease.
- About 10% of patients with phenotypic T2DM actually have LADA, while up to another 5% have autosomal dominantly inherited forms such as MODY and

mitochondrial diabetes. The remaining 85% patients have "garden variety" T2DM which is a polygenic disorder.

1. **Abnormalities of insulin secretion and β-cell defects in T2DM:**
   - Until recently, it was thought that insulin resistance preceded β-cell dysfunction and was the primary genetic factor
   - But studies suggest that during OGTT, elevated 2 h postchallenge plasma insulin level in people with T2DM was accompanied by reduced early (30 min) insulin response
   - This reduction in early insulin response and the resultant hyperglycemia provides a greater stimulus to β cell, explaining the late (2 h) hyperinsulinemia
   - At time of diagnosis, β-cell function is already reduced by 50%.

2. **Pattern of insulin release in T2DM:**
   - Basal insulin secretion is usually normal in nonobese and high in obese T2DM patients but commonly found insulin secretion abnormalities:
     - Absent first phase and diminished second phase release
     - Response to ingestion of mixed meals and to nonglucose stimuli is reduced with a ↓ maximal secretory capacity
     - The secretory pulses are smaller and less regular
     - The ratio of proinsulin to insulin release is also elevated (normally 10%–20% of secreted insulin is proinsulin).

3. **Causes of abnormalities of insulin secretion and β-cell defects in T2DM:**
   - **Genetic factors:** The concordance rates for T2DM approach 100% in monozygotic twins. Over 20 genes are associated with T2DM, the largest effect is seen with transcription factor 7 like 2 (TCF7L2) gene
   - **Malnutrition in utero and early childhood:** Malnutrition in utero and during first few months of life may damage β-cell development
   - **Glucotoxicity:** Prolonged and acute hyperglycemia causes increased production of reactive O_2 species within β cell and increased β-cell apoptosis
   - **Lipotoxicity:** Prolonged elevation of plasma free fatty acid (FFA), for example, in obese patient inhibits glucose stimulated insulin secretion, impair insulin gene expression and promote β-cell apoptosis
   - **Obesity**
   - **Inadequate stimulation by incretins:** Incretin effect is impaired in T2DM
   - **Islet amyloid:** Islet amyloid is found in 90% of patients with T2DM, but also in 20% elderly individuals with normal glucose tolerance
   - **Cytokines.**

4. **Histopathology of islets in T2DM:**
   - Abnormal extracellular deposits of islet amyloid found in 90% patients with T2DM
   - β-cell mass is reduced by 30%–50%

- α-cell mass is either unchanged or slightly increased. Abnormal α-cell function includes impaired suppression by hyperglycemia, excessive response to amino acid or mixed meals and diminished response to hypoglycemia.

Q. Discuss about insulin resistance.

Ans.
- Inability of insulin to produce its usual biologic actions at circulating concentrations that are effective in normal subjects
- Insulin resistance is an early finding in T2DM especially in obese and some nonobese patients. It may exist even 10 years prior to onset of diabetes
- The molecular basis of the resistance seems to reside both at the receptor as well as postreceptor level
- Observation like higher basal insulin level, low glucose–insulin ratio, decreased effect of exogenous insulin, glucose clamp with insulin infusion study support this in T2DM.

1. **Mechanism of insulin resistance in T2DM:**
   - Intra-abdominal central adipose tissue is metabolically active and release FFA which may induce insulin resistance because they compete with glucose as a fuel supply for oxidation in peripheral tissues, for example, muscle
   - Adipose tissue release a number of hormones including a variety of peptides called adipokines which act on specific receptor to influence sensitivity to insulin in other tissues
   - Because visceral adipose tissue drain into portal vein, central obesity may have a potent influence on insulin sensitivity in liver and therapy adversely affect gluconeogenesis and hepatic lipid metabolism.

2. **Insulin resistance in liver:**
   - Impaired ability of insulin to inhibit hepatic glucose production leading to hyperglycemia and stimulation of insulin secretion
   - Failure of insulin suppression of very low-density lipoprotein production which leads to hypertriglyceridemia
   - HDL level decrease due to increased exchange of cholesterol esters for triglyceride (TG), mediated by cholesterol ester transfer protein
   - Small, dense LDL particles also predominate in insulin resistance states and are highly atherogenic
   - Hepatic insulin resistance is directly proportionate to amount of fat in liver.

3. **Insulin resistance in adipose tissue:**
   - It is characterized by decreased production of insulin-sensitizing hormone adiponectin and by impaired ability of insulin to suppress lipolysis
   - Raised nonesterified FA (NEFA) levels are the most important source of intrahepatocellular TG both under fasting and postprandial conditions
   - Adiponectin deficiency may also contribute to fat accumulation in liver.

4. **Insulin resistance in muscle:**
   - Insulin resistance in muscle is associated with defects at multiple postreceptor sites
   - Glycogen synthesis is also decreased
   - Raised NEFA level also interfere with glucose uptake and utilization by muscle.

Q. Draw a flowchart about natural history of T2DM disease spectrum.

Ans. Earliest abnormality is insulin resistance without any glucose intolerance. Glucose intolerance begins with appearance of impaired fasting glucose (IFG) or impaired glucose tolerance (IGT). Ultimately, it reaches diabetic level with increasing glucose intolerance.

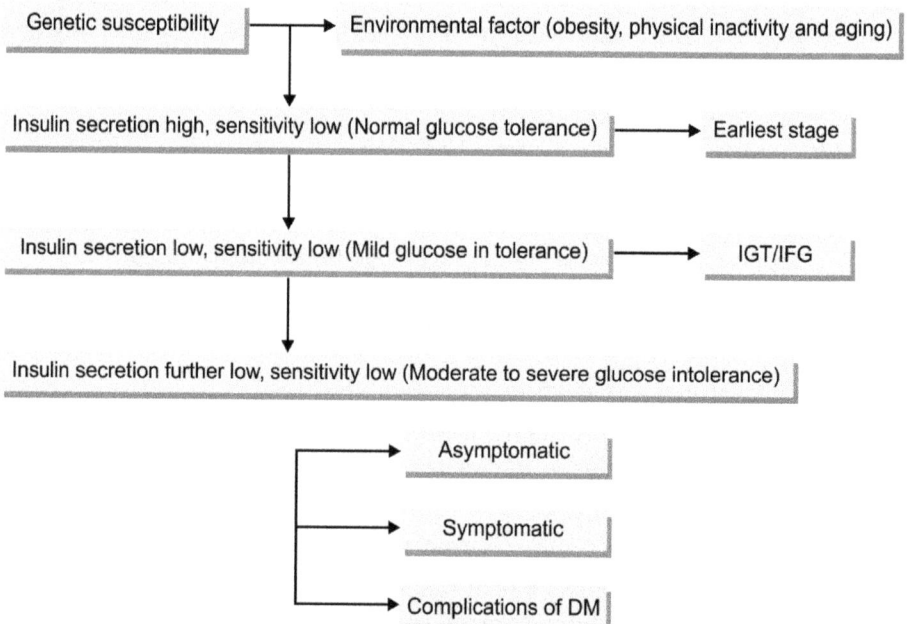

Q. Mention chronic complications of DM.

Ans.
- **Microvascular complication:**
  - Diabetic retinopathy
  - Diabetic nephropathy
  - Diabetic neuropathy
- **Macrovascular complication:**
  - Coronary circulation: Myocardial ischemia/infarction
  - Cerebral circulation: TIA/stroke
  - Peripheral circulation: PVD, ulceration.

Q. Discuss pathogenesis of microvascular complication of diabetes.

Ans.

1. **Increased glucose flux through polyol/sorbitol pathway:**
   - Aldose reductase, an enzyme found in tissues, for example, nerve, retina, lens, glomerulus, blood vessel wall, reduces glucose to sorbitol which is converted to fructose by sorbitol dehydrogenase
   - In hyperglycemia, sorbitol dehydrogenase becomes depleted, and there is intracellular accumulation of sorbitol that results in osmotic damage due to water retention and cell swelling.

2. **Increased intracellular formation of advanced glycation end products (AGE):**
   - Advanced glycation end products are formed by reaction of glucose with proteins that damage cells by
     - Modification of intracellular proteins → Altered function
     - Modification of extracellular matrix
     - Interaction with AGE receptors such as receptor of AGE (RAGE) in endothelial cells and macrophages →↑ production of reactive oxygen species (ROS).

3. **Increased expression of RAGE:** Increased expression of RAGE leads to ↑ production of ROS → oxidative stress.

4. **Increased protein kinase C activation:** Hyperglycemia leads to enhanced de novo synthesis of diacylglycerol (DAG) which ↑ protein kinase C activation that leads to cellular injury.

CHAPTER 3

Fibrocalculous Pancreatic Diabetes

Q. Define fibrocalculous pancreatic diabetes (FCPD).

Ans. In developing countries of tropical world, ketosis resistant, insulin requiring diabetes mellitus (DM) occurring in young lean individual (BMI < 19 kg/m^2) showing evidence of malnutrition and pancreatic calculi present with recurrent abdominal pain said to be suffering from FCPD provided that alcoholism and biliary diseases are excluded.

Q. What is malnutrition-related diabetes mellitus (MRDM) and tropical calcific diabetes (TCD)?

Ans.
- According to World Health Organization (WHO) and American Diabetic Association (ADA) in 1985, MRDM is a type of DM which was again subdivided into FCPD and protein deficient DM (PDDM). In 1997 classification, WHO and ADA expressed that FCPD is secondary diabetes
- TCD is prediabetic stage of FCPD, whereas FCPD is used once diabetes is developed.

Q. Discuss epidemiology of FCPD.

Ans.
- Geographical distribution: On both sides of equator and is restricted to tropical countries between 23° north and 23° south
- Four percent of all diabetics below the age of 30 in India (Ramachandaran et al., 1988) and 1% of all diabetic patients
- Nineteen percent of all diabetics below the age of 30 in BIRDEM of Bangladesh and 1% of all diabetic patients.

Q. Discuss etiopathogenesis of FCPD.

Ans.
- **Malnutrition:** Malnutrition particularly protein–energy malnutrition (PEM) with deficient sulfur-containing amino acids like methionine and cystine (needed for detoxification of cyanides) may be causative factor of FCPD. However, this may be consequence rather than cause of pancreatopathy
- **Cassava and other dietary toxins:** Cassava/tapioca/Manihot esculenta is a tuber consumed as staple food by poor people that contains only 0.4% protein and

95% starch. Cassava contains cyanogenic glycosides linamarin. Cyanide is normally detoxified in body by conversion to thiocyanate by sulfur and excreted in urine. In PEM, cyanides cannot be detoxified, accumulate in body and damage pancreas
- **Familial and genetic factors:** FCPD have been found as cluster in families and may be associated with *SPINK 1* gene
- **Antioxidant and micronutrient deficiency and heightened oxidative stress:** Various xenobiotics (cigarettes, alcohol, occupational chemicals) may induce cytochrome P-450, and relative deficiency of antioxidants (ascorbic acid, β carotene, micronutrients) generates free radicals and damages pancreas.

Q. How does calculi form in FCPD?

Ans. Malnutrition or prolonged starvation causes blockage of pancreatic duct by inspissated mucus plug that provides a nidus for stone formation. Pancreatic calculi are composed of calcium carbonate.

Q. Discuss clinical features of FCPD.

Ans.
- **Triad: Abdominal pain, steatorrhea, diabetes**
- Patients are usually poor and below 30 years of age in tropical country
- Recurrent upper abdominal pain, deep seated, radiate to back, aggravated by fatty meal, relieved by leaning forward. Sometimes, pain may persist in spite of all efforts. The severity of pain tends to decrease and usually disappears with onset of exocrine insufficiency and/or diabetes
- Steatorrhea: Pale, bulky, offensive, frothy, oily loose stool, float in pan, difficult to flush away, may contain undigested food particle
- Typical symptoms of diabetes
- Physical examinations reveal that patient is grossly emaciated with evidence of malnutrition. Thin hair with discoloration, bilateral parotid swelling, cyanotic hue of lip, distended abdomen, polyneuropathy and mature cataract.

Q. Mention Mohan's diagnostic criteria of FCPD.

Ans.
- Occurrence in tropical country
- Diabetes as defined by WHO
- Evidence of chronic pancreatitis: Pancreatic calculi on plain X-ray abdomen or at least three of the followings:
  - Structural pathology in pancreas, for example, small size of pancreas, dilatation of pancreatic duct or ductal stones as evidenced by ultrasonogram, endoscopic retrograde cholangiopancreatography (ERCP), computed tomography (CT) scan or histopathology
  - Recurrent abdominal pain

- Steatorrhea
- Exocrine pancreatic insufficiency—by PABA or fecal chymotrypsin test
  - Exclusion of other causes of chronic pancreatitis for example alcoholism, hepatobiliary disease.

Q. Mention heterogenecity of FCPD.

Ans.
- Asymptomatic, symptomatic
- Carbohydrate intolerance: Normal oral glucose tolerance test (OGTT), impaired glucose tolerance (IGT), and overt DM
- β-cell preserve: Good, poor, negligible
- Response to therapy: Diet alone, oral agents, insulin
- Proneness to ketosis: Ketosis resistant, ketosis prone
- Exocrine dysfunction: Only after provocative test, clinical steatorrhea
- Pancreatic pathology: Mild ductal change, gross ductal change, no stone, one or more stones.

Q. Mention complications of FCPD.

Ans.
- Chronic pancreatitis
- Pancreatic carcinoma
- Complications related to diabetes:
  - Microvascular complications: Similar to type 2 DM
  - Macrovascular complications: Less common as patients are young, lean, have lower lipid levels.

Q. Why FCPD patients are ketosis resistant?

Ans.
- Low body fat cause reduced supply of NEFA, so less ketosis, but when these cases are well feed and when they gain weight, they may develop ketosis
- Inability of hepatic production of ketones
- Damage of pancreas lead to α-cell damage leading to decreased glucagon production
- Partial preservation of β-cell function as shown by C peptide studies
- Resistance of subcutaneous adipose tissue lipolysis to epinephrine
- Carnitine deficiency affecting transfer of NEFA across mitochondrial membrane.

Q. Why abdominal pain occurs in FCPD?

Ans. Intraductal calcification causes duct obstruction leading to abdominal pain.

Q. How will you investigate a case of FCPD?

Ans.
- **Blood sugar/OGTT**
- **Urine routine microscopic examination (R/M/E):** Glycosuria but no ketonuria

- **Plain X-ray abdomen:** Pancreatic calculi, usually on right side of first and second lumbar vertebra or overlapping it but in long standing case, calculi may present in body and tail of pancreas. Stones are large, dense, rounded with discrete margin in contrast to small, speckled with ill-defined margins in alcoholic chronic pancreatitis. However, calculi develop after several years of abdominal pain, and 10% patients do not develop calculi
- **Tests of pancreatic structure:**
  - USG of whole abdomen: Volume of pancreas/degree of fibrosis, dilated pancreatic duct with intraductal calculi
  - CT abdomen/ERCP/Endoscopic ultrasound
- **Exocrine pancreatic function tests:**
  - Para aminobenzoic acid (PABA) test: After ingestion of PABA, PABA is eliminated in urine. In FCPD, PABA excretion is less as it is not absorbed from intestine
  - Fecal chymotrypsin test: Fecal chymotrypsin level <6 U/g of fecal mass
- **Endocrine pancreatic function test (C peptide estimation):** In FCPD, C peptide level is higher than IDDM (partial preservation of β-cell) but lower than nondiabetics and NIDDM.

Q. Discuss management of FCPD.

Ans.

1. **Diet:**
   - Because these patients are underweight, there should be no calorie restriction; rather, high calorie should be given with high protein content
   - If steatorrhea present, fatty food may be restricted
   - Vitamin supplements should be given, preferably parenteral.

2. **Abdominal pain:**
   - Analgesic: Nonopioid or opioid (risk of addiction)
   - Oral pancreatic enzyme supplement: Decrease pain as suppression of pancreatic secretion reduces intraductal pressure. Pancreatin up to 2 g daily given. As pancreatin is inactivated by gastric acid; it should be taken with food or immediately before or after food. Concurrent H_2 blocker or PPI decreases inactivation of enzyme by acid
   - Celiac plexus neurolysis
   - Intervention:
     - Endoscopic therapy: Dilatation or stenting of pancreatic duct, removal of calculi
     - Surgical method: Pancreaticojejunostomy, partial or total pancreatectomy.

3. **Steatorrhea:** Low fat diet, oral pancreatic enzyme supplement.

4. **Diabetes:** More than 80% patients need insulin often in larger doses—1.5–2 U/kg body weight/day. Some cases may be treated with oral agents (10%) or diet alone.

Q. Mention indications of intervention in FCPD patients.
Ans.
- Chronic pain not responsive to medical treatment
- Pain hampering everyday life
- Obstruction, for example, pancreatic duct >7 mm dilated or obstructive jaundice
- Multiple stones.

Q. Mention role of pancreaticojejunostomy in FCPD patients.
Ans. Main pancreatic duct is connected to jejunum. Pain relieved by reduction of obstruction even if stones are not gone. No need to remove stones.

CHAPTER 4

Exercise in Diabetes Mellitus

Q. Define exercise.

Ans. Physical activity that involves planned, structured and repetitive bodily movement performed for the purpose of improving or maintaining physical fitness.

Q. What are the types of exercise?

Ans.

1. **Aerobic exercise:** Exercise that uses primarily aerobic energy-producing systems and involves the repeated and continuous movement of same large muscle groups for extended periods of time ($\geq$10 min at a time). It is a type of exercise that overloads the heart and increases cardiorespiratory fitness. For example, walking, cycling, jogging, swimming.

2. **Anaerobic exercise:** Short, high-intensity exercise supported by energy sources already stored in the muscles that do not require oxygen. For example, sprinting at very fast speed.

3. **Resistance exercise:** Also known as strength training or weight training exercise. Resistance exercise involves the use of muscular strength to work against a resistive load or move a weight. For example, lifting free weights or using weight machines.

Q. What are the benefits of exercise in diabetic patients?

Ans.

- Improved blood glucose, lipid profile and blood pressure control
- Increases peripheral insulin sensitivity
- Weight reduction
- Increases physical work capacity
- Increases sense of well-being and quality of life
- Prevents atherosclerosis and thereby macroangiopathic complications of diabetes mellitus (DM).

Q. What are the benefits of aerobic exercise?

Ans.

- Increases maximal O_2 consumption
- Improves cardiovascular and respiratory function

- Increases blood supply to muscles and their ability to use O_2
- Lowers systolic and diastolic blood pressure
- Increases HDL cholesterol, decreases LDL cholesterol, increases mean LDL particle diameter (less atherogenic), decreases triglyceride (TG) of blood
- Decreases body fat and helps in weight reduction
- Increases peripheral insulin sensitivity.

Q. What are the benefits of anaerobic and resistance exercises?

Ans.
- Increase muscular strength
- Increase strength of tendons and ligaments
- Potentially improves flexibility (range of motions of joints)
- Decrease body fat and increase lean body mass (muscle mass)
- Improve blood glucose control and increase peripheral insulin sensitivity
- Improve strength, balance and functional ability in older adults.

Q. Discuss about fuel metabolism in aerobic exercise.

Ans.
- Muscle glycogen is the main source of energy during first 5-10 min of exercise
- Blood borne substrates like glucose and nonesterified fatty acid (NEFA) become increasingly important with prolongation of exercise
- If exercise of moderate intensity continues for several hours, the contribution of glucose diminishes and NEFA become the major fuel.

Q. Discuss about fuel metabolism in anaerobic exercise.

Ans.
- Such exercise is fueled by energy generated from breakdown of stored intramuscular ATP and phosphocreatine
- Glycolytic anaerobic energy production leads to blood lactate accumulation.

Q. Discuss about guidelines for exercise in diabetic patients.

Ans.
- Exercise plan should be individualized according to patient's physical status, meal, antidiabetic medication, lifestyle, interest, profession, etc.
- People with diabetes should be advised to perform at least 150 min/week of moderate intensity aerobic physical exercise (50%–70% of maximum heart rate) or 75 min/week of vigorous exercise or equivalent combination of both types with no more than two consecutive days without exercise
- Maximum heart rate = (220 – age) or 200% of basal heart rate or simple when feel palpitation
- In absence of contraindications, people with type 2 diabetes should be encouraged to perform resistance training two to three sessions per week

- Multiple shorter exercise sessions lasting at least 10 min each in the course of a day are probably as useful as a single longer session of equivalent length and intensity
- An exercise program should include a proper warm-up and cool-down period. A warm up should consist of 5–10 min of aerobic activity (for example, walking) at low-intensity level. It prepares the heart for exercise. After a short warm-up period, muscles should be gently stretched for another 5–10 min for preparing the muscles and preventing muscle injury. A cool down period of 5–10 min should follow main activity session. It gradually brings the heart rate down to pre-exercise level
- Use proper footwear and if appropriate, other protective equipment
- Avoid exercise in extreme heat or cold
- Inspect feet before and after exercise.

Q. What are the contraindications of exercise in diabetic patients?

Ans.
- Unstable coronary artery disease
- Uncontrolled hypertension
- Severe autonomic neuropathy
- Severe peripheral neuropathy
- Foot lesions (weight bearing exercise contraindicated)
- Unstable proliferative retinopathy
- Ketosis/ketonuria
- Any significant acute illness or uncompensated major chronic illnesses.

Q. Discuss caution and advice of diabetic patients during exercise.

Ans.

1. **Hypoglycemia in type 1 diabetes:**
   - Persons with type 1 DM who do not have complications and have good blood glucose control can do all levels of exercise including leisure activities, recreational sports and competitive professional performance. The emphasis must be given on adjusting the therapeutic regimen with the level of exercise, diet and avoiding hypoglycemia
   - Avoiding heavy exercise during peak insulin action
   - Using nonexercising sites for insulin injection, for example, around umbilicus
   - If using multiple daily injections, reduce pre-exercise insulin dosages by 20%–50% or more if necessary. These reductions should be individualized and based on blood glucose monitoring
   - Monitor glycemia before, during and after exercise as necessary
   - It is recommended to take approximately 15 g carbohydrate before and 15–30 g carbohydrate at every 30–60 min interval during longer exercise sessions (1 g carbohydrate/kg body weight/h of activity)
   - Extracarbohydrate should be advised if pre-exercise blood glucose level <5.6 mmol/L.

2. **Hypoglycemia in type 2 diabetes:**
   - Hypoglycemia is less common during exercise than in type 1 DM and extra carbohydrate is, therefore, usually not necessary
   - Patient taking insulin or sulfonylurea may need to reduce the doses of these medications during days when they exercise. Such adjustments should be guided by glucose monitoring.
3. **Diabetic autonomic neuropathy:** People with diabetic autonomic neuropathy should undergo cardiac investigation before beginning physical activity that is more intense than to which they are accustomed. Autonomic neuropathy increases the risk of exercise induced injury by:
   - Decreased cardiac responsiveness to exercise
   - Postural hypotension
   - Impaired thermoregulation
   - Impaired night vision due to impaired pupillary reaction
   - Unpredictable carbohydrate delivery from gastroparesis predisposing to hypoglycemia
   - Strongly associated with cardiovascular disease.
4. **Diabetic peripheral neuropathy:**
   - Decreased pain sensation in the extremities results in increased risk of skin breakdown, infection and Charcot joint destruction
   - All individuals with peripheral neuropathy should wear proper footwear and examine their feet daily to detect lesions early
   - Non-weight bearing exercise, for example, swimming, cycling, arm exercises are better. However, moderate intensity walking may not lead to increased risk of foot ulcers in patient with peripheral neuropathy
   - Anyone with a foot injury or open sore should be restricted to non-weight bearing activities.
5. **Diabetic retinopathy:** In patient with proliferative diabetic retinopathy or severe nonproliferative diabetic retinopathy, vigorous aerobic or resistance exercise is contraindicated due to increased risk of vitreous hemorrhage or retinal detachment.
6. **Diabetic cardiac patient:**
   - Patient with stable coronary artery disease should perform exercise of moderate intensity
   - Patient with history of or suspected coronary artery disease should be screened by electrocardiogram (ECG) and exercise tolerance test (ETT).
7. **Diabetic nephropathy:**
   - Physical activity acutely increases urinary protein excretion
   - There is no evidence that vigorous exercise increases the rate of progression of diabetic kidney disease
   - There is likely no need for any specific exercise restrictions for people with diabetic kidney disease

Q. Discuss exercise of diabetic patients in special situations.

Ans.
- **Exercise during pregnancy:** During pregnancy, moderate exercise (e.g., walking at moderate speed for 30 min a day at a time or in divided fashion) is advised. Vigorous exercise or exercise causing pressure in abdomen should be avoided
- **Exercise during sick days:** Diabetic patients are asked to avoid exercise or strenuous physical activity in sick days
- **Exercise during ramadan:**
  - Normal level of physical activity should be maintained
  - Exercise or excessive physical activity during day time should be avoided, particularly at late evening
  - Exercise can be performed 2 h after iftar
  - Tarawih prayer should be considered as a part of daily exercise program.

CHAPTER 5

Oral Antidiabetic Drugs

Q. Define oral antidiabetic drugs (OAD).

Ans. Drugs that can be administered orally and help to reduce plasma glucose if there is some β-cell reserves that have the ability to secrete endogenous insulin. They are not useful in type 1 and type 2 diabetes mellitus (T1DM and T2DM) with advanced β-cell failure. No OAD can reduce HbA_1C >2%.

Q. Mention indication and contraindication of OAD.

Ans.

1. **Indications:**
   - Mild to moderate hyperglycemia (HbA_1C >7% but <10%, FBS <14 mmol/L, PPG <16.7 mmol/L)
   - Without complications either diabetes related or nondiabetes related
   - No symptoms of hyperglycemia.

2. **Contraindications:**
   - H/o ketosis/ketoacidosis [diabetic ketoacidosis (DKA)/hyperglycemic hyperosmolar nonketotic coma (HONC)]
   - Pregnancy
   - Acute stress, for example, infection, trauma, MI
   - Preferably without the following diabetic complication
     - Eye disease: Proliferative retinopathy
     - Renal failure: Serum creatinine >2 mg/dL (few OADs can be given with adjusted dose)
     - Acute metabolic neuropathy.

Q. Mention goals of glycemic control in T2DM.

Ans.
- Relief of symptoms
- Prevent acute complications, for example, HONC

- Prevent, defer or reduce severity of microvascular complications
- Provide some benefit against macrovascular complications
- Restoration of sense of well-being
- Maintenance of ideal body weight
- Good pregnancy outcome
- Correction of blood chemistry value.

Q. What are the types of antidiabetic drugs?

Ans.
- Insulin
- Insulin secretagogues
  - Sulfonylureas (SU): Gliclazide, glipizide, glibenclamide/glyburide, glimepiride
  - Nonsulfonylureas: Meglitinides (repaglinide, nateglinide)
- Insulin sensitizers: Metformin, thiazolidinediones (pioglitazone, rosiglitazone)
- α-Glucosidase inhibitors: Acarbose, voglibose, miglitol
- Dipeptidyl peptidase 4 (DPP-4) inhibitors: Vildagliptin, sitagliptin, linagliptin, saxagliptin, alogliptin
- Glucagon like peptide-1 (GLP-1) receptor agonists: Exenatide, liraglutide, albiglutide, lixisenatide, dulaglutide
- Sodium glucose co-transporter 2 (SGLT2) inhibitor: Dapagliflozin, canagliflozin, empagliflozin
- Amylin mimetics: Pramlintide
- Dopamine-2 agonist: Bromocriptine
- Bile acid sequestrants: Colesevelam.

Q. What factors to be considered before selection of antidiabetic agent?

Ans.
- Glycemic status
- Efficacy of medication
- Hypoglycemia risk
- Comorbid disease
- Life style of patient
- Impact on weight
- Delivery method (oral vs subcutaneous)
- Cost
- Potential side effects
- Safety impact of kidney, heart or liver disease
- Patient preference.

Q. Classify OAD with duration of action, dose and excretion.

Ans.

Group	Class	Duration of action (h)	Dose (mg/day)	Excretion
Sulfonylureas	Gliclazide	8–12	40–320	Urine 65%
	Gliclazide MR	18–24	30–120	Urine 65%
	Glipizide	6–16	2.5–40	Urine 70%
	Glibenclamide/glyburide	10–24	1.25–20	Bile 50%
	Glimepiride	12–24	1–8	Urine 60%
Meglitinides	Repaglinide	4–6	0.5–16	Bile 90%
	Nateglinide	3–5	60–360	Urine 80%
Insulin sensitizers	Metformin	8–12, half-life 6 h	500–2,500 XR: 2,000	Not metabolized, excreted unchanged in urine
	Pioglitazone	24	15–45	Bile 60%
	Rosiglitazone	24	4–8	Urine 64%
α-Glycosidase inhibitors	Acarbose	4	25–300	Stool and urine
	Miglitol	4	25–300	Urine
Incretin	Vildagliptin	12–24	50–100	Urine
	Sitagliptin	18–24	25–100	Urine
	Linagliptin	18–24	5	Not metabolized, 90% excreted unchanged in stool
SGLT2 inhibitors	Dapagliflozin	Half-life 12.9 h	5–10	Urine
	Canagliflozin	Half-life 10.6 h	100–300	Stool and urine

Q. Discuss about sulfonylurea.

Ans.

- **Generations:**
  - First generation: Tolbutamide, chlorpropamide (not used now)
  - Second generation: Gliclazide, glipizide, glibenclamide, glimepiride
- **Mechanism of action:**
  - Sulfonylurea ↑ release of insulin from pancreatic β cell
  - Sulfonylurea bind to cytosolic surface of sulfonylurea receptor 1 (SUR1) of pancreatic β-cell leading to closure of ATP dependent K^+ channel, depolarizing plasma membrane
  - Localized membrane depolarization open adjacent Ca^{++} channel leading to ↑ Ca^{++} influx and translocation of secretary granules on the cell surface and secretion of insulin by exocytosis

- Extra pancreatic effects are
  - Reduce hepatic glucose output
  - ↑ insulin stimulated glucose uptake in muscle
  - Stimulate lipogenesis in adipose tissue
- **Advantages:** Potent, reduce pre and postprandial blood glucose
- **Adverse effects:**
  - Hypoglycemia: 20% of SU treated patients have one or more hypoglycemic symptoms annually
  - Weight gain (1-4 kg) common after initiation of SU, stabilizes by 6 months. Weight gain is due to anabolic effect of ↑ plasma insulin with reduced loss of glucose in urine
  - Hypersensitivity reaction like rashes
- **Contraindications:**
  - Hepatic impairment with alanine transaminase (ALT) >two to three times × upper limit of normal (ULN)
  - Reduced dose or avoidance in chronic kidney disease (CKD) (avoid long acting SU in CKD stage 3-5)
- **Facts about sulfonylurea:**
  - SU rapidly absorbed from gut more in empty stomach. So advised to take 1/2 h before meal
  - SU expected to reduce fasting plasma glucose (FPG) 2-4 mmol/L (↓ HbA_1C 1%-2%)
  - Single-dose schedule is preferable particularly in the morning. When morning dose is more than two tab, add small dose in evening
  - SUR2A (cardiac muscle) receptor discovered. Glipizide, glibenclamide, glimepiride bind to these receptors and interfere with myocardial ischemic preconditioning with ↑ cardiovascular (CV) mortality and morbidity during acute events. Gliclazide show little interference with these receptors.

Q. Discuss about meglitinides.

Ans.

- They are without sulfonylurea moiety
- Also called prandial glucose regulator/short acting prandial insulin releasers
- **Advantages:**
  - Reduce postprandial hyperglycemia
  - Lower risk of hypoglycemia in between meal
  - Suitable for individuals with irregular meal habit with unpredictable or missed meals, also in elderly who are reluctant to take food in adequate amount and number
  - No meal, no pill
- Low dose if eGFR <30 mL/min/1.73 m²
- **Disadvantage:** Weight gain.

Q. Define insulin sensitizers.

Ans. Insulin sensitizers are drugs which improve insulin action or reduce insulin resistance.

Q. Discuss about biguanides.

Ans.

- History: In 1920, guanidine rich herb (goat's rue) used to treat diabetes
- Phenformin, Buformin withdrawn due to ↑ risk of lactic acidosis
- Metformin is first line drug to treat diabetes
- Taken with or just after meal to minimize possible GI side effects
- **Mechanism of action:** Not known but possibilities include
  - ↓ Hepatic gluconeogenesis
  - ↑ Insulin sensitivity with ↑ peripheral glucose uptake
  - Delay in absorption of glucose
  - ↑ Insulin action
- **Other metabolic and vascular effects of metformin:**
  - Insulin resistance (↓): ↑ Receptor–postreceptor signaling pathway of insulin action
  - Hyperinsulinemia (↓): ↓ Fasting and often postprandial insulin
  - Obesity: ↓ or stabilizes body weight
  - Impaired glucose tolerance (IGT): ↓ Progression to T2DM
  - Dyslipidemia: Modest benefit if abnormal, ↓ triglyceride (TG), LDL, ↑ HDL
  - Procoagulant state (↓): Antithrombotic (↓ fibrinogen, ↓ platelet aggregation)
  - Endothelial function (↑): ↓ Vascular adhesion molecules
  - Atherosclerosis (↓): ↓ Myocardial infarction (MI), Stroke, ↓ carotid intima-media thickness, ↑ life expectancy
- **Advantages:**
  - Improve insulin sensitivity
  - Weight reduction
  - Reduce pre- and postprandial blood glucose
  - Favorable effect on lipid profile and nonalcoholic fatty liver disease (NAFLD).
- **Adverse effects:**
  - GI upset: Anorexia, nausea, vomiting, diarrhea, abdominal discomfort, metallic taste, ↑ passage of flatus. These are transient and can be prevented by taking the drugs with meals, start at low dose and increase the dose slowly, can try extended release formulation. But 10% patient cannot tolerate metformin at any dose
  - Lactic acidosis: Rare. Predisposing factors are renal failure, impaired hepatic function, any hypoxic condition, alcohol
  - ↓ GI absorption of vitamin B_{12}.
- **Contraindications:**
  - Renal impairment. Avoid if serum creatinine ≥ 1.5 (M) or ≥ 1.4 (F) or eGFR <30 mL/min/1.73 m². Avoid initiation of metformin if eGFR <45 mL/min/1.73 m²

Chapter 5: Oral Antidiabetic Drugs

- Impaired hepatic function (ALT >two to three times × ULN)
- Alcohol abuse
- Acute or chronic acidosis or any hypoxic condition or reduced tissue perfusion (heart failure, respiratory insufficiency, hypotension, septicemia)
- Not used in pregnancy due to risk of ↑ anorexia, vomiting and Metformin may slightly increase prematurity and nearly half of patients with gestational diabetes mellitus (GDM) on metformin ultimately need insulin for glycemic control and they lack long-term safety data.

- **Facts about metformin:**
  - Temporary withdrawn in CV collapse, acute MI, CCF, septicemia, IV radiographic contrast media
  - Stopped 48 h before surgery with GA
  - Metformin exert insulin dependent and independent effect on glucose metabolism
  - The glucose lowering efficacy requires presence of at least some insulin
  - Metformin expected to reduce FPG 2–4 mmol/L (↓ HbA_1C 1%–2%)
  - Lower risk of hypoglycemia
  - Does not lower blood glucose level in non-diabetic persons like as in person with diabetes
  - Metformin not used in <10-year children.

Q. Discuss about Thiazolidinediones.

Ans.

- **Members:** Pioglitazone, rosiglitazone
- **Mechanism of action:**
  - Stimulate nuclear peroxisome proliferator activated receptor γ (PPAR-γ) in adipose tissue, also in muscle and liver
  - ↑ insulin sensitivity with ↑ peripheral glucose uptake
  - ↓ hepatic glucose output
  - Glucose lowering effect need presence of adequate insulin
  - No effect on insulin secretion
  - Dose-dependent effect.
- **Advantages:**
  - Improve insulin sensitivity
  - Reduce pre- and post-prandial blood glucose
  - Favorable effect on lipid (Pioglitazone: ↑ HDL, ↓ TG) and NAFLD.
- **Adverse effects:**
  - Fluid retention (edema, heart failure)
  - Weight gain
  - Anemia (↓ Hb%)
  - Osteoporosis/bone fractures
  - Bladder cancer (pioglitazone)

- ↑ LDL cholesterol (rosiglitazone)
- FDA warning on congestive heart failure of pioglitazone, rosiglitazone.
- **Contraindications:**
  - Impaired hepatic function (ALT >two to three times × ULN)
  - Any water logging condition, for example, heart failure, renal failure
  - Pregnancy and lactation
  - Unexplained anemia
  - Osteoporosis.
- **Facts about thiazolidinedione:**
  - No biological difference in empty or full stomach but peak concentration slightly delayed when taken with food
  - Antihyperglycemic effect of thiazolidinediones usually require 2-3 months to reach maximum effect
  - ↓ Occurrence of new onset DM in individuals with IGT or h/o GDM.

Q. Discuss about α-glucosidase inhibitors.

Ans.

- **Members:** Acarbose, Voglibose, Miglitol
- Should be crushed with first mouthful of food
- **Mechanism of action:** Competitively inhibits activity of α-glucosidase enzyme in brush border of enterocytes lining intestinal villi which breaks down disaccharides and oligosaccharides into monosaccharides, thus inhibiting complete digestion of carbohydrate
- **Advantages:**
  - Reduce postprandial blood glucose
  - Weight neutral
- **Adverse effects:** Flatulence, abdominal discomfort, diarrhea (due to fermentation of unabsorbed carbohydrate in colon)
- **Contraindications:** Impaired hepatic and renal function, IBD, malabsorption syndrome.

Q. Discuss about incretin-based therapy.

Ans.

- **Incretin:** The secretion of insulin in response to rise in blood glucose is greater when glucose is given by mouth than by intravenous infusion. This is caused by secretion of gut hormones or incretins which potentiate glucose-induced insulin secretion. Incretin effect is impaired in patient with type 2 DM
- **Incretin hormones:**
  - Glucagon like peptide-1 (GLP-1): Secreted by L cells of ileum
  - Glucose dependent insulinotropic polypeptide/gastric inhibitory polypeptide (GIP): Secreted by K cells of duodenum

Chapter 5: Oral Antidiabetic Drugs

- **Effect of incretin hormones:**
  - **Effect on pancreatic islets:**
    - Potentiation of glucose/meal-induced insulin secretion
    - Stimulate β-cell proliferation, also enhance differentiation of new β-cell from progenitor cells and prevention of β-cell apoptosis →↑ β-cell mass
    - Suppress glucagon secretion
    - ↑ Somatostatin secretion → inhibition of α-cells
  - **Extra pancreatic effects:**
    - Slow gastric emptying → reduce postprandial hyperglycemia
    - Reduce appetite and food intake, ↑ satiety
    - CV effects: Protection of ischemic heart, improve endothelial dysfunction
  - **Neurotropic effects:** Display neuroprotective effect, proposed as new therapeutic agent for neurodegenerative disease, for example, Alzheimer's disease.

Q. Discuss about GLP-1 receptor agonists/Incretin mimetics.

Ans.
- **Members:**
  - Exenatide: Not used if eGFR <30 mL/min/1.73 m^2
  - Liraglutide: 0.6 mg/day S.C., ↑ weekly to 1.2 mg/day and to maximum 1.8 mg/day. Can be given in renal failure or liver failure as metabolized by tissue endopeptidase
  - Albiglutide, Lixisenatide, Dulaglutide
- **Adverse effects:**
  - GI disturbance: Anorexia, nausea, vomiting, diarrhea
  - Acute pancreatitis
  - C cell hyperplasia/medullary carcinoma of thyroid in animals (Liraglutide)
  - Long-term safety unknown
- **Advantage:** Weight reduction.

Q. Discuss about DPP-4 inhibitor/gliptins/incretin enhancers.

Ans.
- **Members:** Vildagliptin, Sitagliptin, Linagliptin, Saxagliptin, Alogliptin
- **Mechanism of action:** Half-life of incretin hormone is 1–2 min, rapidly degraded by DPP-4 (Dipeptidyl peptidase 4) enzyme and only 8% of secreted incretin reach pancreas as intact peptide. DPP-4 inhibitor inhibits DPP-4 enzyme →↓ degradation of endogenously secreted incretin hormones →↑ incretin effect
- **Advantages:**
  - No hypoglycemia
  - Weight neutral
- **Adverse effects:**
  - ↑ Liver enzymes (Vildagliptin)

- Occasional reports of urticaria/angioedema
- Pancreatitis
- Joint pain
- Long-term safety unknown
- **Dose in CKD:**
  - Vildagliptin: 50 mg daily if eGFR <50 mL/min/1.73 m^2
  - Sitagliptin: 50 mg daily if eGFR 30–50 mL/min (creatinine 1.7–3 in male, 1.5–2.5 in female), 25 mg daily if eGFR <30 mL/min (creatinine >3 in male, >2.5 in female) or dialysis
  - Linagliptin: No dose adjustment in CKD
  - Saxagliptin: 5 mg daily if eGFR >50, 2.5 mg daily if eGFR <50 mL/min/1.73 m^2.

Q. Discuss about sodium glucose cotransporter 2(SGLT2) inhibitors.

Ans.

- **Members:** Dapagliflozin, canagliflozin, empagliflozin
- **Mechanism of action:** Inhibit SGLT2 (involved in reabsorption of glucose in proximal tubules of kidney) → reduce hyperglycemia by ↑ excretion of glucose in urine
- **Adverse effects:**
  - Osmotic diuresis, dehydration, electrolyte imbalance, UTI
  - DKA
  - Bone fractures, risk of amputation (canagliflozin)
  - ↑ LDL cholesterol
- **Dose in CKD:**
  - Dapagliflozin: Not used if eGFR <60 mL/min/1.73 m^2
  - Canagliflozin: Not used if eGFR <45 mL/min/1.73 m^2
  - Empagliflozin: Not used if eGFR <30 mL/min/1.73 m^2.

Q. What is OAD failure?

Ans.

- **Definition:** Failure is said to occur when an orally administered antidiabetic agent does not produce desired fall in blood glucose level in T2DM
- **Primary failure:** Occurring from initiation of treatment when maximum dose of OAD does not produce desired fall in blood glucose level within 3 months. These patients have been diagnosed late in the course of the disease and have advanced β-cell failure
- **Secondary failure:** Maximum dose of OAD fails to produce desired fall in blood-glucose level adequately enough to meet target glycemic value though it has been effective earlier. Occur 5%–10% per year
- Before defining failure of any particular agent, the agent should be used in maximum dose for adequate time period to produce its full effect and other components of treatment (e.g., diet, exercise) should be practiced properly
- Dose response of all sulfonylurea is steepest at low doses, and little additional benefit is obtained when the dose is increased to maximum levels.

CHAPTER 6

Insulin

Q. Mention facts about insulin.

Ans.
- Insulin was discovered at 1921 by Banting, Macloid and Best for which they shared the Nobel Prizes for medicine in 1923
- Purified animal insulin still in market
- Bovine insulin differs from human insulin in orientation of three amino acids (AAs)
- Porcine insulin differs from human insulin in orientation of one AA
- Problems with animal insulin: Immune-mediated side effects
- Human insulin is produced by recombinant DNA technology (insertion of human proinsulin gene into a host cell, usually Baker's cyst or bacteria *Escherichia coli*, allowing it to synthesize insulin)
- Molecular weight: 5,808 Da
- Contain 51 AAs arranged in A (21 AAs) and B chains (30 AAs) linked by disulfide bridges
- In one molecule of insulin, three disulfides bridge, two of them connect A and B chains and the remaining one connects two AAs in A chains
- Granules within β-cell store insulin in the form of crystal consisting of two atoms of zinc and six molecules of insulin
- Half-life of insulin: 3–5 min
- Metabolism of insulin: By liver (60%–80%), kidney (10%–20%), skeletal muscle and fat tissue (10%–20%), also placenta
- Insulin ↓ glucagon secretion but glucagon ↑ insulin secretion. Glucagon is used in treatment of severe hypoglycemia in type 1 DM but avoided in type 2 DM as glucagon itself is an insulin secretagogue producing further hypoglycemia.

Q. Discuss about Islands of Langerhans.

Ans.
- Islets of Langerhans comprise 2%–3% of total pancreatic volume with exocrine (80%), and rest is formed by ducts, blood vessels and connective tissue
- Human pancreas contains 1–2 million islets distributed throughout pancreas, more at tail

- **Cells of islets:**
  - β cell (60%): Secrete insulin. In islets, β cell form a central core surrounded by α cell and δ cell
  - α cell (20%–30%): Secrete glucagon
  - δ cell (10%): Secrete somatostatin, inhibitor of secretory cell but somatostatinoma cause diabetes
  - PP cell/F cell (<5%): Secrete pancreatic polypeptide, facilitate digestive process by unknown mechanism
  - ε cell (1%): Secrete ghrelin. The level is low in overweight people suggesting it may have role in controlling appetite and weight gain
  - Amylin is cosecreted with insulin from β cell; its function is to delay gastric emptying, suppression of postprandial glucagon secretion and increase satiety.

Q. How insulin synthesis occur in our body?

Ans.
- Gene encoding prepoinsulin is located in 11p
- First formed as prepoinsulin in rough endoplasmic reticulum (contain 81 AA)
- In <1 min, it is cleaved into proinsulin and transported to Golgi apparatus where packages as secretory granules
- During exocytosis, it is further cleaved into insulin and C peptide (connecting peptide, 35 AAs)
- C peptide has no known physiological effects. C peptide assay provide an index of β-cell function.

Q. Write down about mechanism of insulin secretion.

Ans.
- Blood glucose enters into β cell through glucose transporter protein type 2 (GLUT- 2) of cell membrane. This does not require insulin because this is an insulin-independent cell
- Within the cell, adenosine triphosphate (ATP)/adenosine diphosphate (ADP) ratio goes up due to increase production of ATP from glycolysis
- ATP sensitive K^+ channels get blocked
- Membrane becomes depolarized
- Voltage gated Ca^{++} channels get opened
- Entry of Ca^{++} within β cell. Insulin is released by exocytosis.

Q. Describe pattern of insulin secretion in healthy subjects.

Ans.
- Blood glucose is principal stimulator of β cell to secrete insulin
- There is continuous low-level secretion of insulin between meals and throughout night. It is called basal insulin (24 U/day)
- Following meals, there is sharp rise called prandial or bolus insulin release. The rate and amount of secretion is influenced by amount and composition of meals (on average 24 U/day).

Chapter 6: Insulin

Q. Describe mechanism of action of insulin.

Ans.
- Insulin binds with insulin receptor which is a glycoprotein and has four subunits (2 α and 2 β)
- α Subunit lies outside the cell membrane, whereas β subunit is transmembrane. Intracellular portion of β subunit has tyrosine kinase activity
- Binding of insulin with α subunit → autophosphorylation of β subunit → activation of tyrosine kinase → phosphorylation of some cytoplasmic proteins (enzymes) which perform all the activities of insulin.

Q. Mention metabolic effects of insulin.

Ans.
- **Carbohydrate metabolism**
  - ↑ Glucose uptake (muscle, adipose tissue)
  - ↑ Glycogenesis and glycolysis
  - ↓ Gluconeogenesis and glycogenolysis
- **Protein metabolism:**
  - ↑ AA transport, protein synthesis
  - ↓ Protein degradation
- **Lipid metabolism:**
  - ↑ Fatty acid and glycerol synthesis
  - ↓ Lipolysis, ketogenesis
  - ↓ Lipoprotein lipase activity (muscle)
  - ↑ Lipoprotein lipase activity (adipose tissue)
- K^+: IV insulin causes K^+ to enter cell.

Q. What are the adverse effects of insulin?

Ans.
- Hypoglycemia
- Weight gain
- Peripheral edema: Initiation of insulin treatment cause transient salt and water retention
- Local/systemic allergy: Rare with human insulin
- Lipodystrophy:
  - Lipoatrophy: Due to immune reaction. Rare nowadays due to advent of human insulin
  - Lipohypertrophy: Due to lipogenesis. Avoid injection at same site repeatedly
- Hypokalemia (IV insulin)
- Pain at injection site: Minimized now with newer devices with ultrafine needle. Pain may be due to faulty techniques also (? intradermal)
- Acute painful neuropathy/insulin neuritis: Due to fast improvement of blood glucose control which is reversible
- Temporary worsening of vision due to osmolarity changes of lens.

Q. What are the routes of insulin administration?

Ans.
- Subcutaneous route: Commonly used
- IV route: Useful in emergency, for example, hyperglycemic crisis
- Intramuscular route: Useful in emergency situation when IV access is difficult
- Continuous subcutaneous insulin infusion (CSII) pump
- Inhaled route
- Newer route in future:
  - Intraperitoneal route: May be useful in patients receiving RRT
  - Oral route: With techniques, for example, insulin modification to prevent degradation by peptide.

Q. Mention insulin injection sites.

Ans.
- Abdomen (periumbilical area): Preferred site for faster absorption, less affected site by muscle activity and exercise
- Front or lateral aspect of both upper thighs: Preferred site for easy access and well-visualized site for self-insulin administration
- Arms (front and lateral aspect of both upper arms, 2 inches above elbow joint): Needs help from another person for injection.

Q. What are the factors affecting insulin absorption?

Ans.
- Age: Young children → less subcutaneous fat → faster absorption
- Obesity: More subcutaneous fat → slower absorption
- Site: Abdomen >arm >leg (rate of absorption)
- Route: Intramuscular faster > subcutaneous route
- Exercise: Faster absorption
- Fever/high body temperature/hot climate/sitting in sauna: Faster absorption.

Q. Is cleaning of insulin injection sites necessary?

Ans.
- Cleaning is not essential unless hygiene is a real problem
- Insulin syringe or pen needle may be used multiple times for same person only till the head end becomes blunted or injection is more painful.

Q. What is the technique of insulin administration?

Ans.
- Pinch the skin fold and elevate slightly (to avoid IM injection)
- Inject at 90° angle to the skin
- Keep the needle in site for 5–10 s to prevent backflow of insulin
- Do not rub the area of injection given.

Chapter 6: Insulin

Q. How can you mix regular insulin with NPH?

Ans.
- Push the desired amount of air in NPH vial and withdraw the needle
- Push the desired amount of air in soluble insulin vial and draw the amount of insulin as required, then withdraw the needle
- Then reinsert the syringe in NPH vial and draw the desired amount of insulin from vial
- Both the insulin in syringe do not need shaking
- Always take the soluble insulin in syringe first.

Q. How to store insulin?

Ans.
- Insulin may be kept at room temperature (below 25°C) for 4 weeks
- Currently using vial and pen do not need storage at refrigerator, if temperature is below 25°C always
- When stored at 2–8°C in refrigerator, shelf life is 30 months
- If patients have no refrigerator, insulin can be kept in cool and dark places, and he is advised not to buy >1 month insulin needed.

Q. Discuss about vial syringe mismatch of insulin.

Ans.
- A volume of 40 U insulin vial and 100 U insulin vial has 40 and 100 U of insulin in 1 mL, respectively. A volume of 40 U syringe have red cap and marked up to 40, while 100 U syringe have orange cap and marked up to 100
- Same unit of insulin taken from 40 or 100 U vial with corresponding syringe is equal. For example, 10 U insulin from 40 U vial with 40 U syringe = 10 U insulin from 100 U vial with 100 U syringe
- If 40 U vial and 100 U syringe → 2.5 times less of desired insulin taken → poor glycemic control
- If 100 vial and 40 syringe → 2.5 times more of desired insulin taken → hypoglycemia.
- Always advice patient to buy 100 U vial and syringe (cost effective). In USA, mainly 100 U insulin vial and 100 U syringes are available, but in India and Bangladesh both are available
- All insulin in pen is of 100 U/mL.

Q. Define 1 U insulin.

Ans.
- Previous definition: Amount of insulin that reduces blood glucose level 45 mg/dL in a fasting rabbit

- New definition: 1 IU corresponds to 0.035 mg of anhydrous human insulin (28 IU/mg insulin).

Q. Mention indications of insulin.

Ans.
- Type 1 DM
- Severe acute complication/illness, for example, MI, acute infection
- Uncompensated chronic complication/illness
- Pregnancy and lactation
- At least 3–5 months prior to planned conception
- Major surgery
- Poor glycemic status (HbA$_1$C ≥10% or FBS 14–16.7 mmol/L with symptoms of hyperglycemia or FBS >16.7 mmol/L with or without symptoms)
- Oral antidiabetic drug (OAD) failure (FBS >6 mmol/L, PPG >8 mmol/L, HbA$_1$C >7% in spite of >50% of maximum dose of SU) and maximum tolerable dose of sensitizer
- Adverse effect of OAD.

Q. Discuss about inhaled insulin.

Ans.
- Inhaled insulin (Afrezza) has got US FDA approval
- Inhaled insulin administered by specific inhaler at the beginning of meal to control postprandial glucose, and it is not a substitute for long-acting insulin
- Onset of action is 12 min, peak at 35–45 min and duration of action 1.5–3 h
- Perform a detailed medical history, physical examination and spirometry (FEV1) to identify potential lung disease in all patients prior to start inhaled insulin
- Contraindicated in patients with chronic lung disease like asthma, COPD and in patients who smoke or recently stopped smoking
- Adverse effects:
  - Acute Bronchospasm in patients with asthma and COPD
  - Decline in Pulmonary function: Perform spirometry before initiating, after 6 months of therapy and annually, even in the absence of pulmonary symptoms
  - Lung cancer
  - Diabetic ketoacidosis
  - Hypersensitivity reactions
  - Hypokalemia
- How to switch to inhaled insulin from subcutaneous premixed insulin: Estimate the mealtime injected dose by dividing half of the total daily injected premixed insulin dose and distribute among three meals of the day. Administer half of the total daily injected premixed dose as injected basal insulin dose.

Q. Classify insulin.

Ans. Insulins are classified and explained in detail in the table given below:

Class	Name	Trade name	Onset of action	Peak action	Duration	Time relation with meals	Color	Color of insulin leveling
A. Human insulin								
Short-acting	Regular	Actrapid	30–60 min	2–4 h	6–8 h	30 min before	Clear	Yellow
Intermediate-acting	NPH Lente	Insulatard	2–4 h	6–8 h	12–18 h	30 min before	Cloudy	Light green
Long-acting	Ultralente		6–8 h	8–14 h	24–36 h	No specific time	Cloudy	
B. Analog insulin								
Rapid-acting analog	Lispro Aspart Glulisine	Humalog Novorapid Apidra	5–15 min	1–1.5 h	3–4 h	5 min before to 15 min after	Clear	Orange
Long-acting analog	Glargine Detemir	Lantus, Basaglar Levemir	2–4 h	No peak Small peak at 6–8 h	24 h 18 h	No specific time, not related to meals but same time everyday	Clear	Green
	Insulin degludec	Tresiba			Beyond 42 h			
C. Premixed insulin								
Human: Various combination 30/70, 25/75, 50/50 (short acting/intermediate acting) Analogs: Biphasic aspart (Novomix), Insulin lispro protamine mix (Humalog mix), insulin degludec/insulin aspart (Ryzodeg)								

Q. Discuss about different types of insulin regimen.

Ans.

1. **Basal only regimen:** NPH insulin given once or twice a day according to need or long-acting insulin analog given once daily. It serves as supplement of basal insulin.
   - Example:
     - Inj. NPH 6 + 0 + 6 or
     - Inj. NPH 0 + 0 + 6 or
     - Inj. Glargine/Detemir 0 + 0 + 6
   - Use:
     - Common regimen of initiation of insulin therapy

- To remove anxiety and stress associated with shift of treatment from tablet to insulin, also to make patient confident about self-injection of insulin.

2. **Basal plus regimen:** This is the combination of basal insulin with one or more doses of short-acting insulin or rapid acting insulin analog before meal as needed.
   - Example:
     - Inj. Regular 0 + 6 + 0
     - Inj. NPH 6 + 0 + 6
     Or
     - Inj. Aspart 0 + 6 + 0
     - Inj. Glargine 0 + 0 + 6.
   - Use: Useful regimen in elderly and CKD patients.

3. **Premixed insulin:** Here combination of short and intermediate acting insulin given twice a day before breakfast and before dinner. Morning and predinner dose is adjusted according to predinner and fasting blood glucose level, respectively. Premixed analog also can be used.
   - Example: Inj. Premixed insulin 30/70 6 + 0 + 6
   - Advantage:
     - Worldwide most commonly prescribed insulin regimen
     - Convenient for patient, so more patient compliance to the regimen
   - Disadvantage:
     - Difficult to achieve glycemic control at all points of day
     - Risk of hypoglycemia when meal time is irregular.

4. **Split mixed regimen:** Short-acting insulin given two or three times daily as needed with intermediate acting insulin given one or two times daily according to blood sugar level.
   - Example:
     - Inj. Regular 6 + 6 + 6
     - Inj. NPH 6 + 0 + 6
     Or
     - Inj. Regular 6 + 0 + 6
     - Inj. NPH 6 + 0 + 6
     Or
     - Inj. Regular 6 + 6 + 6
     - Inj. NPH 0 + 0 + 6
   - Advantage: Easier to achieve glycemic control at all points of day
   - Disadvantage:
     - Not convenient for patient/need for multiple injections
     - Dose adjustment is sometimes difficult for patient

5. **Basal bolus regimen:** Long-acting insulin analog given at bedtime as basal dose and rapid acting insulin analog given before each meal as bolus doses
   - Example:
     - Inj. Aspart 6 + 6 + 6
     - Inj. Glargine 0 + 0 + 20
   - Advantage:
     - Ideal insulin regimen as it mimics normal physiological insulin secretion pattern
     - This is very flexible and ideal for those who are very active and cannot comply with rigid meal plan or in whom diabetes control is difficult with other regimen
   - Disadvantage: Need for multiple injections.

6. **CSII pump:** Insulin pump is a medical device used to deliver insulin at basal rate throughout 24 h and patient activated boluses during meal times through a subcutaneous cannula. Some of the devices are also equipped with real-time continuous glucose monitoring (RT-CGM) system
   - Uses:
     - Used only in selected patients, for example, history of recurrent hypoglycemia and hypoglycemic unawareness
     - HbA_1C above goal despite best attempts of physician and health-care team
     - Postrenal transplant diabetic patients on steroid
   - Advantages:
     - Improved metabolic control in type 1 DM
     - Better reduction in HbA_1C without associated increase in hypoglycemia
     - Easy delivery of multiple insulin injections
     - Accurate delivery of more precise amount of insulin
     - Insulin pump user reports better quality of life
   - Disadvantages:
     - Expensive
     - Restriction from activities that may damage pump, for example, rough sports, activities in water
     - Some user finds it uncomfortable to wear pump all the time
     - Risk of insulin pump malfunction
   - Complication:
     - Infusion site scarring
     - Infusion catheter kinking or dislodgement
     - Need to change the pump reservoir and infusion system on regular basis
     - Insulin instability in pump infusion system
     - Pump malfunction or failure.

Q. Draw a flowchart about insulin initiation guideline (ADA 2018) in type 2 DM.

Ans.

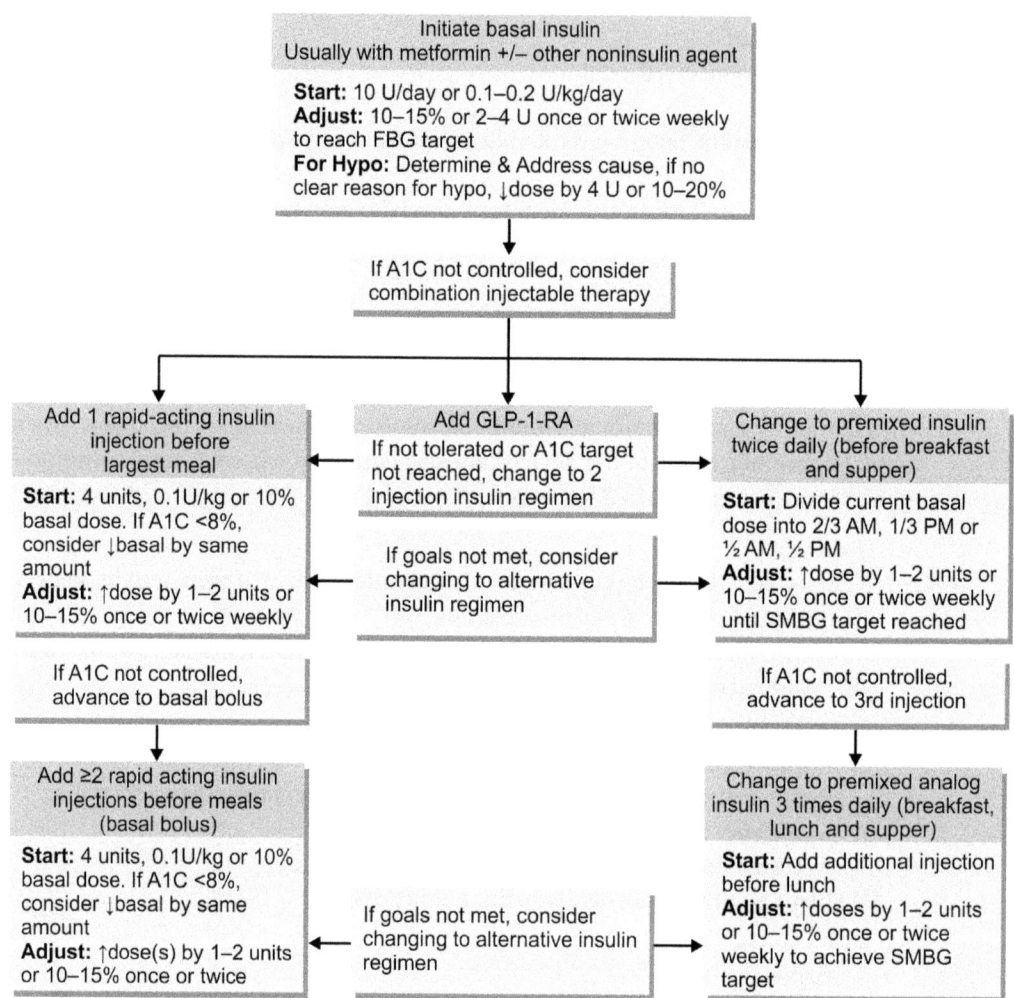

Q. What are the indications of intravenous insulin infusion?

Ans.

- Diabetic ketoacidosis and hyperosmolar nonketotic coma
- Critical illness, for example, acute MI, stroke
- Prolonged (>12 h) nil per os (NPO) status
- Total parenteral nutrition
- Perioperative period
- During delivery

Chapter 6: Insulin

- Uncontrolled hyperglycemia exacerbated by illness or steroid
- Any condition requiring prompt lowering of blood glucose.

Q. How to initiate insulin in OAD failure?

Ans.
- Continue metformin (if not contraindicated) at maximum tolerable dose
- To replace secretagogue with insulin, some prefer to taper OAD with simultaneous initiation and increment of insulin dose with some period overlapping, but some authors advocate not using secretagogue with insulin
- Start with basal insulin and increase dose and add bolus insulin, if needed.

Q. How to switch split mixed regimen from premixed regimen?

Ans.
- Regular insulin and NPH dose is calculated from premixed regimen and NPH given before breakfast and dinner and regular insulin given two or three times before meal
- **Example:** If patient getting Inj. premixed insulin 30 + 0 + 20. So total regular insulin 15 U, NPH 35 U
- So split-mixed regimen will be
  - Inj. Regular 10 + 0 + 6
  - Inj. NPH 20 + 0 + 14.

Q. How to switch basal bolus regimen from premixed regimen?

Ans.
- Calculate total dose of regular insulin and NPH
- Total NPH dose is reduced by 30% and given as basal insulin at bed time
- Total dose of regular insulin distributed as rapid acting analog
- **Example:** If patients getting Inj. premixed insulin 30 + 0 + 20. So total regular insulin 15 U, NPH 35 U. Thirty percent of 35 U = 10 U to reduced
- So basal bolus regimen will be
  - Inj. Aspart 6 + 6 + 6
  - Inj. Glargine 0 + 0 + 26.

Q. Discuss about insulin analogs.

Ans.
- **Definition:** AA sequence of human insulin is altered to produce insulin analogs with altered pharmacokinetic properties.
- **Types:**

1. **Rapid acting analogs:**
   - Insulin lispro: Proline at position B28 moved to B29, and lysine at position B29 moved to B28
   - Insulin aspart: Substitution of B28 proline with negatively charged aspartic acid
   - Insulin glulisine: Substitution of B3 lysine with asparagine and B29 lysine with glutamic acid.

- **Advantages of rapid acting analogs:**
  - Rapid onset and early peak action of rapid acting analogs more closely mimic normal endogenous prandial insulin secretion and control postprandial hyperglycemia more effectively than regular insulin
  - Fewer episodes of between meal hypoglycemia than regular insulin
  - Their very rapid onset of action allows them to be injected immediately before meals or even after meals which is especially useful in patient with erratic eating patterns, for example, young patient, elderly, CKD
  - Lowest variability of absorption (5%) with 25% for regular insulin
  - Preferred insulin for use in CSII pump
  - Insulin lispro and aspart can be administered IV and used as alternative to soluble insulin for diabetic emergency and at the time of surgery
- **Disadvantage of rapid acting analogs:** Shorter duration of action than regular insulin can cause preprandial hyperglycemia.

2. **Long-acting analogs:**
   - Insulin glargine: Attachment of two arginine molecule to B chain carboxyl terminal and substitution of A21 asparagine with glysine
   - Insulin Detemir: Terminal threonine is removed from B30 position, and FA chain is attached to B29 lysine
   - Insulin degludec: Terminal threonine is removed from B30 position, and a side chain consisting of glutamic acid and fatty acid has been attached to B29 lysine.
   - **Advantages of long-acting analogs:**
     - More reproducible absorption than conventional long-acting insulin
     - A flat dose profile with low peak of action provides more predictable control than NPH
     - Long-acting analogs reduce the risk of nocturnal hypoglycemia.
   - **Comparison between long-acting analogs:**
     - Duration of action of glargine (24 h), detemir (18 h), insulin degludec (beyond 42 h)
     - Detemir is weight friendly, so choice in obese patient
     - As detemir has short duration of action, so choice in CKD patients (less risk of hypoglycemia).

CHAPTER 7

Hypoglycemia

Q. Define hypoglycemia.

Ans.
- All episodes of abnormally low plasma glucose concentration expose the individual to potential harm
- Hypoglycemia is defined biochemically with blood glucose level <2.5 mmol/L with clinical features of adrenal overactivity and neuroglycopenia
- Glycemic threshold for symptoms shifts to lower plasma glucose concentration in people with tightly controlled diabetes or recurrent hypoglycemia and to higher plasma glucose concentration in those with poorly controlled diabetes (relative hypoglycemia).

Q. Mention clinical features of hypoglycemia.

Ans.

1. **Whipple's triad:**
   - Patients had symptoms of hypoglycemia
   - Low plasma glucose at the time of symptoms
   - Symptoms resolved on correction of hypoglycemia

2. **Autonomic/adrenergic features:** Also called warning symptoms, caused by sympathoadrenal discharge.
   - Sweating, palpitation, tremor
   - Anxiety, hunger, paresthesia

3. **Neuroglycopenic features:** Caused by deprivation of glucose in brain.
   - Headache
   - Visual disturbance
   - Behavioral changes
   - Cognitive impairment
   - Convulsion, confusion, drowsiness, coma

Q. Discuss defense against hypoglycemia.

Ans.

Response	Glycemic threshold (mmol/L)	Role
↓ Insulin	4.4–4.7	First defense against hypoglycemia
↑ Glucagon	3.6–3.9	Second line defense against hypoglycemia
↑ Epinephrine	3.6–3.9	Third defense against hypoglycemia
↑ Cortisol and GH	3.6–3.9	Involved but not critical
Symptoms	2.8–3.1	Prompt behavioral defense (food ingestion)
↓ Cognition	<2.8	Compromises behavioral defense

- **First defense against hypoglycemia:** ↓ Insulin secretion →↑ gluconeogenesis in liver and kidney, ↓ glucose utilization by insulin sensitive tissues, for example, muscle
- **Second defense against hypoglycemia:** ↑ Glucagon secretion caused by ↓ in intra-islet insulin and ↑ autonomic nervous system—sympathetic, parasympathetic and adrenomedullary inputs. Glucagon ↑ hepatic glycogenolysis
- **Third defense against hypoglycemia:** ↑ Adrenomedullary epinephrine secretion. Epinephrine ↑ gluconeogenesis in liver and kidney, ↓ glucose utilization by insulin sensitive tissues, mobilization of gluconeogenic substrate, for example, lactate and amino acid from muscle, glycerol from fat
- Glucagon and epinephrine act rapidly (within minute) to raise plasma glucose concentration. ↑ Cortisol and GH ↓ glucose utilization by insulin sensitive tissues and ↑ gluconeogenesis over a longer time frame (hours)

Q. Discuss about hypoglycemia unawareness/hypoglycemia-associated autonomic failure.

Ans.

- **Definition:** In certain conditions, diabetic patients may not have adrenergic symptoms in response to falling blood glucose, so appropriate actions cannot be taken with risk of severe hypoglycemia known as hypoglycemia unawareness
- **Risk factors:**
  - Long-standing type 1 diabetes
  - Type 2 diabetes with predominant β-cell destruction
  - Autonomic neuropathy
  - Diabetic person on beta blocker
  - During sleep
  - Persons with strict glycemic control
- **Pathogenesis:**
  - In long-standing type 1 diabetes mellitus (T1DM) or type 2 diabetes mellitus (T2DM) with predominant β-cell destruction, circulating insulin concentration cannot decrease in response to falling plasma glucose due to therapeutic/exogenous hyperinsulinemia. There is also loss of increase in circulating glucagon concentration. So both first and second line defenses against hypoglycemia are lost

Chapter 7: Hypoglycemia

- Epinephrine secretory response to falling plasma glucose is attenuated that causes defective glucose counter regulation and attenuated sympathetic neural response cause reduced adrenergic/warning symptoms of developing hypoglycemia. As it compromises behavioral defense against developing hypoglycemia (e.g., ingestion of food), hypoglycemia awareness is associated with ↑ risk of severe hypoglycemia
- **Treatment:** Frequent blood sugar monitoring to prevent and treat severe hypoglycemia.

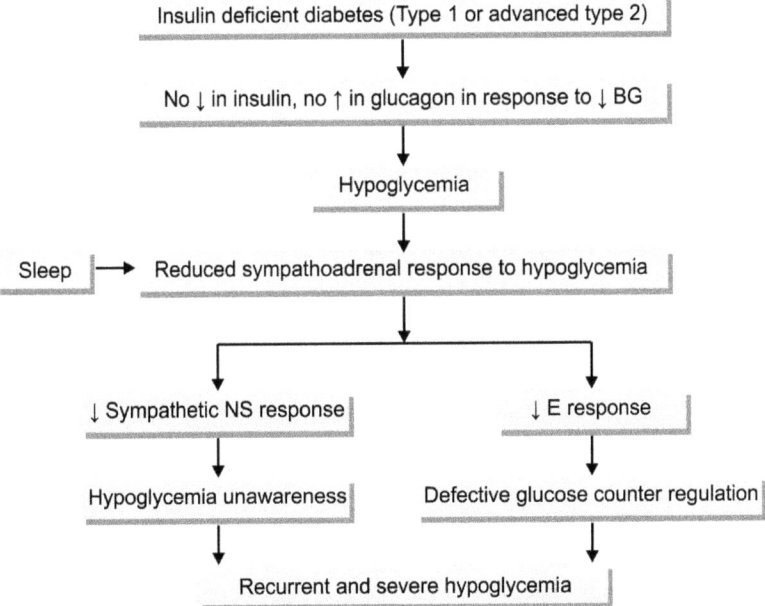

Q. Mention causes of hypoglycemia.

Ans.

- Missed, delayed or inadequate meal
- Error in oral antidiabetic drugs or insulin dose/schedule/administration, for example, insulin vial and syringe mismatch
- Unexplained or unusual exercise
- Alcohol
- Severe liver or kidney function impairment
- Poorly designed insulin regimen
- Lipodystrophy at injection site causing variable insulin absorption
- Gastroparesis due to autonomic neuropathy
- Malabsorption, for example, celiac disease, gastroenteritis
- Unrecognized other endocrine disorder, for example, Addison's disease, hypopituitarism
- Factitious/deliberately induced.

Q. What are the risk factors for severe hypoglycemia?

Ans.
- C-peptide negativity (absolute endogenous insulin deficiency)
- Strict glycemic control/aggressive glycemic therapy
- Hypoglycemia unawareness
- Age (very young and elderly)
- Increasing duration of diabetes
- Sleep
- H/o previous severe hypoglycemia
- Renal impairment.

Q. Mention complications of hypoglycemia.

Ans.
- **CNS:** Convulsion, coma, intellectual decline, transient ischemic attack/stroke, hypoglycemic encephalopathy/brain damage
- **Heart:** Cardiac arrhythmia, myocardial infarction
- **Eye:** Vitreous hemorrhage, worsening of retinopathy
- **Others:** Accident/road traffic accident.

Q. Discuss about nocturnal hypoglycemia.

Ans.
- Night time hypoglycemia usually occur between 2 AM and 4 AM
- As hypoglycemia may not waken a person, the warning symptoms are not perceived
- Sometimes, patients may have poor quality of sleep, vivid dream, nightmare, morning headache, hangover, forgetfulness, chronic fatigue
- Sometimes partner may observe sweating, restlessness, twitching or even seizure
- Diagnosis is by measuring blood glucose at night.
- Treatment:
  - Reduction of evening dose of intermediate/long acting $\pm$ regular/rapid acting analog
  - Ensure a carbohydrate snack before going to bed
  - A long acting insulin analogue should be taken with breakfast instead of at bed time so that its action will be waning at night.

Q. Classify hypoglycemia.

Ans.
- **Mild hypoglycemia:** Self-treated
- **Severe hypoglycemia:** Require assistance of another person for recovery
- **Relative hypoglycemia:** Hypoglycemia-like symptoms with measured plasma glucose concentration >3.9 mmol/L but approaching that level. Glycemic threshold for symptoms shift to higher plasma glucose concentration in those with poorly controlled diabetes.

Chapter 7: Hypoglycemia

Q. How will you prevent hypoglycemia in a diabetic patient?

Ans.
- Patient education about potential cause and risk of hypoglycemia including management
- Relative and friends should also be familiar with the symptoms and signs of hypoglycemia and management
- Carry a supply of fast acting carbohydrate
- If strenuous exercise is anticipated, the preceding dose of insulin should be reduced or extra carbohydrate ingested
- Perform frequent blood sugar testing
- Flexible and appropriate insulin or other drug regimens
- Individualized glycemic goals
- Ongoing professional guidance and support
- Use rapid acting insulin analog for long distance air travel.

Q. How you treat hypoglycemia?

Ans. Treatment depends on severity and whether patient in conscious and able to swallow.
- **Mild hypoglycemia:**
  - Oral fast acting carbohydrate, for example, 15–20 g glucose for patient with glucose alert value (<3.9 mmol/L) or equivalent food, for example, snack or meal. It usually raises blood glucose to safe limit (5.5 mmol/L)
  - The food/drink repeated every 15 min until patient is stable
- **Severe hypoglycemia:**
  - Administer 25–50 mL 25% dextrose IV
  - Inj. Glucagon 1 mg IM or SC may be given in T1DM but avoided in T2DM as glucagon itself is an insulin secretagogue
  - Glucose gel, jam or honey may be applied to buccal mucosa
  - When patient is conscious and able to swallow, give oral refined glucose as drink or sweets
  - If hypoglycemia occurs due to long or intermediate acting insulin or long acting sulfonylurea, for example, glibenclamide, 10% dextrose infused to prevent recurrent hypoglycemia
  - Antidiabetic medication should be started later with the dose reduced by 10%–20% of previous dose
  - If patient fails to regain consciousness after blood glucose is restored to normal, cerebral edema and other causes of impaired consciousness should be considered
  - Cerebral edema require urgent treatment with mannitol and high dose O_2.

Q. Discuss about early morning hyperglycemia/prebreakfast hyperglycemia.

Ans.

1. **Etiology:**
   - Waning of circulating insulin level by morning (common cause)

- Somogyi effect/posthypoglycemic hyperglycemia: Nocturnal hypoglycemia leads to surge of counter regulatory hormones to produce high-blood glucose level at morning
- Dawn phenomenon: Reduce tissue sensitivity to insulin between 5 AM and 8 AM.

2. **Investigations:**

	Blood glucose		
	10 PM	3 AM	7 AM
Waning of insulin	N	High	High
Somogyi effect	N	Low	High
Dawn phenomenon	N	N	High

3. **Treatment:**
   - Waning of insulin: ↑ Evening dose of insulin or shifting it from dinner time to bed time or both
   - Somogyi effect: ↓ Dose of intermediate/long insulin at dinner time and snacks at bed time
   - Dawn phenomenon: Dose of intermediate insulin divided between dinner time and bed time or ↑ evening dose of insulin or shifting it from dinner time to bed time.

Q. What are causes of unconsciousness in a diabetic patient?

Ans.
- **Related to DM:**
  - Hypoglycemia
  - Hyperosmolar nonketotic coma and diabetic ketoacidosis
  - TIA/stroke
- **Not related to DM:**
  - **Metabolic:**
    - Electrolyte imbalance commonly hyponatremia
    - Hepatic failure
    - Uremia
    - Respiratory failure
    - Drug or alcohol intoxication
    - Thiamine deficiency/Wernicke encephalopathy
  - **Endocrine:**
    - Myxedema coma
    - Adrenal crisis
    - Hypercalcemic crisis
  - **Infection:** Meningitis, meningoencephalitis, brain abscess, malaria, septicemia
  - **Others:** Syncope, head injury, ICH.

CHAPTER 8

Diabetic Ketoacidosis and Hyperosmolar Nonketotic Coma

Q. Mention acute complications of diabetes mellitus (DM).

Ans.
- Hypoglycemia
- Diabetic ketoacidosis (DKA)
- Hyperosmolar nonketotic coma (HONC)
- Lactic acidosis.

Q. Define diabetic ketoacidosis.

Ans. It is a medical emergency in diabetic patients defined as presence of all three of the following:
- Hyperglycemia (blood glucose >15 mmol/L)
- Acidosis (arterial pH <7.3, plasma bicarbonate <15 mEq/L)
- Ketosis.

Q. Discuss pathophysiology of diabetic ketoacidosis.

Ans.
- DKA commonly found in type 1 DM, but it also occurs in other types of diabetes during stressful situations
- It results from lack of insulin and rise in counter regulatory hormones, which leads to hyperglycemia and subsequent lipolysis
- Insulin deficiency may be relative (e.g., in the setting of severe infection) where normal amount of insulin is insufficient or absolute when insulin therapy is neglected
- Many patients have infection but present with normothermia or even hypothermia caused by peripheral vasodilation due to acidosis
- Despite potassium depletion, serum K^+ either normal or even elevated initially due to disproportionate loss of water, intracellular to extracellular shift caused by insulin deficiency, acidosis (H^+ displace intracellular K^+)
- However, soon after insulin treatment, there is likely to be a precipitous fall in plasma K^+ due to dilution of extracellular K^+ by administration of intravenous fluids, movement of K^+ into cells as a result of treatment with insulin

- DKA may present with normal or moderately elevated glucose concentrations (euglycemic ketoacidosis in 1%–3% cases) particularly when ketones are produced early in patients with reduced carbohydrate intake, for example, patients with gastrointestinal disease.

Q. Discuss about hormonal regulation of ketogenesis and glucose metabolism.

Ans.

Hormone	Ketogenesis	Gluconeogenesis	Glycogenolysis	Glycolysis	Glycogenesis
Insulin	↓	↓	↓	↑	↑
Glucagon	↑	↑	↑	↓	↓
Catecholamine	↑	↑	↑	↓	↓
GH	↑	↑	↑	↓	↓
Cortisol	↑	↑	↑	↓	↓

Q. How will you differentiate stress ketosis, DKA and HONC?

Ans.

Points	Stress ketosis	DKA	HONC
Plasma glucose	Variable	>15 mmol/L	>30 mmol/L
Arterial pH	Normal	<7.3	Usually normal
Serum HCO_3^-	Normal	<15 mmol/L	>15 mmol/L
Urine/blood ketones	↑	↑	Normal/marginally ↑
Anion gap	Normal/marginally ↑	>10	Variable
Mental status	Normal	Usually conscious, may be drowsy, coma in severe cases	Drowsy, coma

Q. Mention precipitating factors of DKA.

Ans.

- Undiagnosed diabetes (up to 20% type 1 DM may present with DKA)
- Omission of insulin dose
- Injudicious reduction of insulin dose
- Intercurrent illness, especially acute infection (20%–40%)
- Cardiovascular events, for example, MI, stroke
- Trauma, pregnancy, pancreatitis
- Alcohol, corticosteroid, drug abuse.

Q. Mention average amount of fluid and electrolyte loss in DKA.

Ans.

- Water: 6 L (3 L extracellular-replace with saline, 3 L intracellular-replace with dextrose)
- Na^+: 500 mEq
- Cl^-: 350 mEq

- K^+: 300–1,000 mEq
- Ca^+: 50–100 mmol
- PO_4^{++}: 50–100 mmol
- Mg^{++}: 25–50 mmol.

Q. Mention clinical features of DKA.

Ans.

1. **Symptoms:**
   - DKA usually develops rapidly (hours to days)
   - Symptoms of uncontrolled diabetes precedes (polyuria, polydipsia)
   - Weakness
   - Nausea, vomiting, abdominal pain, leg cramps
   - Visual disturbance.

2. **Signs:**
   - Dehydration: Dry skin, tongue, sunken eyeball, hypotension, rapid weak pulse
   - Rapid respiration leads to air hunger/acidotic breathing/Kussmaul breathing (deep and sighing respiration) in severe cases
   - Acetone breath in smell (nail varnish remover)
   - Hypothermia
   - Confusion, drowsiness, coma (10%). The state of consciousness is very variable in DKA. A patient with dangerous ketoacidosis may walk into consulting room.

Q. How will you investigate DKA?

Ans.

- Blood glucose, urea, creatinine, electrolytes (↑ urea: dehydration)
- Arterial blood gas
- Blood/urine for ketone body (3-hydroxybutyrate in blood/acetoacetate in urine)
- ECG
- Infection screen: Full blood count, blood and urine culture, C-reactive protein, chest X-ray (leukocytosis may occur in DKA in absence of infection, may represent a stress response)
- HbA_1C
- Serum amylase and lipase levels may be elevated even in absence of pancreatitis.

Q. Mention calculations in DKA.

Ans.

- Calculation of serum osmolality (mOsm/kg): $2 Na^+ + 2 K^+ + glucose + urea$ (mmol/L)
- Glucose in (mg/dL)/18 = mmol/L, urea in (mg/dL)/2.8 = mmol/L
- Calculation of anion gap: $(Na^+ + K^+) - (Cl^- + HCO_3^-)$
- Correction of serum Na^+ for hyperglycemia: For each 100 mg/dL glucose above 100 mg/dL, add 1.6 mEq Na^+, for example, measured Na-120 mmol/L, RBS-600 mg/dL
   So, corrected Na^+ = measured Na^+ + (RBS-100/100) × 1.6 = 128 mmol/L

Q. How you will manage a case of DKA?

Ans.

1. **Principles of management:**
   - Fluid replacement for correction of dehydration
   - Short acting/soluble insulin
   - Potassium replacement
   - Treatment of infection, if present
   - Proper nursing care
   - Monitoring.

2. **Fluid replacement:**
   - 0.9% normal saline IV
     - One liter over 30 min
     - One liter over 1 h
     - One liter over 2 h
     - One liter over next 2-4 h
   - Subsequent choice of fluid replacement depends on state of dehydration, serum electrolytes, urine output and blood glucose level
   - If serum Na^+ >155 mmol/L, 0.45% NS should be used
   - When blood glucose comes to 14 mmol/L, switch to 5% dextrose 1 L IV 8 hourly depending on frequent blood sugar monitoring
   - Typical requirement is 6 L in first 24 h but avoid fluid overload in elderly patients
   - Subsequent fluid requirement should be based on clinical response including urine output.

3. **Short acting/soluble insulin:**
   - If infusion pump available: 50 U soluble insulin in 50 mL 0.9% saline (0.5 mL inj. Actrapid 100 + 49.5 mL NS) IV via infusion pump 6 U/h initially
   - Or 10-20 U of soluble insulin IM followed by 5-10 U IM hourly
   - When blood glucose comes to 14 mmol/L: 2-3 units/h
   - Hourly fall of blood glucose should be 3-4 mmol/L
   - In limited facility: 50 U inj. Actrapid 100 + 500 mL NS IV by microburette at 60 µdrop/min (6 U insulin/h) initially
   - "Sliding scales" of insulin administration (in which insulin is prescribed according to blood glucose levels immediately before injection) should not be used as sliding scale insulin therapy treat hyperglycemia after it has already occurred, instead of preventing the occurrence of hyperglycemia. This reactive approach leads to rapid changes in blood glucose level exacerbating both hyper- and hypoglycemia
   - Transition from IV to SC insulin therapy if
     - Patient is clinically stable
     - Patient is biochemically stable
     - Patient is able to take oral food

Chapter 8: Diabetic Ketoacidosis and Hyperosmolar Nonketotic Coma

- Formula:
  - Calculate total insulin required in last 6 h. For example, if patient getting 2 U/h, so in last 6 h, he got $2 \times 6 = 12$ U. So 24 h insulin requirement $12 \times 4 = 48$ U
  - Eighty percent of last 24 h insulin requirement given $= 40$ U/day
    - For example, inj. Regular insulin 100 6+6+6 and
    - Inj. NPH 100 0+0+20

    Or
    - Inj. Aspart 6+6+6 and
    - Inj. Glargine 0+0+20
- The very short half-life of IV insulin necessitates administering the first dose of SC insulin before discontinuation of IV insulin
- If short or rapid acting insulin is used, SC insulin started 1–2 h before stopping the infusion
- If intermediate or long acting insulin is used, it should be started 2–3 h before
- A combination of short/rapid and intermediate/long acting insulin is preferred
- Basal insulin can be initiated any time of the day and should not withhold to a specific dosing time, for example, bed time.

4. **Potassium replacement:** Depends on blood level of K^+

Serum K^+ (mmol/L)	K^+ infusion (mmol/L)
<3.5	40
3.5–5.5	20
>5.5 or patient is anuric	Not to be given

- Potassium should be added to any bicarbonate given
- ECG monitoring or periodic tracing helpful to look cardiac toxicity
- After correction of K^+, oral supplementation should be continued for 1 week.

5. **Sodium bicarbonate:** Rarely indicated as it causes hypokalemia and paradoxically worsen intracellular acidosis. If pH <7, 100 mL sodium bicarbonate 1.26% IV over 45–60 min added with 20 mmol KCl.

6. **Proper nursing care:**
   - Catheterization if no urine passed after 3 h
   - NG tube to keep stomach empty in unconscious or semiconscious patients or if vomiting is protracted
   - CV line if cardiovascular system compromised to allow fluid replacement to be adjusted accurately
   - Antibiotic if infection demonstrated or suspected.

7. **Monitoring:**
   - Clinical condition (Pulse, BP, temperature, respiratory rate, urine output) hourly
   - Blood glucose, urea, creatinine, electrolyte, ABG 2–4 hourly until stable
   - Blood/urine ketone
   - Other tests as required.

Q. What are the complications of DKA.

Ans.
- Cerebral edema: Caused by very rapid reduction of blood glucose, use of hypotonic fluids or bicarbonate. Treat with mannitol
- Acute circulatory failure
- Thromboembolism
- Disseminated intravascular coagulation (DIC).

Q. What are the causes of death of DKA?

Ans.
- Before treatment is initiated: Cardiovascular collapse, acidosis
- After initiation of treatment: Cerebral edema, hypokalemia (insulin induced K$^+$ flux and unnecessary HCO_3^- infusion).

Q. What are the prognostic factors of DKA?

Ans.
- Severity of acidosis/HCO_3^- level/anion gap (pH <7, HCO_3^- level <10 and anion gap >12: poor prognosis)
- Severity of dehydration
- Shock
- Hypokalemia
- Thromboembolism
- DIC
- Extremes of age, comorbidity
- Coma
- Mortality: 5%–10% in specialized centers and 15%–25% in other hospitals.

Q. Define hyperosmolar nonketotic coma.

Ans. It is a medical emergency usually seen in elderly type 2 DM patients with presence of the following:
- Hyperglycemia (blood glucose >30 mmol/L)
- Hyperosmolality (effective serum osmolality >320 mOsm/kg)
- No acidosis (arterial pH >7.3, plasma bicarbonate >15 mEq/L)
- Absence of significant ketonemia/ketonuria (residual insulin reserve prevent ketosis)
- DKA and HONC are not mutually exclusive, and in fact, one third of patients admitted for hyperglycemia exhibit characteristics of both DKA and HONC better termed hyperosmolar hyperglycemic state (HHS).

Q. What are the precipitating factors of HONC?

Ans.
- Long period of poor control or undiagnosed type 2 DM
- Any acute stress, for example, infection, MI, stroke, trauma

Chapter 8: Diabetic Ketoacidosis and Hyperosmolar Nonketotic Coma

- Underlying chronic disease (renal, cardiac, old stroke)
- Compromised fluid intake
- Drugs, for example, glucocorticoids, diuretics.

Q. Mention clinical features of HONC.

Ans.
- Develops slowly (days to weeks)
- Symptoms of uncontrolled DM precede
- Dehydration is profound
- Impairment of consciousness is common, when osmolality >340 mOsm/kg (normal 280–295 mOsm/kg).

Q. How will you treat HONC?

Ans.
- 0.45% NS given until osmolality comes to normal, then 0.9% NS can be used
- These patients are relatively sensitive to insulin and approx. half of the dose recommended for DKA is given (3 U/h)
- Thromboembolic complications are common. So prophylactic low-molecular weight heparin given
- Mortality rate high (20%–50%).

Q. What are ketone bodies?

Ans.
- **Name:** Acetoacetate, β hydroxybutyrate, acetone
- **Site of formation:** Liver (solely), in mitochondria
- **Function:** Serve as a fuel for skeletal muscle, cardiac muscle, renal cortex. Even brain can utilize them during prolonged period of fasting
- **Routes of excretion:** Urine except acetone (excreted by lung as volatile).

Q. What are the causes of ketosis?

Ans.
- DKA
- Eclampsia
- Prolonged starvation
- High fat, low carbohydrate diet.

Q. Write down the procedure of Rothera's test.

Ans.
- A volume of 3 mL urine saturated with ammonium sulfate taken in a test tube
- Three drops of freshly prepared 5% sodium nitroprusside added to it and shake well
- A volume of 2 mL concentrated ammonium hydroxide is added by the side of test tube
- A permanganate/purple-colored ring at the junction of two solutions indicate ketone body present in urine (acetoacetate).

CHAPTER 9

Diabetic Retinopathy

Q. What is diabetic retinopathy?

Ans.
- **Definition:** It is a specific form of microangiopathy of retina with one or more of the following lesions:
  - Microaneurysm
  - Hemorrhage
  - Exudate
  - New vessel formation
- **Epidemiology:**
  - Leading cause of blindness
  - Strongly related to duration of diabetes and level of glycemic control
  - Some degree of retinopathy is evident after 15–20 years in nearly all type 1 diabetes mellitus (T1DM) and in >60% of type 2 diabetes mellitus (T2DM)
  - Up to 20% of people with T2DM have retinopathy at the time of diagnosis of DM.

Q. Mention risk factor for diabetic retinopathy.

Ans.
- Prolonged duration of DM
- Poor glycemic control
- Hypertension (HTN)
- Dyslipidemia
- Nephropathy
- Smoking
- Pregnancy.

Q. Describe pathogenesis of diabetic retinopathy.

Ans.
- Chronic hyperglycemia ↑ retinal blood flow also impairs vascular autoregulation and causes loss of pericyte
- The resulting increased blood flow initially dilates capillaries, but due to ↑ production of vasoactive substance and platelet stickiness leads to capillary closure

- This causes chronic retinal hypoxia and stimulates production of vascular endothelial growth factor (VEGF)/angiogenic factor that causes new vessel formation
- These new vessels are fragile, leaking and liable to rupture causing hemorrhage (intraretinal, preretinal or vitreous). Serous protein leakage from these new vessels stimulate connective tissue reaction called retinitis proliferans, later on retinal detachment may occur.

Q. How will you assess a patient of diabetic retinopathy?

Ans.

1. **Protocol:**
    - Initial dilated and comprehensive eye examination by an ophthalmologist should be done at diagnosis and then
        - Yearly in T2DM
        - Yearly after 5 years in T1DM
        - Less frequent examination (2 yearly) if one or more annual eye examinations reveal normal and glycemia is well controlled or at least annually if retinopathy is documented and more frequently if retinopathy is progressing or sight threatening
    - Eye examination should be done before pregnancy or in first trimester with monitoring in each trimester and for 1 year postpartum.

2. **History:** Duration of DM, treatment history, any ocular complaints.

3. **Examination:**
    - Ptosis
    - Cataract
    - Visual acuity (Snellen chart): Visual acuity testing may be misleading in uncontrolled DM. So assessment for refraction should be done after controlling blood sugar. A temporary deterioration of vision may occur following control of blood sugar due to osmolarity change of lens
    - Field of vision
    - Color vision (Ishihara chart)
    - Movement of eyeball, diplopia
    - Pupil examination: Size, shape, light and accommodation reflex
    - Dilated ophthalmoscopy
    - Slit lamp biomicroscopy of retina: To diagnose retinal disease, macular edema.

4. **Lab test:**
    - Color fundus photography
    - Fundus fluorescein angiography (FFA): To detect retinal disorder and to evaluate ischemic retinal leakage, neovascularization, unexplained reduction of vision
    - Optical coherence tomography (OCT): To detect macular disorder

- Ultrasound B scan: To examine the density and extent of vitreous hemorrhage and presence or absence of retinal detachment where the retinal view is obscured
- Perimetry: For visual field analysis.

5. **Referral to ophthalmologist:** Severe nonproliferative diabetic retinopathy (NPDR), PDR, any level of macular edema.

Q. **Classify diabetic retinopathy.**

Ans.

1. **Early NPDR:** Microaneurysm, dot and blot hemorrhage, hard exudate.
   - Microaneurysm: Earliest and hallmark of diabetic retinopathy. Dilation of capillary due to loss of supporting pericyte and localized increased hydrostatic pressure appear as small red dot along the vessel wall
   - Dot and blot hemorrhage: Red round or blot-shaped hemorrhage in inner nuclear layer/deeper hemorrhage. Superficial flame-shaped hemorrhage particularly if patient is hypertensive
   - Hard exudate: Small yellowish deposit with sharp margin results from serous protein leakage from vessels.

2. **Moderate to severe NPDR:** ±Lesions of early NPDR.
   - Cotton wool spot/soft exudate: Fluffy white patches composed of axoplasm and organelles of nerve fibers indicative of retinal ischemia
   - Venous loops and beading
   - Intraretinal microvascular abnormalities

3. **Proliferative diabetic retinopathy:** ±Lesions of NPDR
   - Neovascularization of disc (NVD): Large bundles of new vessels on the optic nerve head
   - Neovascularization elsewhere (NVE): Large bundles of new vessels on the periphery of retina
   - Vitreous hemorrhage: Vitreous is cloudy or opaque and often has a reddish hue
   - Fractional retinal detachment: Loss of vision if macula is detached.

4. **Maculopathy:** Edema, exudate or hemorrhage in and around the macula. Patient complaint of visual impairment.

Q. **How you treat a patient of diabetic retinopathy?**

Ans.

- **Metabolic control:** Good glycemic control ↓ incidence and progression of diabetic retinopathy
- **Control of HTN:** As uncontrolled HTN cause rapid progression of diabetic retinopathy
- **Argon laser phototherapy:** ↓ Risk of vision loss in patients with PDR, severe NPDR, clinically significant macular edema. Laser treatment is beneficial in ↓ risk of further

visual loss but generally not beneficial in reversing already diminished acuity. Patient with PDR treated with pan retinal photocoagulation (PRP). In this procedure, a series of 1,200–1,600 laser burns of 500 μm diameter are applied in midperipheral retina, avoiding macular region. Pregnancy is not contraindication to laser treatment
- **Vitrectomy:** Done in advanced PDR where visual loss is caused by recurrent vitreous hemorrhage
- **Pharmacotherapy:**
  - Aldose reductase inhibitor
  - Intravitreal injection of VEGF inhibitor. Bevacizumab (Avastin) is recombinant monoclonal antibody against VEGF cause some regression of neovascularization and reduction of leakage from vessels but effect is transient (2–11 weeks)
  - Aspirin can be given for cardioprotection (no ↑ risk of retinal hemorrhage).

Q. Mention complications of laser treatment.

Ans.
- Loss of peripheral areas of visual field
- Unintended laser absorption, for example, to lens
- Inadvertent coagulation, for example, to the fovea
- Choroidal detachment.

Q. Mention complications of PDR.

Ans.
- Vitreous hemorrhage
- Retinal detachment
- Glaucoma
- Rubeosis iridis (new vessel formation in iris).

Q. Classify hypertensive retinopathy

Ans.

Keith–Wagener–Barker classification:
- Grade 1: Arteriolar thickening, tortuosity and increased reflectiveness (Silver wiring)
- Grade 2: Grade 1 + constriction of veins of arterial crossing (arteriovenous nipping)
- Grade 3: Grade 2 + retinal ischemia (flame shaped or blot hemorrhage and cotton wool exudate)
- Grade 4: Grade 3 + papilledema.

Q. Mention ocular complication of diabetes.

Ans.
- Prone to infection: Orbital cellulitis, mucormycosis (fungal), dacrocystitis
- Third, fourth and sixth nerve palsy
- Diabetic retinopathy
- Cataract: Senile cataract comes 10–15 years earlier in diabetic patient. Very rarely, diabetic specific "snow flake cataract" in young patient

- Glaucoma: Secondary/angle closure glaucoma develops due to blockage of aqueous flow by new vessels on anterior surface of iris
- Rubeosis iridis.

Q. What are the causes of loss of vision in DM?

Ans.

1. **Gradual:**
   - Diabetic retinopathy
   - Cataract
   - Glaucoma
   - Rubeosis iridis
2. **Sudden loss of vision:**
   - **Related to DM:**
     - Vitreous hemorrhage
     - Retinal detachment
     - Central retinal vein occlusion (stormy sunset appearance)
     - Amaurosis fugax (transient monocular blindness due to vascular occlusion in retina)
     - Acute ischemic optic neuropathy
     - Acute glaucoma
   - **Not related to DM:**
     - Methanol poisoning
     - Ethambutol, quinine toxicity
     - Pituitary apoplexy
     - Cortical blindness (stroke), bilateral occipital lobe infarction
     - Migraine
     - HCR.

CHAPTER 10

Diabetic Nephropathy

Q. Define diabetic nephropathy.

Ans. It is one of the microvascular complications of diabetes mellitus (DM) which is a specific form of microangiopathy of kidney with the characteristic hall mark of:
- Persistent loss of albumin in urine and
- Progressive renal insufficiency with or without hypertension (HTN).

Q. Mention epidemiology of diabetic nephropathy.

Ans.
- Leading cause of end-stage renal failure (ESRF) in the world
- Approximately 30%–40% of type 1 diabetes mellitus (T1DM) will eventually develop diabetic nephropathy
- Nephropathy is less common in type 2 diabetes mellitus (T2DM) than in T1DM, but due to greater number of T2DM, majority of patients with ESRF are T2DM.

Q. Discuss natural history of diabetic nephropathy.

Ans.
- Approximately 30%–40% of T1DM will develop diabetic nephropathy after 20 years in contrast to T2DM, where 15%–20% will develop clinical kidney disease
- It passes through several stages which differ with respect to renal hemodynamics, systemic BP, urinary findings and susceptibility to therapeutic interventions
- At the onset, kidneys are usually enlarged with hyperfiltration. Glomerular filtration rate (GFR) may be as high as 40% above normal. In the next stage, the first evidence of nephropathy is detected by appearance of microalbuminuria (urinary albumin excretion 30–299 mg/day)
- Once microalbuminuria is established, blood pressure starts to rise. In the next stage, there is overt proteinuria (urinary albumin excretion ≥300 mg/day) where BP continues to rise
- There is a progressive decline in renal function with reduction of GFR and retention of nitrogenous waste product in body
- Ultimately, patients progress to ESRF with features of azotemia
- Histologically, the changes associated with diabetic nephropathy is thickening of glomerular basement membrane and accumulation of matrix material in the mesangium (nodular glomerulosclerosis/Kimmelstiel-Wilson nodule).

Q. What are the stages of chronic kidney disease (CKD)?

Ans.
- Stage 1: kidney damage with normal or increased eGFR ≥ 90 mL/min/1.73 m^2
- Stage 2: kidney damage with eGFR 60–90
- Stage 3: eGFR 30–59
- Stage 4: eGFR 15–29
- Stage 5: eGFR <15 or dialysis

Kidney damage means pathological abnormalities of blood, urine tests or imaging studies. Two eGFR values 3 months apart are required to assign a stage.

Q. Mention normal protein excretion in urine.

Ans. Less than 150 mg/day (Tamm–Horsfall protein secreted by tubule).

Q. Discuss about microalbuminuria.

Ans.
- Identifies incipient nephropathy in T1DM and T2DM and an independent predictor of macrovascular disease in T2DM
- Urinary albumin excretion 30–299 mg/day or 20–199 µg/min or albumin–creatinine ratio (ACR) 2.5–30 (M) or 3.5–30 mg/mmol (F)
- Risk factor include HTN, poor glycemic control, smoking
- Who to screen:
  - T1DM: Annually from 5 years after diagnosis
  - T2DM: Annually from time of diagnosis
- Abnormal results:
  - Exclude recent (24 h) vigorous exercise, fever, heart failure, urine infection, menstruation, marked hyperglycemia, marked HTN
  - If microalbuminuria is present, perform two additional measurements in next 3–6 months. Diagnosis of microalbuminuria is established if two out of three measurements are abnormal as microalbuminuria may be intermittent or persistent.

Q. Mention risk factors associated with development and/or progression of diabetic nephropathy.

Ans.
- Long duration of diabetes
- Poor glycemic control
- HTN, dyslipidemia, smoking
- Urinary tract obstruction
- Urinary tract infection

Chapter 10: Diabetic Nephropathy

- Nephrotoxic medications
- Reduced renal perfusion, for example, renal artery stenosis, poor cardiac function
- Presence of other microvascular complications
- Genetic factors.

Q. How will you screen for diabetic nephropathy?

Ans. Annual serum creatinine, calculate estimated GFR (eGFR), serum K^+, urine R/M/E (early morning urine sample/dipstick for proteinuria).

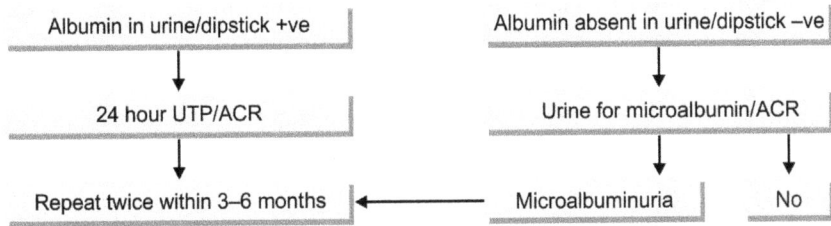

Q. How to calculate creatinine clearance rate (CCR)?

Ans. Cockcroft and Gault equation reasonably accurate at normal to moderately impaired renal function, require age, sex, serum creatinine, body weight

$$CCR = \frac{(140 - \text{age in years}) \times \text{lean body weight (kg)} \times 1.22 \text{ (male) or } 1.04 \text{ (female)}}{\text{Serum creatinine } (\mu mol/L)}$$

Serum creatinine mg/dL × 88.4 = µmol/L.

Q. How you investigate a patient of diabetic nephropathy?

Ans.

- Blood urea, creatinine, electrolytes
- Blood glucose profile, HbA_1C
- Urine R/M/E: UTI (may be asymptomatic)
- 24 h UTP/ACR, CCR and eGFR estimation
- Serum albumin (low in nephrotic syndrome, also malnutrition, inflammation)
- USG of W/A with PVR: Kidney size, progressive ↑ in echogenicity of cortex
- CBC with ESR
- Ca^{++}, PO_4^{++}, intact parathyroid hormone (iPTH), X-ray hand (renal osteodystrophy)
- Fasting lipid profile: Cardiovascular risk
- ECG: IHD, electrolyte imbalance
- If patient is anemic: PBF, iron profile, vitamin B_{12}, folate
- HBsAg, HIV: If dialysis or transplantation planned, HBV vaccination if sero –ve

- Renal biopsy: Indicated in uncertainty in etiology of renal disease (absence of retinopathy, RBC cast in urine, nephrotic range proteinuria, unexplained rapid deterioration of renal function in absence of renal papillary necrosis).

Q. How you will manage a case of diabetic nephropathy?

Ans.

1. **Aim of management:**
   - Prevent further renal damage, for example, by glucose control, control of HTN
   - Identify reversible factors which are making renal function worse, for example, UTI, urinary tract obstruction, nephrotoxic medication
   - Limit adverse effects of loss of renal function
   - Address any associated cardiovascular risk/disease
   - Institute renal replacement therapy (RRT) when appropriate.

2. **Diet and nutrition:**
   - **Protein restriction:**
     - Reduce glomerular hyperperfusion and albuminuria
     - Low-protein diet does not alter the progression of nephropathy significantly but reduce uremic symptoms (risk of malnutrition)
     - No more than moderate protein restriction
     - 0.8 g/kg/day (nondialysis dependent), 1–2 g/kg/day when on dialysis
     - At least 50% of dietary protein should be of high biological value
   - **Carbohydrate intake:**
     - Adequate calorie intake (30–35 kcal/kg/day) is essential for patient with CKD, especially those on protein restriction
     - Source: Mainly complex carbohydrate
   - **Potassium restriction:**
     - With deteriorating renal function, K^+ restriction needed (<70 mmol/day), especially patient taking angiotensin-converting enzyme inhibitor (ACEI) or angiotensin receptor blocker (ARB)
     - K^+ rich food: Fruit, fruit juice, tomato, raw tea
     - Low K^+ fruit: Apple, guava, papaya
   - **Phosphate restriction:**
     - Target serum PO_4^{++} in CKD <4.6 (stages 3 and 4) and <5.5 mg/dL (stage 5)
     - Phosphate rich food: All protein containing food, for example, milk, cheese, egg, meat. So it is difficult to balance dietary phosphate restriction against adequate protein intake
     - Phosphate binder used if dietary restriction alone fails
   - **Salt restriction:** If BP ↑ ± volume overload. Aim <6 g/day (<100 mmol/day)
   - **Fluid restriction:** In CKD stages 4–5, fluid and salt restriction is needed to prevent volume overload. Depends on urine output. Previous day output + 500 mL (insensible loss) is to be advised

- **High uric acid containing food restriction:** Red meat, sea fish, liver, kidney, brain
- **Avoid fatty food:** ↑ Risk of cardiovascular disease.

3. **Glycemic control:**
   - Good glycemic control reduces incidence and progression of diabetic nephropathy significantly
   - HbA_1C target <7% without undue hypoglycemia
   - Red cell turnover is abnormal in CKD. So HbA_1C may be misleading, more reliance on SMBG
   - Sulfonylurea: Reduced dose or avoidance. Avoid long acting SU in CKD stages 3–5
   - Meglitinides: Low dose if eGFR <30 mL/min/1.73 m²
   - Metformin: Risk of lactic acidosis. Avoid if serum creatinine ≥1.5 (M) or ≥1.4 (F) or eGFR <30 mL/min/1.73 m². Avoid initiation of metformin if eGFR <45 mL/min/1.73 m²
   - TZDs: Use limited due to fluid retention
   - Insulin: Excreted by kidney, may need reduced dose or switch to shorter acting preparation
   - GLP-1 receptor agonist: Exenatide not used if eGFR <30 mL/min/1.73 m² Liraglutide is probably safe
   - DPP-4 inhibitor:
     - Vildagliptin: 50 mg daily if eGFR <50 mL/min/1.73 m²
     - Sitagliptin: 50 mg daily if eGFR 30–50 mL/min (creatinine 1.7–3 in male, 1.5–2.5 in female), 25 mg daily if eGFR <30 mL/min (creatinine >3 in male, >2.5 in female) or dialysis
     - Linagliptin: No dose adjustment in CKD
     - Saxagliptin: 5 mg daily if eGFR >50, 2.5 mg daily if eGFR <50 mL/min/1.73 m².

4. **Control of HTN:**
   - Target BP: <140/90 and <130/80 mm Hg if high risk of cardiovascular disease, albuminuria or CKD (eGFR <60 mL/min/1.73 m²)
   - Drug of choice: ACEI, ARB, thiazide like diuretics or dihydropyridine CCB, for example, amlodipine
   - If albuminuria is present, drug of choice is ACEI or ARB. Dilate efferent arteriole →↓ glomerular perfusion pressure →↓ proteinuria and also retard the progression of renal failure (renoprotective action)
   - If ACEI or ARB used, check creatinine, eGFR and serum K⁺ periodically. If GFR ↓ >20% or creatinine ↑ >25% from baseline or creatinine >5 mg/dL → stop ACEI/ARB → investigate to exclude bilateral RAS
   - If BP ≥160/100 mm Hg, start with two antihypertensive medications.

5. **Others management:**
   - Weight reduction for obese patients and keep BMI <25 kg/m²
   - Dyslipidemia: Statin

- Stop smoking
- Aspirin 75 mg/day
- Muscle cramp: Quinine sulfate
- Restless leg syndrome: unpleasant sensation in leg at night relieved by movement, treated with clonazepam
- Treatment of anemia
- RRT: If indicated.

6. **Referral to nephrologist:**
   - eGFR <30 mL/min/1.73 m²
   - Uncertainty about etiology of kidney disease
   - Rapidly declining renal function
   - Difficult management issue (anemia, secondary hyperparathyroidism, metabolic bone disease, resistant hypertension).

Q. Discuss relationship between erythropoietin (EPO) and CKD.

Ans.
- EPO is produced by peritubular interstitial fibroblasts in outer medulla and deep cortex of kidney
- EPO is essential for terminal maturation of erythrocytes
- CKD and renal scarring →↓ EPO synthesis →↓ RBC production and anemia
- Anemia occur in most forms of advanced CKD (eGFR <30 mL/min/1.73 m²) except adult polycystic kidney disease, renal cell carcinoma where EPO may be overproduced (So anemia is less severe or absent).

Q. What are the causes of anemia in CKD?

Ans.
- Relative deficiency of EPO
- Toxic effect of uremia on marrow precursor cells
- ↓ Red cell survival
- Blood loss (capillary fragility, poor platelet function)
- ↓ Iron and other hematinics intake, absorption and utilization
- Hyperparathyroidism/bone marrow fibrosis.

Q. How to evaluate anemia of CKD?

Ans.
- EPO deficiency is not only the cause of anemia in CKD. Patient with CKD are susceptible to all other causes of anemia
- So initial laboratory evaluation therefore aimed at identifying other factors that may cause or contribute to anemia or lead to EPO hyporesponsiveness
- Initial assessments of anemia include full blood count with film, reticulocyte count, iron profile, vitamin B_{12} and folate, C-reactive protein (CRP)
- Anemia of CKD is normochromic and normocytic (MCV, MCH, MCHC: ↔).

Q. What are the treatment modalities of anemia?

Ans.
- Erythropoiesis stimulating agent (ESA)/EPO
- Iron.

Q. Discuss about erythropoietin (EPO) therapy in CKD.

Ans.
- **Indications of EPO:**
  - Any anemic CKD patient, assuming other causes of anemia have been excluded
  - Consider EPO when Hb% <10 g/dL
- **Preparation before EPO therapy:**
  - Have other causes of anemia excluded, especially iron deficiency
  - Is the patient likely to respond to EPO? Inflammatory cytokines associated with infection or chronic inflammatory state inhibits the effect of EPO. Treat these first (↑ CRP often predict poor response)
  - Is BP controlled? EPO tends to ↑ BP, especially in early days of EPO use
- **EPO preparation and dose:**
  - Epoetin (recombinant human EPO) α: Start with 50 U/kg (3,000–4,000 U/dose) once or twice a week, adjusted according to response at interval of 4 weeks
  - Epoetin β
  - Epoetin Δ
  - Darbepoetin α (Hyperglycosylated derivative of EPO)
  - Methoxy polyethylene glycol epoetin β (continuous EPO receptor activator): Start with .6 µg/kg every 2 weekly, adjusted according to response at interval of at least 4 weeks. Once Hb% 11 g/dL is reached, maintenance dose may be given every 4 weeks
- **Routes of administration of EPO:**
  - Subcutaneous (SC) route: In nonHD–CKD patients
  - Intravenous (IV) route: In HD–CKD patients
  - SC route is preferable to IV route as it requires 33% lower dose for same effect
- **Monitoring of EPO therapy:**
  - Measure Hb% and BP weekly at first
  - Hb% should raise no >1 g/dL every 4 weeks
  - ↓ EPO dose by 25% if rise of Hb% exceeds 2 g/dL over 4 weeks or if Hb% approaches or exceeds 12 g/dL
  - Iron stores likely to rapidly deplete, monitor and replace as necessary
  - Once in steady state, monitor Hb% and iron stores 1–2 monthly in predialysis patients and monthly in dialysis patients
- **EPO therapy target:**
  - Target Hb: 11–12 g/dL
  - Hematocrit: 33–36%
  - Overzealous correction (>12 g/dL) associated with ↑ thrombotic risk, cardiac risk and mortality

- **Adverse effects of EPO:**
  - Hypertension: In 20% patients. Intensify antihypertensive medication, reduce or even withhold of EPO dose may be necessary
  - Blood coagulability and thrombosis of AV fistulae
  - Fit
  - Thrombocytosis
- **Hyporesponse to EPO:** Failure to ↑ Hb% >11 g/dL despite EPO dose equivalent to epoetin >500 IU/kg/week. Causes are
  - Iron deficiency
  - Infection/inflammation (measure CRP)
  - Chronic blood loss (particularly GI)
  - Severe hyperparathyroidism (Cause BM fibrosis-check PTH)
  - Aluminum toxicity (in dialysis patients)
  - Hemoglobinopathies
  - Vitamin B_{12} or folate deficiency
  - Occult malignancy
  - Pure red cell aplasia
  - Malnutrition
  - Inadequate dosing
  - Poor compliance.

Q. Write down about normal iron profile?

Ans.

- Serum iron: 10–32 μmol/L
- Serum ferritin: Male—20–300, female—15–150 ng/L (ferritin is an acute phase protein. So if inflammation presents, it will be misleadingly high. So measure CRP simultaneously)
- Total iron binding capacity: 45–70 μmol/L
- Percentage saturation of iron binding protein/transferrin saturation (TSAT): 33%

$$TSAT = Iron/TIBC \times 100.$$

Q. Discuss about iron therapy in CKD.

Ans.

- **Indication of iron replacement:** Patient with serum ferritin <100 ng/mL or TSAT <20% should receive iron supplementation
- **Targets of iron therapy:**
  - HD-CKD (Hemodialysis dependent CKD): Serum ferritin >200 ng/mL and TSAT >20%
  - ND-CKD (nondialysis dependent CKD) and PD-CKD (peritoneal dialysis dependent CKD): Serum ferritin >100 ng/mL and TSAT >20%
  - Upper level of ferritin: >500 ng/mL not routinely recommended

Chapter 10: Diabetic Nephropathy

- **Oral iron preparations:**
  - Ferrous sulfate 300 mg (elemental iron 60 mg), ferrous fumarate 200 mg (elemental iron 65 mg)
  - Ferrous fumarate is better as elemental iron is higher and more absorbable than other forms
  - Iron absorption decreases with antacid, phosphate binder, tea, milk and tetracycline
  - Iron rich food: Liver, meat, banana, apple (fruits that become black on cutting)
- **Parenteral iron preparations:**
  - Iron dextran: Risk of anaphylactic reaction more, so not used nowadays
  - Iron sorbitol: Commonly used
  - Dose calculation in mg: Weight (kg) × (target Hb – patients Hb) × .24 + 500–1000 mg (for stores)
  - Precaution: Anaphylactic reaction can occur. So patients should be given a small test dose initially (1 mL + 20 mL NS IV over 15 minutes) and facilities for dealing with anaphylaxis and cardiopulmonary resuscitation should be available
  - Normal dosage is 1–2 ampules one to three times a week depending on iron status
  - Full blood count, reticulocyte count and iron profile should be checked 3–4 weeks after final dose of IV iron.

Q. Define renal bone disease/renal osteodystrophy.

Ans. It is a heterogeneous disorder leading to diminished bone strength in patients with impaired kidney function.

Q. Mention components of renal osteodystrophy.

Ans.
- **Secondary hyperparathyroidism/hyperparathyroid bone disease/osteitis fibrosa cystica:** PTH secretion (and parathyroid gland proliferation) is stimulated by ↓ Ca^{++}, ↓ $1,25(OH)_2D$ and ↑ PO_4 in CKD. ↑ PTH causes increased bone resorption and formation (high turnover disease) causing haphazardly organized and weak bone
- **Osteomalacia:** Refers to defect in mineralization related to ↓ $1,25(OH)_2D$ but Al intoxication and uremic acidosis are also risk factors
- **Osteoporosis**
- **Osteosclerosis.**

Q. What is low turnover disease?

Ans. Low PTH causes ↓ bone resorption and formation may be observed in patients over treated with vitamin D metabolites, also known as adynamic bone disease.

Q. How tertiary hyperparathyroidism occur in CKD?

Ans. After prolonged secondary hyperparathyroidism, hyperplastic parathyroid glands become autonomous and continue to secrete PTH causing tertiary hyperparathyroidism.

Q. Write down the clinical features of renal bone disease.

Ans.
- Usually asymptomatic
- Bone pain and arthralgia
- Muscle weakness (esp. proximal)
- ↑ Fracture risk
- Marrow fibrosis contributes to anemia and poor response to EPO
- Increased cardiovascular risk.

Q. How will you investigate renal bone disease?

Ans.
- Serum Ca^{++}, PO_4^{++}, ALP, iPTH
- X-ray lumbosacral spine lateral view: ↑ Bone density at upper and lower part of vertebral body with translucency in the middle part giving rise to rugger jersey spine (osteosclerosis).

Q. Discuss about treatment of renal bone disease.

Ans.

1. **Goals:**
   - Keep serum Ca^{++} within normal range (normal serum Ca^{++} 8.5–10.5 mg/dL)
   - Keep serum 25(OH) Vitamin D within normal range (>30 ng/mL or >75 nmol/L)
   - Keep serum PO_4^{++} within normal range (normal serum PO_4^{++} 1.7–4.5 mg/dL). Target serum PO_4^{++} in CKD <4.6 (stages 3 and 4) and <5.5 mg/dL (stage 5)
   - Keep serum iPTH (intact PTH) appropriate to above objectives. Target serum iPTH in CKD 35–70 (stage 3), 70–110 (stage 4), 150–300 pg/mL (stage 3),
   - Keep bone turnover and strength as near normal as possible
   - Prevent development of parathyroid hyperplasia.

2. **Measures to ↑ serum Ca^{++} and suppress PTH synthesis and secretion:**
   - Calcium salts (e.g., calcium carbonate) also acts as phosphate binder
   - Vitamin D analogs (calcitriol .25–1 μg/day, alfacalcidol)
   - Parathyroidectomy (in tertiary hyperparathyroidism when persistent plasma iPTH >800 pg/mL with hypercalcemia refractory to medical therapy).

3. **Measures to reduce serum PO_4^{++}:**
   - Dietary PO_4^{++} restriction (milk, cheese, egg, protein rich foods)
   - Phosphate binders: Take just before meals to bind phosphate in gut. Aluminum hydroxide, calcium carbonate, sevelamer, lanthanum
   - Removal through adequate dialysis.

4. **Measures to suppress PTH synthesis and secretion directly:** Calcimimetic agents/calcium sensing receptor agonist Cinacalcet bind to parathyroid calcium sensing receptor and mimic the effect of ↑ extracellular Ca^{++} →↓ PTH. Indicated in tertiary hyperparathyroidism when parathyroidectomy is unsuccessful or not possible.

Chapter 10: Diabetic Nephropathy

Q. What is calciphylaxis?

Ans.
- Calciphylaxis (calcific uremic arteriopathy) is small vessel vasculopathy involving mural calcification with initial proliferation, fibrosis and thrombosis. It occurs in CKD and results in ischemia and necrosis of skin, soft tissue, viscera, skeletal muscle
- No treatment is of proven benefit. Wound care, avoid calcium-based binder and daily hemodialysis.

Q. Compare between primary and tertiary hyperparathyroidism.

Ans.

Points	*Primary hyperparathyroidism*	*Tertiary hyperparathyroidism*
Renal Function	Usually normal renal function but may have renal impairment	Stages 3–5 CKD
Phosphate	Low normal/low	High
25(OH) Vitamin D	Normal	↓
Renal osteodystrophy	Uncommon but may progress through CKD.	Common
Pathology	Single adenoma 85%	All parathyroid gland hyperplasia
iPTH	↑↑↑	↑↑

CHAPTER 11

Diabetic Neuropathy

Q. Define diabetic neuropathy.

Ans. Presence of symptoms and/or signs of peripheral or autonomic nerve dysfunction in people with diabetes after exclusion of other causes of neuropathy. Diabetic neuropathy (DN) is a diagnosis of exclusion.

Q. Discuss epidemiology, pathogenesis and histopathology of diabetic neuropathy.

Ans.

- **Epidemiology:**
  - DN is the most common neuropathy
  - Affects approximately 30% of diabetic patients
- **Pathogenesis:** DN is associated with long duration of diabetes, poor glycemic control, visceral obesity, smoking, hypertension (HTN) and dyslipidemia
- **Histopathology:**
  - Axonal degeneration of both myelinated and unmyelinated fibers
  - Thickening of schwann cell basal lamina
  - Patchy, segmental demyelination
  - Abnormalities of intraneural capillaries, thickening of basement membrane and microthrombi in intraneural capillaries.

Q. Why early diagnosis and management of diabetic neuropathy is important?

Ans.

- Non-DN may be present in patients with diabetes
- A number of treatment options exist for symptomatic DN
- Up to 50% of DN may be asymptomatic, and patients are at ↑ risk of foot lesions
- Autonomic neuropathy may involve every system in the body
- Autonomic neuropathy cause ↑ mortality and morbidity particularly if cardiac autonomic neuropathy (CAN) is present.

Chapter 11: Diabetic Neuropathy

Q. Classify diabetic neuropathy.

Ans.
1. Somatic:
   - Polyneuropathy:
     – Symmetrical, mainly sensory and distal
     – Asymmetrical, mainly motor and proximal (including amyotrophy)
   - Mononeuropathy including mononeuritis multiplex
2. Autonomic neuropathy.

Q. What is hyperglycemic neuropathy/acute sensory neuropathy?

Ans. Following periods of poor metabolic control, for example, diabetic ketoacidosis or sudden change in glycemic status (e.g. insulin neuritis following institution of insulin treatment), acute onset of severe sensory symptoms like continuous burning pain in soles (walking on burning sand) with marked nocturnal exacerbation with few neurological signs on examination is known as acute sensory neuropathy. A characteristic feature is cutaneous contact discomfort to clothes, for example, hypersensitivity to tactile (allodynia) or painful stimuli (hyperalgesia).

Q. Discuss about chronic sensorimotor diabetic peripheral neuropathy.

Ans.
- Most common presentation of DN
- Present with paresthesia or pain in lower limb and feet (burning, electric, sharp, stabbing, tingling, deep aching) typically worse at night and when tired or stressed
- Fifty percent of patients may be asymptomatic and diagnosed only by examination, and patients may present with painless foot ulcer. Longer axons to lower limbs are more vulnerable to lesion by diabetes
- Examination reveals loss of vibration, light touch, pain (glove and stocking) and absent ankle reflexes
- Other cause of neuropathy like chronic inflammatory demyelinating polyneuropathy (CIDP), vitamin B_{12} deficiency, hypothyroid, chronic renal failure should be ruled out.

Q. What is diabetic amyotrophy/Bruns–Garland syndrome?

Ans. Sudden onset of severe neuropathic pain, usually unilateral or bilateral muscle weakness and atrophy of proximal thigh muscles. Sometimes, there may be marked loss of weight (neuropathic cachexia). Usually no sensory loss. Often begins during hyperglycemia, may improve with good glycemic control.

Q. Discuss about diabetic autonomic neuropathy.

Ans. It may or may not be associated with peripheral neuropathy. Either sympathetic or parasympathetic nerve may be affected in one or more of the systems. The development of autonomic neuropathy is less clearly related to poor metabolic control than somatic neuropathy, and improved glycemic control rarely results in amelioration of symptoms. CAN have 5-year mortality rate 16%–50% with high proportion attributed to sudden cardiac death.

1. **Clinical features of autonomic neuropathy:**
   - **Cardiovascular:**
     - Postural hypotension: Fall in SBP >20 mm Hg or DBP >10 mm Hg in response to postural change from supine to standing. Patient may be asymptomatic or experience lightheadedness, dizziness, visual blurring, syncope. It is due to efferent sympathetic vasomotor denervation causing reduced vasoconstriction at splanchnic and other peripheral vascular beds. It is aggravated by vasodilator, diuretics
     - Resting tachycardia: Resting HR >100 beats/min. It is due to relative ↑ in sympathetic tone associated with vagal impairment. It may be due to anemia or thyroid disorder also
     - Fixed heart rate/impaired heart rate variability: Earliest clinical indicator of CAN. Normally HR fluctuates with respiration, ↑ with inspiration and ↓ with expiration. This variability is lost in CAN. A fixed HR that is unresponsive to moderate exercise, stress or sleep indicates CAN
     - Abnormal BP regulation: Normal subject exhibit predominance of vagal tone and ↓ sympathetic tone at night. In CAN, this pattern is altered resulting in sympathetic predominance at night leading to nocturnal HTN and cardiovascular events
     - Silent myocardial ischemia/cardiac denervation syndrome
     - Intraoperative and perioperative cardiovascular instability
   - **Gastrointestinal:**
     - Dysphagia due to esophageal atony
     - Abdominal fullness or discomfort, early satiety, nausea, vomiting, belching, bloating, unstable glycemia due to delayed gastric emptying (gastroparesis)
     - Nocturnal diarrhea due to bacterial overgrowth from stasis in gastrointestinal tract (GIT)
     - Fecal incontinence
     - Constipation due to colonic atony
   - **Genitourinary:**
     - Frequency, urgency, nocturia, urinary retention, incontinence, recurrent urinary tract infection (UTI) due to atonic bladder
     - Erectile dysfunction, retrograde ejaculation
     - Vaginal dryness and dyspareunia
   - **Sudomotor:**
     - Gustatory sweating: Profuse sweating of face during eating
     - Nocturnal sweats without hypoglycemia

Chapter 11: Diabetic Neuropathy

- Anhidrosis, fissures in the feet
- **Vasomotor:**
  - Feet feel cold due to loss of vasomotor response
  - Dependent edema due to loss of vasomotor tone and ↑ vascular permeability
- **Pupillary:**
  - Decreased pupil size
  - Resistant to mydriatics
  - Delayed or absent reflexes to light.

Q. How will you test cardiac autonomic neuropathy at bedside.

Ans.
- **Resting heart rate:** Resting HR >100 beats/min
- **Postural hypotension:** Measure supine BP after patient rests quietly on bed for 15 min and when the patient stands, measure BP after 1-2 min. Normal response is fall of <10 mm Hg. Fall in SBP >20 mm Hg or DBP >10 mm Hg indicates postural hypotension
- **Heart rate response to deep breaths:** With the patient at rest and supine, record pulse rate, and the patient is asked to take six deep breaths in 1 min. Pulse rate decrease >15 is normal and <10 indicate autonomic dysfunction
- **Heart rate response to valsalva manoeuvre:** Patient closes the glottis and attempts maximal expiratory efforts for 15 s; the resultant reduced venous return should reflexly lower pulse rate via vagus. The ratio of highest pulse rate in rest period to lowest pulse rate during the test >1.2 in normal subject and <1.2 in autonomic dysfunction. Not done in proliferative diabetic retinopathy (PDR) or severe non-PDR
- **Diastolic BP response to sustained handgrip:** With the patient lying flat, he/she grips a sphygmomanometer cuff as hard as possible to establish a maximum. Grip is then squeezed at 30% maximum for 5 min. Normal response is the rise of DBP >16 mm Hg in other arm.

Q. Write down management of diabetic neuropathy.

Ans.
- **Painful diabetic peripheral neuropathy:**
  - **Good glycemic control:** Neuropathic symptoms improve not only with good control but also avoidance of blood glucose fluctuations. Good glycemic control may halt progression of neuropathy
  - **Tricyclic antidepressants:** Amitriptyline (25–150 mg/day), Imipramine, (25–150 mg/day)
  - **SSRIs:** Duloxetine (60 mg/day), citalopram (40 mg/day)
  - **Anticonvulsants:** Gabapentin (900–1,800 mg/day), pregabalin (150–600 mg/day), carbamazepine (200–400 mg/day), topiramate (up to 400 mg/day)
  - **Opioids:** Tramadol (50–400 mg/day), oxycodone controlled release (CR)
  - **Topical capsaicin (substance P depletor):** For burning feet syndrome
  - **Aldose reductase inhibitor:** Epalrestat

- **Antioxidant:** α-Lipoic acid and linolenic acid
- **Postural hypotension:**
  - Gradual rise from bed or chair
  - Movement of leg prior to rising
  - Sleeping with elevated foot end of bed (20–30 cm)
  - Use of full length support stocking
  - Fludrocortisone: Risk of fluid overload and hypokalemia
  - Midodrine (α_1 adrenoreceptor agonist)
  - Others: Erythropoietin (EPO), salt loading, nonsteroidal anti-inflammatory drugs (NSAIDs)
- **Gastroparesis:**
  - Dopamine antagonist: Domperidone (10–20 mg 4–6 times/day) or metoclopramide
  - Percutaneous enteral (jejunal) feeding
- **Diabetic diarrhea:**
  - Loperamide (2 mg 3–4 times/day) or codeine phosphate
  - Tetracycline, erythromycin may act upon bacterial overgrowth in intestine
- **Constipation:** Stimulant laxatives (senna)
- **Atonic bladder:** Intermittent self-catheterization
- **Excessive sweating:** Anticholinergic (propantheline bromide), clonidine, topical antimuscarinic agent (glycopyrrolate cream)
- **Erectile dysfunction:**
  - Oral selective phosphodiesterase 5 inhibitor: Sildenafil, tadalafil
  - Intracavernosal injection of alprostadil (PGE_1)
  - Intraurethral alprostadil
  - External vacuum devices
  - Penile prosthesis
  - Vascular surgery
  - Psychosexual therapy.

Q. How to screen peripheral neuropathy in DM.

Ans. All patients with DM should be screened for peripheral neuropathy at diagnosis of T2DM or 5 years after diagnosis of T1DM and at least annually thereafter if no peripheral neuropathy is present.

Q. Discuss about neuropathic/charcot joints.

Ans.
- **Definition:** It is a rapidly destructive arthropathy of joints
- **Etiology:**
  - DN
  - Syringomyelia
  - Leprosy

- Tabes dorsalis
- **Pathogenesis:**
  - Repetitive microtrauma following sensory loss (neurotraumatic hypothesis)
  - Altered blood flow secondary to impaired sympathetic nervous system control (neurovascular hypothesis)
- **Clinical features:**
  - Subacute or insidious monoarthritis or dislocation
  - Pain is minimal
  - Joint grossly swollen with effusion, crepitation, marked instability and deformity (classic rocker-bottom dislocation of midfoot)
  - Sign disproportionally greater than symptoms
  - No ↑ warmth
  - Ultimately flail joint
- **Investigations:**
  - X-ray: Disorganization of normal joint architecture. Multiple loose bodies either no (atrophic) or gross (hypertrophic) new bone formation (sucked candy appearance)
  - MRI
  - Bone scintigraphy
- **Management:**
  - In acute phase: Immobilization, orthoses and shoes
  - Surgical management: Ostectomy, arthrodesis
- **Indication of surgery:**
  - Instability
  - Deformity
  - Recurrent ulceration
  - Refractory to conservative treatment
  - Must be quiescent
  - Circulation intact
  - No active infection
  - Medically stable.

CHAPTER 12

Diabetic Foot

Q. What is diabetic foot?
Ans. A variety of pathologic conditions that might affect the feet of people with diabetes.

> "Superior doctors prevent the disease, middle doctors treat the disease before evident and inferior doctors treat the full blown disease."

Q. Mention prevalence of diabetic foot.
Ans.
- Foot ulceration affects up to 25% of patients with diabetes during their lifetime
- Diabetes is the most common cause of nontraumatic foot amputation
- A leg is lost to diabetes somewhere in the world every 30 s.

Q. What are the risk factors of diabetic foot ulceration?
Ans.
- Peripheral neuropathy (somatic, autonomic)
- Peripheral vascular disease
- History of foot ulcer
- Previous amputation
- Severe foot deformity
- Limited joint mobility
- Plantar callus
- Visual impairment
- Diabetic nephropathy (especially patient on dialysis/end-stage renal disease)
- Poor glycemic control
- Cigarette smoking.

Q. Define high-risk foot of diabetics.
Ans. A foot is labeled as high-risk foot if one or more of the six factors are present:
- Loss of protective sensation
- Absent pedal pulses
- History of foot ulcer
- Previous amputation
- Severe foot deformity (claw toes, prominent head of metatarsal, loss of planter arch, callus, bunion, bunionette, Charcot joint, bony prominence)

- Limited joint mobility

(Coming events cast their shadow before)

Q. Discuss about pathogenesis of diabetic foot lesions.

Ans.
- Diabetic foot is due to
  - Loss of protective sensation (neuropathy)
  - Poor circulation (peripheral vascular disease)
  - Higher likelihood of developing infections
- Patient may or may not have neuropathic symptoms, but both groups may have significant sensory loss
- Neuropathic symptoms correlate poorly with sensory loss, and their absence never means lack of foot ulcer risk
- Assessment of foot ulcer risk must always include a careful foot examination after removal of shoes and socks, whatever the neuropathic history.

(Pain is God's greatest gift to mankind)

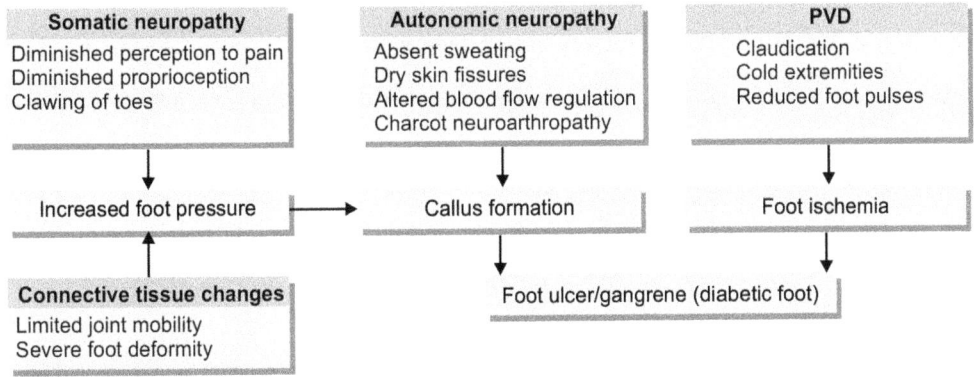

Q. How will you examine a diabetic foot?

Ans.

1. **Inspection:**
   - Evidence of past/present ulcer
   - Evidence of infection or increased pressure, for example, erythema, callus formation on weight bearing areas, discoloration of skin (ischemia), hemorrhage under a callus
   - Presence of thick nails, limited joint mobility, foot deformity
   - Fungal infection may affect skin between toes and nails.

2. **Neurological:**
   - Light touch: 10-g monofilament (Semmes–Weinstein nylon monofilament) at four sites on each foot + 1 of the following:

- Vibration using 128 Hz tuning fork
- Vibration perception threshold: Biothesiometer
- Pinprick sensation
- Ankle reflexes.

3. **Vascular:**
   - Peripheral pulses
   - Skin temperature and capillary refill
   - Doppler test (ankle brachial pressure index—ABPI)—if age >50 years or age <50 years with other peripheral arterial disease (PAD) risk factors (e.g., smoking, hypertension, dyslipidemia, duration of DM >10 years)
   - Pressure stat: Footprint mat able to identify areas of high foot pressures. The higher the pressure, the darker the color of footprint.

Q. What are the examination findings of PAD?

Ans.

1. **Inspection:**
   - Thin shiny skin with loss of hair
   - Nail: Brittle/falling
   - Ulcer (ischemic) at dorsum of foot, lateral malleolus
   - In gangrene: Black color.

2. **Palpation:**
   - Temperature: Cold extremity
   - Pulses: Diminished or absent
   - Pallor on elevation and rubor on dependency (Buerger's sign)
   - Superficial vein empty (gutter) on minimal elevation
   - Capillary refill time of fingertip >3 s.

Q. Mention anatomical position of leg arteries.

Ans.

- **Arteria dorsalis pedis:** At the proximal part of groove of first intermetatarsal space lateral to extensor hallucis longus tendon. It may be absent or abnormally sited in 10% normal subjects
- **Posterior tibial artery:** 2 cm below and behind of medial malleolus.

Q. Classify diabetic foot lesions according to Meggitt–Wagner.

Ans.

- Grade 0: No ulcer but high-risk foot
- Grade 1: Superficial ulcer
- Grade 2: Deep ulcer but no bony involvement, no abscess
- Grade 3: Deep ulcer with bony involvement or abscess
- Grade 4: Localized gangrene (at toe, heel)
- Grade 5: Gangrene of whole foot.

Chapter 12: Diabetic Foot

Q. Why wound healing is delayed in diabetic foot?

Ans.
- Inadequate tissue perfusion
- Altered bactericidal and chemotactic properties of phagocyte
- Abnormalities in cytokines and growth factors in tissues
- Repetitive pressure on the wound.

Q. What are the indicators of bony involvement or osteomyelitis?

Ans.
- Ulcer area $>2 \times 2$ cm
- Positive probe to bone test
- Elevated erythrocyte sedimentation rate
- Abnormal radiograph (negative MRI makes the diagnosis much less likely).

Q. What investigations should be done in a diabetic foot patient?

Ans.
- CBC: Evidence of infection
- Blood glucose
- Urine R/E (glycosuria)
- Serum creatinine
- Fasting lipid profile (atherosclerosis)
- Culture from deep wound and blood culture if indicated
- X-ray foot
- Doppler USG of lower limb vessels: To assess arterial circulation by measuring ABPI (normal >1, arterial disease/intermittent claudication <0.8, critical limb ischemia <0.5)
- Angiography: If plan of percutaneous transluminal angioplasty (PTA).

Q. How will you treat a patient of diabetic foot?

Ans.
- Team approach in collaboration of endocrinologist, podiatrist and vascular surgeon
- Good glycemic control with insulin
- Control of infection with broad spectrum antibiotic. Initial antibiotic regimen may be flucloxacillin + ampicillin + metronidazole or clindamycin + ciprofloxacin. Antibiotic changed according to culture report. Features of infection include—purulent discharge, rapid extension, cellulitis, local warmth, swelling, patient febrile or toxic
- Pressure offloading by various means
- Minor noninfected wound is treated with dressing and foot rest
- Infected lesions and more severe lesions need intensive therapy at hospital with wound debridement and dressing
- Wide surgical incision and drainage of deep infection is almost
- Debridement of devitalized tissue is must
- Deroofing of all the cavities should be done

- Diabetic foot will tolerate extensive incision far better than undisturbed deep infection
- Extent of devitalized tissue invariably greater than that of clinical external appearance
- No corrosive or detergent should be used in the wound
- Diluted hydrogen peroxide and diluted povidone iodine can be used when grossly infected, otherwise normal saline wash is best
- Amputation is needed if spreading infection threatening patient's limb or even life
- Consider vascular surgery in appropriate cases
- Newer therapies:
  - Growth factors
  - Hyperbaric oxygen
  - Negative pressure wound therapy
  - Bioengineered skin substitutes.

Q. Discuss foot care education of diabetics.

Ans.

1. **Screening for high-risk foot:** Screening for high-risk foot should be done at initial visit and at least yearly thereafter. Follow-up of high-risk foot should be done every 3-6 months.

2. **How to avoid heat injury to foot?**
   - Do not have very hot baths
   - Avoid sitting too close to the heater or fire
   - Do not use hot fomentations
   - Avoid hot water bottles or electric blankets in bed at night
   - Avoid all possible injuries to foot.

3. **How to inspect feet?**
   - Inspect feet daily—the toes, between the toes and the sole
   - Look and feel for breaks in the skin, cuts, scratches, bruises, blisters, sores and discoloration
   - Use of mirror or friend/relative to aid better viewing.

4. **How to cut nails?**
   - Cut nails after bath when these are soft and pliable
   - Cut nails straight not too deep on the sides
   - Do not use sharp instrument to clean under the nail or in the grooves
   - In case of pain or difficulty in cutting, consult nurse or doctor.

5. **How to choose footwear for a diabetic?**
   - **Shape and size:** Shoes must be of correct shape and size for feet. It is important to draw the outline of feet by placing them on paper. Cut this outline and carry it when buying shoes. The cut paper must fit inside of the shoes properly without folding anywhere. This would be the correct and comfortable shoe size

- **Heel and sole:** Flat shoes should be chosen. Thick soles protect the feet from sharp objects. High heel should be avoided by ladies
- **Toe box:** Rounded wide toe box give more space to feet
- **Material:** Leather shoes help the feet breathe freely
- **Shopping time:** Shopping for shoes should be always in the evening when the feet are the largest
- **Socks:** Woolen/cotton socks are to be used. Knee-high socks or socks with tight tips should be avoided. Check the size of shoes wearing the thickest socks
- **Slippers and sandals:** Slippers and sandals do not provide adequate support to the feet and should be avoided for full-day support. They should be used only for shorts periods like night wear.

6. When to contact with a doctor?
   - Color change of skin of foot (become red or black)
   - Temperature change of skin of foot (raised temperature or cool feet)
   - Swelling of feet
   - Ulcer of foot
   - Ingrowing nail causing lesions
   - Corn/callus in foot
   - Crack in sole.

Q. How can you differentiate an arterial ulcer from a neuropathic ulcer?

Ans. Arterial ulcer and neuropathic ulcer are differentiated as follows:

Points	Arterial ulcer	Neuropathic ulcer
Area	Cold extremity, thin shiny skin with loss of hair	Warm, dry and pink
Pulse	Reduced or absent	Normal
Site of ulcer	Dorsum of foot, lateral malleolus	Heel, ball of great toe (maximum pressure points)
Nature	Painful and punched out ulcer	Painless
Sensation	Normal	Reduced or absent

- Almost all ulcers of diabetic foot is neuroischemic type
- Vasculitis leg ulcer site: Upper leg
- Venous leg ulcer site: Lower leg, lateral malleolus.

Q. What are the other causes of leg ulcer?
- Arterial: PAD/Buerger disease
- Neuropathic: Leprosy, tabes dorsalis, peripheral neuropathy due to any cause
- Venous hypertension
- Infection: Tuberculosis, leishmaniasis
- Malignancy: Squamous cell carcinoma, basal cell carcinoma
- Systemic lupus erythematosus, sickle cell anemia.

CHAPTER 13

Dyslipidemia in Diabetes Mellitus

Q. Define dyslipidemia and hyperlipidemia.
Ans.
- **Dyslipidemia:** Abnormal level of one or more blood lipids
- **Hyperlipidemia:** Misnomer as patient may have isolated low HDL.

Q. Classify dyslipidemia.
Ans.
1. **Primary dyslipidemia:**
   - Polygenic (majority)
   - Familial hypercholesterolemia (LDL receptor defect, defective ApoB 100)
   - Familial hypertriglyceridemia, for example, Lipoprotein lipase deficiency.
2. **Secondary dyslipidemia:**
   - **Secondary hypercholesterolemia:**
     - Hypothyroidism
     - Nephrotic syndrome
     - Pregnancy
     - Cholestatic liver disease
     - Drugs (diuretics, ciclosporin, corticosteroids, androgens, antiretroviral agents)
     - Anorexia nervosa
     - Porphyria
   - **Secondary hypertriglyceridemia:**
     - Diabetes mellitus (Type 2)
     - Chronic renal disease
     - Abdominal obesity/central/apple shaped obesity
     - Excess alcohol
     - Hepatocellular disease
     - Drugs (beta blockers, retinoids, corticosteroids, antiretroviral agents).

Q. Mention cardiovascular risk factors.
Ans.
- Advancing age (male ≥ 45 years, female ≥ 55 years)
- Cigarette smoking

- Dyslipidemia
- Diabetes mellitus
- Hypertension (BP ≥140/90 mm Hg or on antihypertensive medication)
- Obesity, abdominal obesity
- Family history of premature coronary artery disease (CAD) (definite MI or sudden death before age 55 years in father or other male first-degree relative or before age 65 years in mother or other female first-degree relative).

Q. **What are the emerging cardiovascular risk factors?**

Ans.
- Family history of dyslipidemia
- Total cholesterol/HDL cholesterol ratio (normally <6)
- Elevated lipoprotein(a)
- Elevated ApoB (reflect LDL-C particle number)
- Elevated small, dense LDL-C
- Fasting/postprandial hypertriglyceridemia
- Polycystic ovarian syndrome
- Dyslipidemic triad (hypertriglyceridemia, low HDL-C and elevated small, dense LDL-C)
- Elevated clotting factors, for example, plasminogen activator inhibitor-1, fibrinogen
- Inflammation markers (C-reactive protein, lipoprotein-associated phospholipase A2)
- Elevated homocysteine
- Elevated uric acid
- Impaired glucose tolerance/impaired fasting glucose
- Antiphospholipid antibodies
  (HDL cholesterol ≥60 mg/dL counts as a "negative" risk factor, and its presence removes one risk factor from patient's risk profile).

Q. **Mention target lipid profile in diabetic patients.**

Ans.
- Total cholesterol: <200 mg/dL
- LDL cholesterol:
  - Less than 100 mg/dL
  - Less than 70 mg/dL (high-risk patients, e.g., h/o cardiovascular disease (CVD))
  - 30%–40% reduction from baseline LDL-C (If drug treated patients do not reach above targets with maximum tolerated statin)
- HDL cholesterol: As high as possible, >40 (male) and >50 mg/dL (female)
- Non-HDL cholesterol (total cholesterol–HDL-C): 30 mg/dL above patient specific LDL goal
- TG: <150 mg/dL
- Total cholesterol/HDL cholesterol ratio: <6
- ApoB:
  - Less than 90 (patients at risk of CAD, including those with diabetes)
  - Less than 80 (patients with established CAD or diabetes plus ≥1 additional risk factor)

Q. How will you screen for dyslipidemia?

Ans.
- Adult aged 20 years or older: Once every 5 years
- Increasing age or presence of CAD risk factors: More frequent assessment (1–2 yearly)
- Family history of premature CAD: Screen children older than 2 years every 3–5 yearly
- Patient hospitalized for acute coronary syndrome: Lipid profile within 24 h (as there is often a transient fall in blood cholesterol in 3 months following infarction)
- In patients with diabetes: Measure fasting lipid profile at least annually.

Q. What is Friedewald equation?

Ans.
- LDL-C = (total cholesterol – HDL-C) – TG/5 mg/dL
  - This method is valid only for values obtained during fasting state
  - Increasingly inaccurate when TG >200 mg/dL
  - Not valid when TG >400 mg/dL
  - Measure LDL-C directly when fasting TG >250 mg/dL or those with diabetes or known vascular disease
  - Cholesterol in (mg/dL)/38.7 = mmol/L, TG in (mg/dL)/88.6 = mmol/L.

Q. Mention clinical manifestations of dyslipidemia.

Ans.
- **Hypercholesterolemia:**
  - Xanthelasma
  - Tendon xanthoma
  - Corneal arcus
- **Hypertriglyceridemia:**
  - Lipemia retinalis
  - Acute pancreatitis (TG >800 mg/dL)
  - Lipemic blood and plasma
  - Hepatosplenomegaly
  - Eruptive xanthoma.

Q. Mention key features of diabetic dyslipidemia.

Ans.
- Low HDL cholesterol
- High TG
- High small dense LDL (more susceptible to oxidation and more atherogenic).

Q. Mention nonpharmacological management of dyslipidemia.

Ans.
- Therapeutic lifestyle changes diet:
  - Reduce intake of saturated fat (<7% of total calories), transunsaturated fat <1% and cholesterol <200 mg/day

- Increase intake of food containing LDL lowering nutrient, for example, *n*–3 fatty acid, dietary fiber (10-25 g/day or 14 g/1,000 kcal), plant sterols (2 g/day)
- Carbohydrate (50%-60% of daily calorie intake (DCI)). Carbohydrate should be derived predominantly from complex/unrefined carbohydrate, fruits and vegetables ($\geq$5 servings/day)
- Protein: 10%-20% of DCI
- Fat: 25%-35% of DCI, polyunsaturated fat (up to 10% of DCI), monounsaturated fat (up to 20% of DCI)
- Replace saturated fat and cholesterol with alternative foods, for example, lean meat, low fat dairy products, polyunsaturated fat and low glycemic index carbohydrates
- Reduce energy dense foods, for example, soft drinks

- Attain and maintain ideal body weight. Ideal body weight = (height in cm – 100) kg
- Regular physical activity: At least 150 min/week moderate intensity aerobic physical activity or 75 min/week of vigorous exercise or equivalent combination of both types with no more than two consecutive days without exercise (consuming 4-7 kcal/min with expenditure of $\geq$200 kcal/day)
- Stop smoking and alcohol ($\leq$2 drinks/day for adult men and $\leq$1 drink/day for adult women or <21 U/week for men and <14 U/week for women). 1 unit = 8 g of alcohol.

Q. Classify lipid-regulating drugs.

Ans.

Drug class	Agents and daily doses	Lipid/lipoprotein effects
HMG CoA reductase inhibitors (statins)	Atorvastatin (10–80 mg) Rosuvastatin (5–40 mg) Fluvastatin (20–80 mg) Pravastatin (20–40 mg) Simvastatin (20–80 mg) Cerivastatin (0.4–0.8 mg)	LDL ↓ 18%–55% HDL ↑ 5%–15% TG ↓ 7%–30%
Fibric acid derivatives	Gemfibrozil (300–600 mg) Fenofibrate (200 mg)	LDL ↓ 5%–20% HDL ↑ 10%–20% TG ↓ 20%–50%
Niacin/nicotinic acid/vitamin B3	Immediate release (1.5–3 g) Extended release (1–2 g)	LDL ↓ 5%–25% HDL ↑ 15%–35% TG ↓ 20%–50%
Bile acid sequestrants	Cholestyramine (4–16 g) Colestipol (5–20 g) Colesevelam (2.6–3.8 g)	LDL ↓ 15%–30% HDL ↑ 3%–5% TG no change or increase
Cholesterol absorption inhibitors	Ezetimibe (10 mg)	LDL ↓ 10%–18%
Omega 3 FA/omega 3 fish oil	2–4 g	↓ TG

Q. How can you treat dyslipidemia in diabetes?

Ans.
- Drug therapy should be added to lifestyle therapy, regardless of baseline lipid levels for diabetic patients:
  - With overt CVD
  - Without CVD but age >40 years and have one or more other CVD risk factors (family history of CVD, hypertension, smoking or albuminuria) or 10 year risk of coronary heart disease >20%.

1. **Statins:**
   - Statins competitively inhibit HMG CoA (3-hydroxy-3-methylglutaryl CoA) reductase—rate limiting enzyme of cholesterol synthesis in liver
   - Adverse effects:
     - Muscle effects/myopathy: Myalgia, myositis, rhabdomyolysis, asymptomatic increase in creatine kinase (CK)
     - Increase liver enzyme
   - Contraindication: Active liver disease or chronic liver disease, pregnancy
   - Advice to patient: To report if unexplained muscle pain, tenderness or weakness
   - Increase risk of myopathy:
     - High-dose statin or given with fibrate
     - Renal impairment
     - Personal or family history of muscular disorder
     - In those with hypothyroidism
     - With immunosuppressants, for example, ciclosporin
     - In elderly
   - Patient with hypothyroidism should receive adequate thyroid replacement before assessing requirement for lipid regulating drug because correcting hypothyroidism itself may resolve lipid abnormalities. Untreated hypothyroidism increase risk of myositis with lipid regulating drug.

2. **Fibrate:**
   - Mechanism of action:
     - ↑ Activity of lipoprotein lipase →↑ catabolism of TG
     - Stimulate peroxisome proliferator activator receptor (PPAR) α →↓ synthesis of FA, TG, very low-density lipoprotein (VLDL)
   - Adverse effects:
     - Gemfibrozil may ↑ LDL-C 10%–15%
     - Increase fibrinogen level
     - Prolong action of anticoagulant
     - ↑ Homocystiene
     - GI symptoms, cholelithiasis
     - Myopathy, rhabdomyolysis
   - Contraindication: Renal or hepatic disease.

Chapter 13: Dyslipidemia in Diabetes Mellitus

3. **Niacin:**
    - ↓ Hepatic synthesis of LDL-C and VLDL-C, ↓ lipoprotein
    - Most effective drug for raising HDL cholesterol
    - Adverse effects:
        – Flushing (due to prostaglandin-mediated vasodilation)
        – Hyperuricemia/gout
        – Hyperglycemia at higher dosage (>2 g/day)
    - Treatment of flushing: Low-dose aspirin, extended release formulation, Prostaglandin D-2 receptor inhibitor (laropiprant).

4. **Combination therapy:**
    - Increase risk of myositis/rhabdomyolysis, hepatotoxicity/abnormal transaminase
    - Indication:
        – When cholesterol level is markedly increased and monotherapy does not achieve the therapeutic goal
        – When mixed dyslipidemia is present. Therapy with statin and fenofibrate may be considered for men with both triglyceride level ≥204 mg/dL and HDL cholesterol level ≤34 mg/dL.

5. **Isolated low HDL (<40 mg/dL):**
    - Weight loss
    - ↑ Physical activity
    - Smoking cessation
    - If coronary heart disease or 10-year risk of coronary heart disease >20%: Consider drug therapy (nicotinic acid, fibrate).

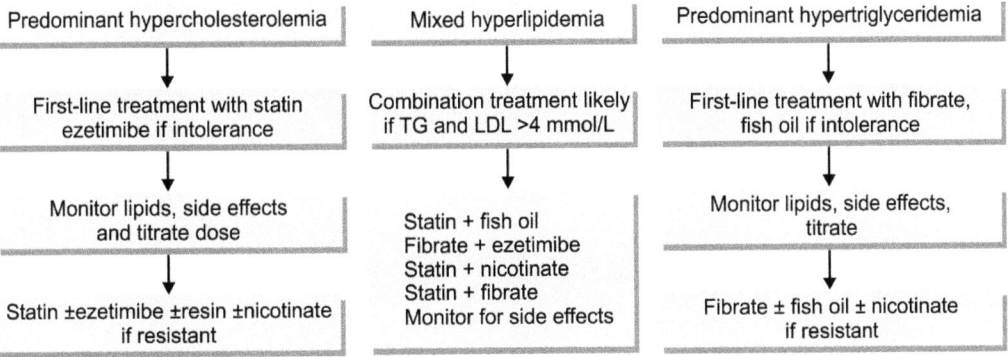

6. **Special consideration:**
    - Women: Statin or fibrate is contraindicated in pregnancy and lactation
    - Children: Statin, colesevelam, cholestyramine can be given in familial hypercholesterolemia of children of 10 years or older.

Q. How will you follow-up a patient on lipid regulating drug?

Ans.
- Assess lipid status 6 weeks after therapy (12 weeks for fibrates) initiation, thereafter every 6–12-month intervals
- Liver transaminase measured before and 3 months after, then repeated semiannually
- Creatine kinase level checked if patient reports clinically significant myalgia or muscle weakness
- Interrupt treatment if CK >5–10 times upper limit of normal or elevated with muscle symptoms or serum glutamic pyruvic transaminase/alanine transaminase more than two to three times upper limit of normal.

CHAPTER 14

Preconceptional Care in Diabetic Patients

Q. Discuss about preconceptional care in diabetic patients.

Ans.

1. **Goals:**
   - Involvement and empowerment of patient in management of her diabetes
   - Achieve HbA_1C as close to normal as is safely possible ($HbA_1C < 6.5\%$) without undue risk of hypoglycemia
   - Effective contraception until stable and acceptable glycemia is achieved
   - Identify, evaluate and treat long-term diabetes complications, for example, retinopathy, nephropathy, neuropathy.

2. **Patient education:**
   - Importance of good glycemic control before and during pregnancy
   - Medical nutrition therapy
   - Skill on insulin injection techniques, home monitoring of blood glucose
   - Need for close and regular follow-up
   - Self-adjustment of insulin doses
   - Treatment of hypoglycemia (patient and family members).

3. **Information to cover during preconceptional care:**
   - Risk of pregnancy to mother, also to fetus and neonate
   - Increased risk of large for gestational age baby with increased risk of birth trauma, induction of labor and cesarean section
   - Need for safe delivery and early feeding of baby to prevent neonatal hypoglycemia
   - Benefit of regular follow-up and good glycemic control.

4. **Contraception:**
   - Use of effective contraception until stable and acceptable Glycemia is achieved
   - There is no contraceptive method that is specifically contraindicated in diabetic women.

5. **Glycemic targets:** When $HbA_1C < 6.5\%$ is achieved, couples are asked to try to conceive.

6. **Advise on diet, exercise and lifestyle:**
   - Obese women encouraged to lose weight through diet and exercise
   - Avoid smoking and alcohol.
7. **Folic acid supplementation:** Women planning to become pregnant advised to take folic acid (5 mg/day) until 12 weeks of gestation to decrease risk of neural tube defect.
8. **Antidiabetic medication:** Oral antidiabetic medication should be changed to insulin at least 3 months before trial for conception (if necessary) to achieve glycemic targets.
9. **Safety of medications:** ACE inhibitor (angiotensin converting enzyme inhibitor), ARB (angiotensin receptor blocker) and statin should be discontinued before conception or as soon as pregnancy is confirmed.
10. **Screening for retinopathy:**
    - Dilated comprehensive eye examination is necessary before conception
    - Patient should be counseled about the risk of development or progression of diabetic retinopathy
    - The risk can be reduced by good glycemic control, and proliferative retinopathy (PDR) should be considered for laser treatment prior to pregnancy.
11. **Screening for nephropathy:**
    - Assessment of renal function by serum creatinine and urine albumin-to-creatinine ratio
    - Serum creatinine >3 mg/dL or creatinine clearance rate <60 mL/min should be referred to nephrologist.
12. **Screening for neuropathy:**
    - Autonomic neuropathy manifested by gastroparesis, urinary retention, hypoglycemic unawareness or orthostatic hypotension may complicate management of diabetes in pregnancy
    - Manifestations of neuropathy should be identified, evaluated and treated before conception
    - Peripheral neuropathy, especially compartmental syndrome, for example, carpal tunnel syndrome may be exacerbated during pregnancy.
13. **Screening for cardiovascular disease:** Women with previous or suspected history of ischemic heart disease should be assessed by electrocardiogram and echocardiogram to ensure that patients will tolerate increased cardiovascular demand of gestation.
14. **Continuing care:** If conception does not occur within 1 year, patient's fertility should be assessed.

CHAPTER 15

Gestational Diabetes Mellitus

Q. Define gestational diabetes mellitus (GDM).

Ans. Any degree of glucose intolerance first recognized during pregnancy, regardless of whether the condition, may have predated the pregnancy or persisted after the pregnancy. GDM affects 2%–8% of all pregnancies. Human placental lactogen is responsible for development of GDM.

Q. Discuss about screening for GDM.

Ans.
- Women with risk factors for GDM should be screened as soon as possible after confirmation of pregnancy/at first prenatal visit using standard diagnostic criteria, and for negative cases, repeat at 24–28 weeks of gestation. Criteria for risk of GDM:
  - Age ≥ 25 years
  - Impaired glucose tolerance or impaired fasting glucose on previous testing
  - Bad obstetric history, for example, abortion, infertility, unexplained still birth, etc.
  - Overweight/obese (BMI >25 kg/m^2)
  - First degree relative with diabetes
  - Prior H/o GDM or delivery of large for gestational age infant (>9 lb or >4 kg)
  - Presence of glycosuria
  - Women with polycystic ovarian syndrome (PCOS)
- If no risk factors for GDM present, screen for GDM at 24–28 weeks of gestation
- Diagnosis of GDM: Perform 75 g oral glucose tolerance test (OGTT) in the morning after an overnight fast of ≥ 8 h with plasma glucose measurement at fasting, at 1 and 2 h When any of the following plasma glucose values
  - Fasting ≥ 5.1 mmol/L
  - 1 h ≥ 10.0 mmol/L
  - 2 h ≥ 8.5 mmol/L.

Q. Mention complications of GDM.

Ans.

1. **Mother:**
   - Pregnancy loss: Abortion/intrauterine death

- PET, eclampsia, polyhydramnios
- Deterioration of preexisting complications, for example, retinopathy.

2. **Baby:**
   - Macrosomia (birth weight above 90th percentile for gestational age): Caused by chronic hyperglycemia causing fetal hyperinsulinism that results in excessive fat deposition and organomegaly
   - Intrauterine growth restriction (IUGR)
   - Neonatal hypoglycemia: Due to sudden withdrawal of maternal glucose at birth in presence of fetal hyperinsulinism
   - Neonatal jaundice
   - Respiratory distress syndrome due to inadequate lung surfactant/phospholipids
   - Congenital malformation, for example, cardiac or renal anomaly, caudal regression syndrome, central nervous system effects, etc.

Q. Mention glycemic targets during pregnancy.

Ans.
- Plasma glucose:
  - Fasting/preprandial ≤5.3 mmol/L and either
  - 1 h postmeal ≤7.8 mmol/L
  - Or
  - 2 h postmeal ≤6.7 mmol/L
- HbA_1C 6%–6.5% (due to increased red cell turnover, HbA_1C is lower in normal pregnancy)
- No hypoglycemia
- Absence of significant or sustained ketonuria
- Target of weight gain: 10–15 kg
- Normal fetal size and wellbeing
- BP: Systolic—120–160, diastolic—80–105 mm Hg.

Q. How will you manage GDM.

Ans.
- Follow up: Once every 2 weeks up to 30th gestational weeks and thereafter weekly
- Treatment team should consist of diabetologist, obstetricians and nutritionists
- Frequent home monitoring of blood glucose and urine ketone testing
- Increase intake of carbohydrate and dose of insulin to eliminate ketonuria
- HbA_1C measurement initially and once in each trimester.

1. **MNT and physical activity:**
   - Daily total calorie intake 30 kcal/kg ideal body weight in first trimester and 38 kcal/kg ideal body weight thereafter
   - Carbohydrate 50%–60%, fat 30%, protein 10%–20% (may be increased in exchange of carbohydrate)

- Meal plan:
  - Major meal—breakfast, lunch, dinner
  - Snacks—midmorning, midafternoon and bedtime
- Bedtime snack is essential to prevent fasting ketonuria
- Moderate physical activity should be encouraged.

2. **Retinal assessment:**
   - A first trimester screen and a repeat screen at 28 weeks (if no retinopathy present) or at 16–20 weeks (if retinopathy is present)
   - Patient should be assured that tropicamide eye drop used to dilate the eye is safe in pregnancy, also photocoagulation therapy if required.

3. **Renal assessment:** At first visit in pregnancy. If serum creatinine is abnormal or 24 h UTP >2 g/day, refer to nephrologist (estimated glomerular filtration rate should not be used during pregnancy).

4. **Screening for congenital malformations:** At 18–20 weeks to detect any anomalies, especially cardiac abnormalities.

5. **Monitoring of fetal growth and wellbeing:** By USG every 4 weeks from 28 to 36 weeks or earlier if any suspicion of IUGR.

6. **Antidiabetic medication:**
   - Insulin is preferred medication in diabetes in pregnancy as it does not cross placenta to a measurable extent
   - Metformin and glyburide both cross placenta with metformin greater extent. Metformin may slightly increase prematurity, and nearly half of patients with GDM on metformin ultimately need insulin for glycemic control and they lack long term safety data so should be avoided in GDM as per American Diabetes Association (ADA) guideline 2018
   - Metformin help PCOS patients to be pregnant by weight reduction, ovulation induction and once thought need to be continued as it decrease risk of abortion, but ADA in 2018 state that metformin need not to be continued once pregnancy is confirmed
   - **Indication of insulin therapy:**
     - If dietary compliance fails to maintain glycemic targets
     - If fasting ketonuria is present
     - If suboptimal weight gain is seen.

7. **Safety of analog insulin in pregnancy:** Rapid acting analogs have been widely used in diabetic pregnancy for over 10 years without any evidence of harm and are recommended in both USA or UK guidelines. Insulin glargine because of its higher binding affinity for the IGF-1 receptor and potential mitogenic potency compared with human insulin still not approved by the United States Food and Drug Administration (US FDA) to be used in pregnancy. Insulin detemir got US FDA approval in 2011 and

has no increased affinity for IGF-1 receptor and may be a more appropriate basal insulin analog than glargine.

8. **Time and mode of delivery:**
   - It is better to allow the pregnancy to proceed to full term
   - Normal vaginal delivery is feasible in most cases
   - Antenatal steroid for lung maturation is not contraindicated in DM
   - Caesarean section is usually required if fetal weight >4 kg or any obstetric complication arise, for example, PET.

9. **Diabetes management during labor and delivery:**
   - Blood glucose should be 4–5.5 mmol/L to prevent neonatal hypoglycemia
   - It is best achieved with continuous insulin infusion. Infusion is stopped immediately after delivery
   - Insulin requirement begin to fall during labor and usually fall rapidly after delivery.

10. **Follow-up:**
    - 65% chance of developing GDM in subsequent pregnancy
    - In all GDM, screen with OGTT at 4–12 weeks postpartum and if normal at least every 3 years thereafter (50% develop DM in 10 years)
    - Insulin treated mother advised to have snack before breastfeeding to reduce risk of hypoglycemia
    - OHA can be resumed if needed after lactation period is over.

Q. What is neonatal hypoglycemia?

Ans. Less than 40 mg/dL in full term baby
Less than 30 mg/dL in preterm baby
- If blood glucose 25–45 mg/dL: 10–15 mL 10% dextrose oral or NG feeding
- If blood glucose <25 mg/dL: IV 10% dextrose @ 6 mL/kg/min.

CHAPTER 16

Diabetes Mellitus and Surgery

Q. Discuss metabolic response to surgery.

Ans.

- **Relative insulin hyposecretion:** Enhanced sympathetic activity together with raised circulating catecholamine tends to inhibit insulin secretion
- **Insulin resistance:** The secretion of counter regulatory or stress hormones, particularly cortisol and catecholamines, is greatly increased, and this can lead to acute decrease in insulin sensitivity.

Q. Mention risk of surgery in diabetes mellitus (DM).

Ans.

- **Hyperglycemia and ketoacidosis:** Surgical stress causes rise in counter regulatory hormones that cause hyperglycemia leading to acute metabolic complications
- **↑ Risk of infection:**
  - The chemotactic, phagocytic and bactericidal activity of neutrophil is deficient
  - Impaired humoral defense mechanism
  - Abnormal complement function
  - Neutrophil function is affected adversely by hyperglycemia
  - The infection if develops tends to become virulent. It further worsens metabolic stability, thus creating a vicious cycle
- **Impaired wound strength and wound healing:**
  - Deficient formation of granulation tissue
  - Poor tensile strength of collagen
  - Deficient capillary growth into wound
- **Cardiac risk:** MI is found to occur in diabetic patients more frequently during surgery particularly in patient with cardiac autonomic neuropathy (CAN).

Q. Discuss preoperative assessment of diabetic patients.

Ans.

- Assess cardiovascular and renal function
- Check for features of neuropathy particularly CAN
- Assess glycemic control:
  - Measure HbA_1C
  - Monitor fasting and postprandial blood glucose

- Review treatment of diabetes:
  - Modify insulin regimen is necessary
  - Stop metformin and long-acting sulfonylurea. Replace with insulin if necessary.

Q. What factors to be considered while planning surgery in DM?

Ans.
- Type of DM
- Treatment: Diet, oral hypoglycemic agent, insulin
- Metabolic status
- Vascular status: Mainly cardiac, also renal and cerebral
- Neurologic status, particularly autonomic nervous system
- Surgery:
  - Emergency or elective
  - Minor or major surgery
  - Type of anesthesia
  - Postoperative oral intake

Q. Discuss general principles of management of surgery in DM.
- **Day prior to surgery:**
  - Long-acting secretagogue and biguanide should be changed prior to surgery
  - For major surgery, patients kept nil per os (NPO) overnight prior to surgery. In patient with gastroparesis, the duration of NPO should be around 10–12 h
- **Day of surgery:**
  - Antidiabetic medications are omitted on the morning of surgery
  - Schedule surgery as early as possible in the morning
  - In all major surgery, start glucose–potassium–insulin (GKI) infusion. The unit of insulin to be added to 5% dextrose is individualized and adjusted as per result of glucometer reading. In utilizing dose, in 1 L 5% dextrose, 20 unit soluble insulin and 20 mmol KCl are added (as 1 unit soluble insulin utilizes 2.5 g glucose)
  - Blood glucose should be monitored 1–2 h and should be 6–11 mmol/L
  - In minor surgery, GKI infusion is required in uncontrolled diabetes but not in stable state
- **During surgery:**
  - The choice of anesthesia best left to the anesthetist. There is no preferred choice of anesthetic agent for diabetes
  - Cardiovascular status should be closely monitored during surgery
- **Postoperative care:**
  - GKI infusion is continued (where required) till the patient is able to take oral food
  - At this time, if blood glucose is not under fair control, short-acting insulin can be given in small doses
  - Once the patient is back to routine diet and is stable, he can be managed with the regimen he was on prior to surgery.

Q. Mention specific strategies of diabetes management during surgery.

Ans.
- **For minor surgery in well-controlled type 2 diabetes mellitus (T2DM):**
  - Patient on short-acting secretagogue or insulin should omit breakfast and the morning dose. The drug is restarted when patient is back to normal routine diet
  - Patient on long-acting secretagogue should be replaced with short-acting secretagogue at least 5 days prior to surgery
  - Per operative GKI infusion may be avoided
- **For major surgery (required overnight NPO) in well-controlled T2DM:**
  - Diabetes controlled with insulin
  - Per operative GKI infusion is essential
  - In postoperative period, once diet is resumed, patient usually do better with short-acting insulin
  - Once patient is fully stable, he can be managed with the regimen he was on prior to surgery
- **For all type 1 diabetes mellitus (T1DM) and poorly controlled T2DM:**
  - Insulin is used to control diabetes in all types of surgery
  - Hospitalize the patient at least 3 days before surgery
  - Short-acting insulin is preferred
- **For emergency surgery in diabetic patients:**
  - Patient is hospitalized
  - GKI infusion started, and frequent monitoring of blood glucose is done
  - Electrolyte, ABG, urine for ketone bodies checked
  - If feasible, surgery is delayed till blood glucose comes below 20 mmol/L and ketonuria disappears
  - If delaying is not possible, operation with intensive management of diabetes is to be done
  - Other management according to general principles of emergency surgery should be followed.

CHAPTER 17

Diabetes Mellitus and Ramadan

Q. Mention health benefits of fasting.

Ans.
- Fasting improves metabolic function
- Helps to lose excess weight
- Better control of hypertension
- Flushes out toxins
- Strengthens immune system.

Q. Mention diabetic patients who cannot fast during Ramadan.

Ans.
- Severe hypoglycemia/diabetic keto acidosis (DKA)/hyperosmolar nonketotic coma (HONC) within last 3 months prior to Ramadan
- Patient with history of recurrent hypoglycemia
- Patient with hypoglycemia unawareness
- Patient with sustained poor glycemic control
- Type 1 diabetes mellitus on multiple insulin injections per day (three or more)
- Acute illness: Overt cardiovascular disease, for example, recent myocardial infarction, hepatic dysfunction
- Pregnancy with poor glycemic control
- Patients on chronic dialysis.

Q. What are the risks associated with fasting?

Ans.
- Hypoglycemia
- Hyperglycemia, for example, DKA/HONC
- Dehydration
- Thrombosis.

Q. How can you manage a diabetic patient during Ramadan?

Ans.

1. **Individualization:**
   - Care must be individualized
   - Management plan differs for each specific patient.

2. **Education and counseling:**
   - Education of diabetic patients and their families regarding
     - Acute complications and their management and how to prevent them
     - Blood sugar monitoring
     - Meal planning
     - Physical activity
     - Drug and dose adjustment.

3. **Diet plan:**
   - Take *sehri* as late as possible
   - Diet should remain same healthy and balanced as before Ramadan
   - Ingestion of foods containing complex carbohydrate that delays in digestion and absorption is good choice for *sehri*, while foods with more simple carbohydrate are more appropriate at iftar
   - Take plenty of fluid after iftar to avoid dehydration
   - Night meal should not be missed
   - Fasting without *sehri* is prohibited
   - Avoid sweet foods, for example, sweets, sugar containing juice or fried foods, for example, fried kabab, pakaura, puri, paratha at iftar.

4. **Exercise:**
   - Normal level of physical activity should be maintained
   - Exercise or excessive physical activity during day time should be avoided, particularly at late evening
   - Exercise can be performed 2 h after iftar
   - Tarawih prayer should be considered as a part of daily exercise program.

5. **Drugs and dose adjustment:**

Before Ramadan	During Ramadan
Patient on medical nutrition therapy	No change is needed (modify time and intensity of exercise) Ensure adequate fluid intake
Once daily sulfonylurea	Dose should be taken at iftar
Sulfonylurea twice daily	Full morning dose at iftar and half of the usual evening dose at *sehri*
Metformin	Two third of total daily dose at iftar and other third at *sehri*
Thiazolidinediones	No change is needed
Meglitinides	No change is needed
Premixed insulin regimen	Usual morning dose at iftar and half of the usual evening dose at *sehri*
Split mixed insulin regimen	Usual morning dose of regular insulin and NPH at iftar and half of the usual evening dose of regular insulin and NPH at *sehri*

(Contd...)

(Contd...)

Before Ramadan	During Ramadan
Basal bolus insulin regimen	Usual morning and lunch dose of rapid acting analogues at iftar and night meal and 50% of dinner dose at *sehri* and half of long acting analogue at fixed time
GLP-1 analog	Same dose preferably at iftar

6. **Blood glucose monitoring:**
   - Blood glucose level during fasting: To recognize subclinical hypo or hyperglycemia
   - Two-h post-*sehri* and 1–2 h pre-iftar: to detect subclinical hypoglycemia
   - Two-h post-iftar, dinner: to detect subclinical hyperglycemia.

7. **Insulin dose adjustment:**
   - Pre-iftar: Adjust basal insulin
   - Two-h post-iftar: Adjust iftar bolus or regular insulin
   - Two-h post-dinner: Adjust dinner bolus or regular insulin
   - Two-h post-*sehri*: Adjust *sehri* bolus or regular insulin
   - Pre-*sehri*: Adjust iftar NPH
   - Basal glucose around midday: Adjust *sehri* NPH.

8. **When to break fasting:**
   - If blood glucose <3.3 mmol/L at any time of day
   - If blood glucose <3.9 mmol/L during first few hours of *sehri*
   - If blood glucose >16.7 mmol/L, check ketones in urine
   - Avoid fasting on sick days.

Q. What are the things that invalidate the fast?

Ans.
- Transfusion of blood
- Receiving via a needle nourishing substances. With regard to injections which do not replace food and drink, rather they are administered for the purpose of medical treatment—such as penicillin or insulin or for the purpose of vaccinations, these do not affect the fast, whether they are intravenous or intramuscular. But to be on the safe side, these injections may be given at night
- Kidney dialysis
- Donating blood, but if a person suffers a nosebleed, his fast is valid because that happened involuntarily
- Vomiting deliberately
- Menstruation
  - If a woman feels that her period has started but no blood comes out until sunset, her fast is still valid
  - If the bleeding of a woman who is menstruating ceases at night and she has the intention of fasting and she does ghusl before dawn, the view of all the scholars is that her fast is valid

- It is preferable for a woman to keep her natural cycle and not to take any medicine to prevent her period. If a woman takes pills and her period stops as a result, her fast is acceptable.

Q. What are the things that do not invalidate the fast?

Ans.
- Enemas, eyedrops, eardrops, tooth extraction and treatment of injuries
- Medical tablets that are placed under the tongue to treat angina but avoid swallowing any residue
- Insertion of anything into the vagina such as pessaries or a speculum or the doctor's fingers for the purpose of medical examination
- Insertion of medical instruments or intrauterine device into uterus
- Anything that enters the urinary tract of a male or female such as catheter tube or medical scopes or opaque dyes inserted for the purpose of X-rays or medicine or a solution to wash the bladder
- Fillings, extractions or cleaning of teeth so long as avoiding swallowing anything that reaches the throat
- Rinsing the mouth, gargling, sprays, etc. so long as avoiding swallowing anything that reaches the throat
- Oxygen or anesthetic gases as long as that do not give the patient any kind of nourishment
- Anything that may enter the body via absorption through the skin such as creams and ointments
- Insertion of a fine tube via the veins for diagnostic imaging or treatment of the veins of the heart or any part of the body
- Taking samples from the liver or any other part of the body so long as that is not accompanied by administration of solutions
- Endoscopy so long as that is not accompanied by administration of solutions or other substances
- Introduction of any medical instruments or materials to the brain or spinal column.

CHAPTER 18

Sick-day Management of Diabetic Patients

Q. Define sick-day management.

Ans. Period of illness, for example, fever, vomiting or diarrhea need special care in diabetic patients known as sick-day management.

Q. What are the risks of sick days?

Ans.
- Hypoglycemia
- Diabetic ketoacidosis (DKA): Increases ketone body formation secondary to inadequate insulin action or inadequate oral intake of carbohydrate
- Dehydration.

Q. Discuss about sick-day management of diabetic patients.

Ans. In brief, S (Sugar testing), I (Insulin dose adjustment), C (Carbohydrate intake), K (Ketone testing).

1. **Antidiabetic medication:**
   - If the person is on insulin, continue intermediate or long-acting insulin, but the dose may need to be reduced (fasting patients still require 40% of usual daily dose as basal to prevent DKA)
   - Short-acting insulin should be adjusted according to blood sugar levels and food intake
   - If the person is on oral antidiabetic drug, the dose is to be readjusted, sometimes the longer-acting oral antidiabetic drug may need to be replaced by shorter-acting one or insulin
   - Never stop antidiabetic medication altogether. Dose may need to be reduced by 20%–50%. Target blood sugar is mildly relaxed in sick days.

2. **Meal plan:**
   - Patient is advised to maintain oral carbohydrate intake to prevent hypoglycemia and maintain energy requirement (aim for 50 g carbohydrate intake every 3–4 h)
   - Patient should eat according to what food he can tolerate. If he cannot eat his usual meals, make sure he has small low fat snacks at regular intervals throughout the day. If he cannot eat food, have sips of fluid frequently.

3. **Fluid intake:**
   - Fluid balance need to be maintained to prevent dehydration (aim for 125–150 mL fluid intake per hour)
   - If blood glucose is low, sweetened fluid, for example, fruit juice to be taken to prevent hypoglycemia. If blood glucose is elevated, low calorie soft drink, soup, broth can be taken.
4. **Exercise:** Avoid exercise or strenuous physical activity in sick days.
5. **Treatment of underlying illness:**
   - Treat the infective focus
   - Treatment of vomiting/diarrhea may also be required
   - Use of sugar-free medicine is not essential.
6. **Monitoring:**
   - **In type 1 diabetes mellitus:** Record blood glucose and urine for ketone body 4 h or more frequently if blood glucose >14 mmol/L or ketonuria present. For greater accuracy, blood ketone testing is preferred, if available
   - **In type 2 diabetes mellitus:** Record blood glucose 6 hourly or more frequently if blood glucose >14 mmol/L and check urine for ketone body if blood glucose >14 mmol/L
   - Maintain temperature and intake-output chart.
7. **When to seek medical assistance:**
   - Vomiting or diarrhea persist >6 h
   - Sick for 2 days and not getting better
   - Blood glucose remains above 14 mmol/L
   - Ketonuria persist despite treatment or blood ketones ≥1.5 mmol/L
   - Signs of DKA or hyperosmolar nonketotic coma: Drowsiness, hyperventilation, dehydration or severe abdominal pain
   - Extremes of age
   - Hypoglycemia
   - Coexisting serious illness
   - Too sick to take any food or drinks.

CHAPTER 19

Skin Manifestation of Diabetes Mellitus

Q. Mention skin manifestations of diabetes mellitus.
Ans.

1. **Cutaneous metabolic manifestations:**
   - Necrobiosis lipoidica diabeticorum (NLD)
   - Diabetic dermopathy/shin spots
   - Diabetic bullae/bullous diabeticorum
   - Granuloma annulare
   - Diabetic thick skin:
     – Diabetic hand syndrome
     – Scleroderma of diabetes
   - Acanthosis nigricans (associated with insulin resistance)
   - Eruptive xanthoma (associated with hypertriglyceridemia).

2. **Vascular changes:**
   - Diabetic rubeosis
   - Erysipelas like erythema
   - Calciphylaxis
   - Ulcer/gangrene of foot.

3. **Cutaneous infections:**
   - Fungal infections:
     – *Candida* infection of mouth (oral candidiasis), genitalia (balanitis, balanoposthitis, vulvovaginitis), nail fold (paronychia), flexural area (groin, axilla)
     – Dermatophyte infection of skin (tinea)
   - Bacterial infection:
     – Boil, abscess, carbuncle, furuncle, styes, folliculitis, cellulitis (*Staphylococcus aureus*)
     – Malignant otitis externa (*Pseudomonas*)
     – Necrotizing fasciitis.

4. **Associated conditions:**
   - Vitiligo
   - Xerosis

Chapter 19: Skin Manifestation of Diabetes Mellitus

- Pruritus
- Lichen planus
- Skin tags.

5. **Due to antidiabetic treatment:**
   - Insulin: Local/systemic allergy, lipodystrophy (lipoatrophy, lipohypertrophy)
   - Sulfonylurea: Skin reaction (rare).

Q. Discuss about necrobiosis lipoidica dibeticorum.

Ans.
- Prevalence: 3% in diabetic patients
- Two-third patients with NLD have diabetes, usually type 1 diabetes mellitus with further 12%–15% have abnormal GTT
- Male:Female = 1:3
- Shiny, atrophic and slightly yellow plaques on shins with underlying telangiectasia. Minor trauma may precipitate slow healing ulcer
- NLD is unrelated to glycemic control
- Treatment is different, but in early stages, topical or intralesional steroid may be beneficial as well as long-term PUVA.

Q. Discuss about diabetic dermopathy.

Ans.
- Most common skin disorder in patients with diabetes, usually in pretibial region
- Usually in long-standing diabetes, associated with other microvascular complication of diabetes
- Usually have four or more lesions as well-circumscribed atrophic brownish scars on the shins
- No effective treatment but resolves over 1–2 years.

Q. Discuss about scleroderma of diabetes.

Ans.
- Marked dermal thickening of posterior aspect of neck and upper part of back
- Found in 2.5% of type 2 diabetes mellitus (T2DM) patients particularly who are overweight with poorly controlled diabetes
- Responds to ultraviolet light.

Q. Discuss about acanthosis nigricans.

Ans.
- Dark, thick, velvety plaque in flexural areas, particularly axilla, neck, inguinal region, inframammary region
- Histology: Thickening of epidermis
- Etiology: T2DM, obesity, polycystic ovarian syndrome, malignancy, for example, gastric (pruritus is a feature of malignancy associated with acanthosis)
- Treatment: Weight reduction, tropical salicylate.

CHAPTER 20

Prevention of Diabetes Mellitus

Q. What measures will you take to prevent diabetes?

Ans.

1. **Primary prevention:** Prevention of occurrence of diabetes mellitus (DM)
   - **Identification of people at risk/criteria for testing for diabetes or prediabetes in asymptomatic adults:**
     - Testing should be considered in overweight or obese [body mass index (BMI) ≥ 25 kg/m² or ≥ 23 kg/m² in Asian] adults who have one or more of the following risk factors:
       - Impaired fasting glucose, impaired glucose tolerance or $HbA_1C \geq 5.7\%$ on previous testing
       - First degree relative with diabetes
       - Women with prior gestational DM (GDM)
       - History of cardiovascular disease
       - Hypertension ($\geq 140/90$ mm Hg or on therapy for hypertension)
       - HDL cholesterol level <35 mg/dL and/or triglyceride level >250 mg/dL
       - Women with PCOS
       - Physical inactivity
       - Other clinical conditions associated with insulin resistance (e.g., severe obesity, acanthosis nigricans)
       - For all patients, testing should begin at age 45 years
     - If results are normal, testing should be repeated at 3-year intervals with consideration of more frequent testing depending on initial results (e.g., those with prediabetes should be tested yearly) and risk status
   - **Intervention:**
     - Attain and maintain BMI <25 kg/m²
     - Regular physical activity, ≥ 150 min/week moderate intensity physical activity
     - Reduce energy dense food: Soft drinks
     - ↑ Consumption of fruits and vegetables also unrefined carbohydrate
     - Prevention or delay of type 2 DM:
       - Achieve and maintain 7% loss of initial body weight

- Metformin should be considered for prevention of type 2 DM in person with prediabetes, especially those with BMI $\geq$35 kg/m^2, age <60 years, women with prior GDM or those with rising HbA$_1$C despite lifestyle intervention.

2. **Secondary prevention:** Early detection of diabetes and prompt initiation of treatment to prevent complications of diabetes.
   - Good glycemic control
   - Education about diabetes, its effects and self-management skills
   - Ongoing clinical care
   - Home blood sugar monitoring and self-adjustment of medications
   - Control of hypertension (HTN)
   - Control of dyslipidemia
   - Weight control
   - Physical activity
   - Cessation of smoking
   - Improved foot care
   - Attain and maintain targets of treatment of DM.

3. **Tertiary prevention:** Delay and/or prevent further deterioration of diabetic complications.
   - Good glycemic control
   - Appropriate treatment of complications
   - Control of HTN, dyslipidemia
   - Psychosocial support and rehabilitation.

SECTION 2

ENDOCRINOLOGY

Part A: Pituitary and Hypothalamic Disorders
21. Hypopituitarism
22. Pituitary Adenoma
23. Acromegaly
24. Prolactinoma
25. Diabetes Insipidus
26. Short Stature

Part B: Thyroid Disorders
27. Thyrotoxicosis
28. Hypothyroidism
29. Thyroid Nodules
30. Thyroid Neoplasm

Part C: Bone and Mineral Disorders
31. Hypercalcemia
32. Hypocalcemia
33. Osteoporosis

Part D: Adrenal Disorders
34. Incidental Adrenal Mass
35. Cushing Syndrome
36. Adrenocortical Insufficiency
37. Judicious Use of Glucocorticoid

38. Endocrine Hypertension
39. Pheochromocytoma
40. Congenital Adrenal Hyperplasia

Part E: Reproductive Endocrinology
41. Puberty
42. Male Hypogonadism
43. Male Infertility
44. Gynecomastia
45. Erectile Dysfunction
46. Hirsutism
47. Polycystic Ovarian Syndrome
48. Female Infertility
49. Amenorrhea
50. Menopause
51. Precocious Puberty
52. Miscellaneous Endocrine Disorders

Part A: Pituitary and Hypothalamic Disorders

CHAPTER **21**

Hypopituitarism

Q. Define hypopituitarism.

Ans. Diminished or absent secretion of one or more anterior and/or posterior pituitary hormones.

Q. Define panhypopituitarism.

Ans. Diminished or absent secretion of two or more anterior and/or posterior pituitary hormones.

Q. What are the causes of hypopituitarism?

Ans. Hypopituitarism may be primary due to pituitary disease or secondary due to hypothalamic pathology. More than 75% of pituitary gland must be destroyed before clinical features are evident.

"9 Is"

1. Invasive: Pituitary adenoma, craniopharyngioma, meningioma, metastasis (breast, lung)
2. Infiltrative: Sarcoidosis, hemochromatosis
3. Infarction: Sheehan syndrome, pituitary apoplexy
4. Infections: Tuberculosis (TB), syphilis, mycotic infections
5. Injury: Head injury, for example, RTA, battered children
6. Iatrogenic: Pituitary surgery, radiotherapy
7. Immunologic: Lymphocytic hypophysitis
8. Idiopathic
9. Isolated, for example, isolated growth hormone (GH) deficiency.

Q. What are the clinical features of hypopituitarism?

Ans.
- Clinical features depend on severity of pituitary hormone deficiency and rate of development, in addition to whether this is intercurrent illness
- Pituitary compression leads to characteristic sequence of loss of hormone secretion. GH → Follicle-stimulating hormone (FSH) and luteinizing hormone (LH) → Thyroid-stimulating hormone (TSH) → Adrenocorticotropic hormone

(ACTH) → finally prolactin (PRL) (rare, except in Sheehan syndrome associated with failure of lactation). Antidiuretic hormone (ADH) deficiency can also occur due to pituitary adenoma, also in head injury or pituitary surgery

1. **Symptoms:**
   - GH:
     - Children: Growth failure
     - Adult:
       - Decreased sense of wellbeing
       - Reduced energy and lower health related quality of life (low mood, fatigue, low motivation, reduced satisfaction)
       - Decreased muscle mass and increased fat mass
       - Increased cardiovascular risk (abnormal lipid profile, insulin resistance, increased inflammatory markers)
   - FSH/LH:
     - Female: Anovulatory cycles, oligo/amenorrhea, vaginal dryness
     - Male: Gynecomastia, reduced frequency of shaving, erectile dysfunction, testicular atrophy
     - Both sex: Loss of libido, infertility, loss of secondary sexual characteristics, for example, hair loss, ↓ bone mass
   - TSH: Similar to primary hypothyroidism. Secondary hypothyroidism excluded if goiter present or incision mark at neck
   - ACTH: In contrast to primary adrenocortical insufficiency, angiotensin II dependent zona glomerulosa function intact and aldosterone secretion maintain normal plasma K^+, also pallor. However, there may be postural hypotension and dilutional hyponatremia (cortisol deficiency) due to failure of vasoconstriction in absence of cortisol (cortisol maintain normal vascular reactivity to catecholamine—permissive effect)
   - PRL: Failure of lactation
   - ADH: Polyuria, polydipsia
   - Houssay phenomenon: Amelioration of diabetes mellitus (DM) in patients with hypopituitarism due to reduction in counter regulatory hormones.

2. **Signs:**
   - Patient with hypopituitarism is usually slightly overweight
   - Skin is fine, pale, smooth with fine wrinkling of the face
   - Body and pubic hair is deficient or absent and atrophy of genitalia
   - Postural hypotension, bradycardia, decreased muscle strength, delayed relaxation of ankle jerk.

Q. How will you investigate hypopituitarism?

Ans.

1. **To identify pituitary hormone deficiency:**
   - ACTH deficiency:
     - Rapid ACTH stimulation test/short synacthen test

- Pituitary stimulation: Insulin tolerance test (ITT), metyrapone stimulation test, corticotropin-releasing hormone stimulation test. Done only if uncertainty in interpretation of rapid ACTH stimulation test. ITT also assess GH reserve
- TSH deficiency:
    - Free T4 (FT4)
    - TSH: No value, as TSH may be low, normal or high due to inactive TSH isoforms in blood
    - TRH stimulation test
- FSH/LH deficiency:
    - In male: Serum testosterone, FSH and LH
    - In premenopausal female: Ask if menses are regular. Regular menstrual cycles is strong evidence that hypothalamic–pituitary–gonadal axis is intact. Low serum estradiol in presence of oligo/amenorrhea is indicative of gonadal failure
    - In postmenopausal female: Measure serum FSH, LH
    - Growth hormone-releasing hormone stimulation test
- GH deficiency: Only investigate if GH replacement therapy is being contemplated
    - ITT
    - Tests with levodopa, clonidine, arginine, glucagon, postexercise and other stimuli
- Prolactin: Serum prolactin, TRH stimulation test
- ADH:
    - It is important to assess and replace ACTH deficiency before assessing ADH deficiency as ACTH deficiency leads to reduced glomerular filtration rate and inability to excrete a water load that may mask diabetes insipidus
    - Exclude other causes of polyuria with RBS, K^+, Ca^{++} level
    - Water deprivation test.

2. **To establish cause:**
   - Pituitary imaging: Magnetic resonance imaging (MRI) of sella and perisellar region with contrast
   - Serum and cerebrospinal fluid (CSF) angiotensin-converting enzyme (neurosarcoidosis)
   - CXR: TB, sarcoidosis.

3. **Supportive investigations:**
   - CBC: Anemia (due to thyroid and androgen deficiency and chronic disease)
   - Hypoglycemia
   - Hyponatremia (related to hypothyroidism) and hypoadrenalism
   - ECG: Low voltage, bradycardia.

Q. How will you treat hypopituitarism?

Ans.
- In acutely ill patients: Initial treatment is similar to adrenal crisis
- In chronic/stable patients: Hormone replacement (in reverse sequence of hormone loss). Steroid → thyroxine → FSH/LH → GH

- Treatment of underlying cause
- **Glucocorticoid replacement:**
  - Hydrocortisone 15–25 mg/day orally or prednisolone 5–7.5 mg/day orally in 2–3 divided doses
  - Minimum effective dosage that provides a proper sense of wellbeing given in order to avoid iatrogenic hypercortisolism
  - ↑ Dose is required during periods of stress, for example, illness, surgery
  - Use clinical assessment of patient's wellbeing rather than biochemical criteria to assess adequacy of glucocorticoid replacement
  - Unlike 1° adrenal insufficiency, ACTH deficiency does not require mineralocorticoid replacement
  - Thyroid hormone replacement before steroid may cause adrenal crisis
- **Thyroid hormone replacement:**
  - Oral levothyroxine 50–150 µg/day
  - Response to therapy is monitored clinically and measurement of FT4, which should be maintained in mid to upper range of normal
  - TSH measurement is of no value in assessing thyroid replacement in hypopituitarism
- **Sex hormone replacement:** Testosterone/estrogen ± progesterone. Gonadotropin therapy is required if fertility is desired
- **GH replacement:** GH.

Q. Discuss about Sheehan syndrome.

Ans. Postpartum ischemic necrosis of anterior pituitary gland.
- **Pathogenesis:**
  - During pregnancy, anterior pituitary enlarges to almost twice of its normal size. This physiological expansion is not accompanied by ↑ blood flow from low-pressure venous system. So there is relative hypoxia of pituitary at pregnancy
  - Following postpartum hemorrhage hypotension along with vasospasm of hypophysial arteries causes compromised arterial perfusion to anterior pituitary
  - Posterior pituitary usually not affected as blood supply directly from arterial branches
- **Clinical features:**
  - Failure of lactation
  - Failure to resume normal menstrual period
  - Clinical features of hypopituitarism are often subtle, and diagnosis may be established many years later
- **Treatment:** Hormone replacement.

Q. Discuss about pituitary apoplexy.

Ans. Spontaneous hemorrhagic infarction of pituitary gland resulting partial or total pituitary insufficiency

Chapter 21: Hypopituitarism

- **Etiology:**
  - Most commonly in patients with pituitary adenoma, usually macroadenoma
  - Postpartum (Sheehan syndrome)
  - DM, hypertension (HTN), anticoagulant, disseminated intravascular coagulation, raised intracranial pressure, sickle-cell anemia
  - Cardiac surgery, dynamic pituitary testing
  - Rarely a normal pituitary gland
- **Clinical features:**
  - Headache, visual impairment, ophthalmoplegia, meningismus
  - Acute hypopituitarism (hypotension, hypoglycemia), rapid mental deterioration, coma and death
- **Investigations:** MRI of sella and perisellar region: Pituitary enlargement with signs of hemorrhage
- **Treatment:**
  - Emergency treatment with corticosteroid, for example, high-dose dexamethasone 4 mg IV twice daily (provide both glucocorticoid support and relief of cerebral edema) or hydrocortisone 50 mg IV 6 h
  - Transsphenoidal decompression of intrasellar contents
- **Prognosis:** Most patients who have survived pituitary apoplexy have developed multiple hormone deficiency but infarction of tumor in some patients may cure hypersecretory pituitary adenoma and its accompanying endocrinopathy.

Q. Describe about empty sella syndrome.

Ans. Herniation of subarachnoid space into sella turcica, partially filling it with CSF that causes compression of pituitary gland.

- **Etiology:**
  - Primary: Congenital incompetence of diaphragmatic sellae
  - Secondary: Pituitary surgery, radiotherapy or pituitary infarction
- **Clinical features:**
  - Most patients are middle-aged women
  - Asymptomatic (incidental diagnosis)
  - Headache
  - Systemic HTN, benign intracranial HTN
  - Spontaneous CSF rhinorrhea
  - Visual field impairment
- **Investigations:**
  - Majority of patients have normal pituitary function
  - Hypopituitarism/hyperprolactinemia found in <10% patients
  - MRI: Sella turcica is empty, filled with CSF (hyperdense) and pituitary gland is compressed below
- **Treatment:** Hormone replacement if hypopituitarism.

CHAPTER 22

Pituitary Adenoma

Q. What are the causes of pituitary adenoma?
Ans.
- Prolactinoma (60%)
- Acromegaly (20%)
- Cushing disease (10%)
- Nonfunctioning pituitary adenoma (10%)
- TSH, gonadotropin secreting pituitary adenomas (rare).

Q. What are the types of pituitary adenoma?
Ans.
- **Pituitary microadenoma:**
  - Less than 1 cm in diameter, present with features of hormone excess without sellar enlargement or suprasellar extension
  - Panhypopituitarism does not occur and such tumors are usually treated successfully
  - Appear as low signal intensity lesion on MRI and do not usually enhance with gadolinium
  - Adenoma <5 mm in diameter may not be visualized in MRI and do not alter normal pituitary contour.
  - Lesion >5 mm in diameter create a unilateral convex superior gland margin and cause deviation of pituitary stalk toward opposite side
- **Pituitary macroadenoma:**
  - More than 1 cm in diameter, cause sellar enlargement with features of hypopituitarism or hormone excess
  - Adenoma >1.5 cm in diameter have suprasellar extension, compression of optic chiasma or lateral extension with invasion of cavernous sinus
  - Large tumor show compression of normal pituitary and distortion of pituitary stalk.

Q. What are the clinical features of pituitary adenoma?
Ans.
- **Local effects**
  - Headache
  - Seizure (temporal lobe)

Chapter 22: Pituitary Adenoma

- Papilledema
- Optic pathway: Visual field defect (bitemporal hemianopia), loss of visual acuity, optic atrophy
- Cavernous sinus: Diplopia, ophthalmoplegia
- Disconnection hyperprolactinemia (compression of pituitary stalk interrupt inhibitory effect of hypothalamic dopamine on prolactin secretion)
- Pituitary apoplexy

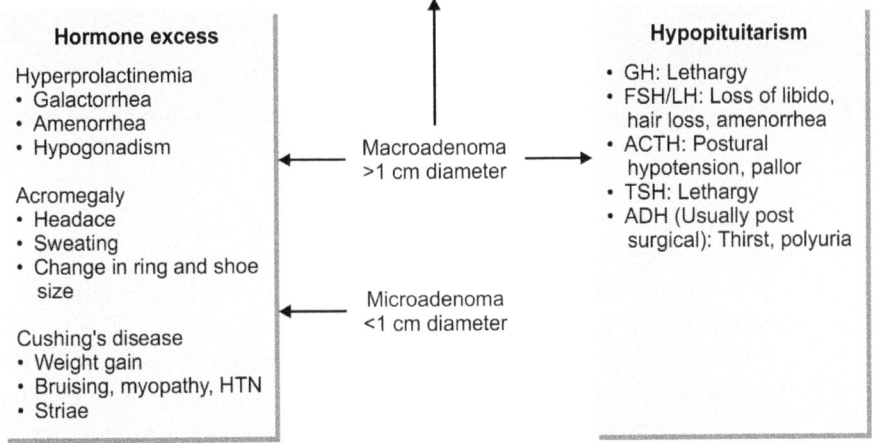

Q. How will you treat pituitary adenoma?

Ans.

- Aim of treatment:
  - To correct hypersecretion of anterior pituitary hormones
  - To preserve normal secretion of other anterior pituitary hormones
  - To remove or suppress the adenoma itself

1. **Surgical treatment:**
   - Trans-sphenoidal microsurgical approach to sella turcica
   - Transfrontal craniotomy: Rare, done in patients of pituitary adenoma with massive suprasellar extension, for example, craniopharyngioma, parasellar tumor, for example, meningioma

- **Procedure:**
  - Surgeon approaches the pituitary from the nasal cavity through sinus, removes the anteroinferior sellar floor, incise the dura and the adenoma is selectively removed. Normal pituitary tissue is identified and preserved
- **Success rate:** 90% in patients with microadenoma, less in patients with large or massive tumors.

2. **Pituitary radiotherapy:**
   - **Indications:**
     - Incomplete resection of large pituitary adenoma
     - Failed medical therapy
     - Invasive sellar mass
     - Tumor recurrence
     - Hormone hypersecretion recurrence
   - **Conventional irradiation:**
     - Daily doses of 180–200 cGy (centigray) for 5–6 weeks
     - Response is slow, 5–10 years may be required to achieve full effect
     - Successful in 80% patient of acromegaly and 55%–60% in patient with Cushing disease
   - **Complications:**
     - Malaise, nausea
     - Hypopituitarism: Incidence ↑ with time following radiotherapy, 50%–60% at 5–10 years
     - Serious otitis media
     - Visual impairment: Damage to optic nerves and chiasma
     - Radionecrosis of brain tissue
     - Second brain tumor, for example, glioma, astrocytoma, meningioma
   - **Focal forms of radiotherapy:**
     - γ Knife radiosurgery: Stereotactic CT guided cobalt-60 γ radiation to narrowly focused area, remission rate 43%–78%. Adequate distance between pituitary tumor and optic chiasma is needed to prevent radiation induced damage
     - Proton stereotactic radiotherapy.

3. **Medical treatment:**
   - Dopamine agonist for prolactinoma
   - Somatostatin analog for acromegaly.

Q. Discuss about trans-sphenoidal pituitary surgery.

Ans.
- **Indications:**
  - **General:**
    - Visual tract or central nervous compression arising from lesion
    - Tumor recurrence after surgery or irradiation

- Pituitary hemorrhage
- Intolerant or resistant to medical therapy
- Desire for immediate pregnancy with macroadenoma
  - **Specific:**
    - Acromegaly
    - Cushing disease
    - Nonfunctioning pituitary adenoma
    - Prolactinoma: Intolerant or resistance to dopamine agonist
    - Nelson syndrome
- **Complications:**
  - **Transient:**
    - DI
    - Peri- or postoperative hemorrhage
    - CSF leak and rhinorrhea
    - Meningitis
    - Visual impairment
  - **Permanent (5%–10%):**
    - DI: Transient DI lasting a few days to 1–2 weeks occurs in 15% patients within 5–14 days of surgery. Permanent DI rare. Mild DI managed with maintenance of adequate oral fluid intake. Severe DI (urine output >4 L) managed with desmopressin/DDAVP (IV, oral, SC, intranasally)
    - Total or partial hypopituitarism
    - SIADH: Managed with fluid restriction, hypertonic saline may be required and ADH receptor antagonist (tolvaptan orally, conivaptan IV)
    - Visual impairment/loss
    - CNS damage, for example, oculomotor palsy
    - Triphasic response: DI (early hypothalamic dysfunction) → SIADH (release of ADH from degenerating pituitary) → DI (depletion of ADH store)
- **Postpituitary surgery follow-up:**
  - Evaluate 4–8 weeks postoperatively to document complete removal of adenoma and correction of endocrine hypersecretion
  - For prolactinoma (serum PRL), acromegaly (glucose suppression test and GH/IGF-1), Cushing disease (24 h UFC, low dose DST) and other anterior pituitary hormone assessment (FT_4, ACTH, FSH/LH)
  - Yearly follow-up for recurrence
  - MRI not needed in patients with normal postoperative pituitary function, done in patients with suspected persistent or recurrent disease.

Q. What are the differential diagnosis of sella and parasellar mass?

Ans.
- Pituitary adenoma
- Benign tumor: Craniopharyngioma, meningioma

- Nonadenomatous pituitary hyperplasia, for example, lactotroph hyperplasia during pregnancy
- Malignant tumor: Sarcoma, chordoma
- Metastatic lesion: Breast, lung
- Glioma: Optic glioma, astrocytoma
- Granulomatous, inflammatory, infections: Lymphocytic hypophysitis, histiocytosis X, TB, pituitary abscess.

Q. Define pituitary incidentaloma.

Ans.

Incidentally detected pituitary lesion that is discovered on imaging study performed for an unrelated reason. Imaging study using MRI demonstrated pituitary microadenoma in 10% of normal individual and macroadenoma in .1% but in autopsy the proportion is 10%–20%.

Q. What are the differential diagnoses of pituitary incidentaloma?

Ans.

- Pituitary adenoma
- Benign tumor: Craniopharyngioma, meningioma
- Nonadenomatous pituitary hyperplasia, for example, lactotroph hyperplasia during pregnancy
- Malignant tumor: Sarcoma, chordoma
- Metastatic lesion: Breast, lung
- Glioma: Optic glioma, astrocytoma
- Granulomatous, inflammatory, infections: Lymphocytic hypophysitis, histiocytosis X, TB, pituitary abscess.

Q. How will you evaluate and manage a case of pituitary incidentaloma?

Ans.

- **Questions to be resolved:**
  - Is the lesion secreting hormones (hyperfunctioning or not)?
  - Size of lesion and any features of compression, for example, visual field defect, hypopituitarism
  - Any ↑ tumor growth in follow-up
- **Clinical assessment:**
  - Complete history and physical examination to assess any features of hormone hypersecretion or hypopituitarism
  - Any features of compression, for example, visual field testing, fundoscopy
- **Investigations:**
  - MRI of sella and perisellar region with contrast (if incidentaloma initially detected by CT)
  - Serum PRL
  - Serum IGF-1, glucose suppression

Chapter 22: Pituitary Adenoma

- 24-h UFC, late night salivary cortisol, overnight 1-mg DST, ACTH
- FT4, FT3, TSH

- **Management:**

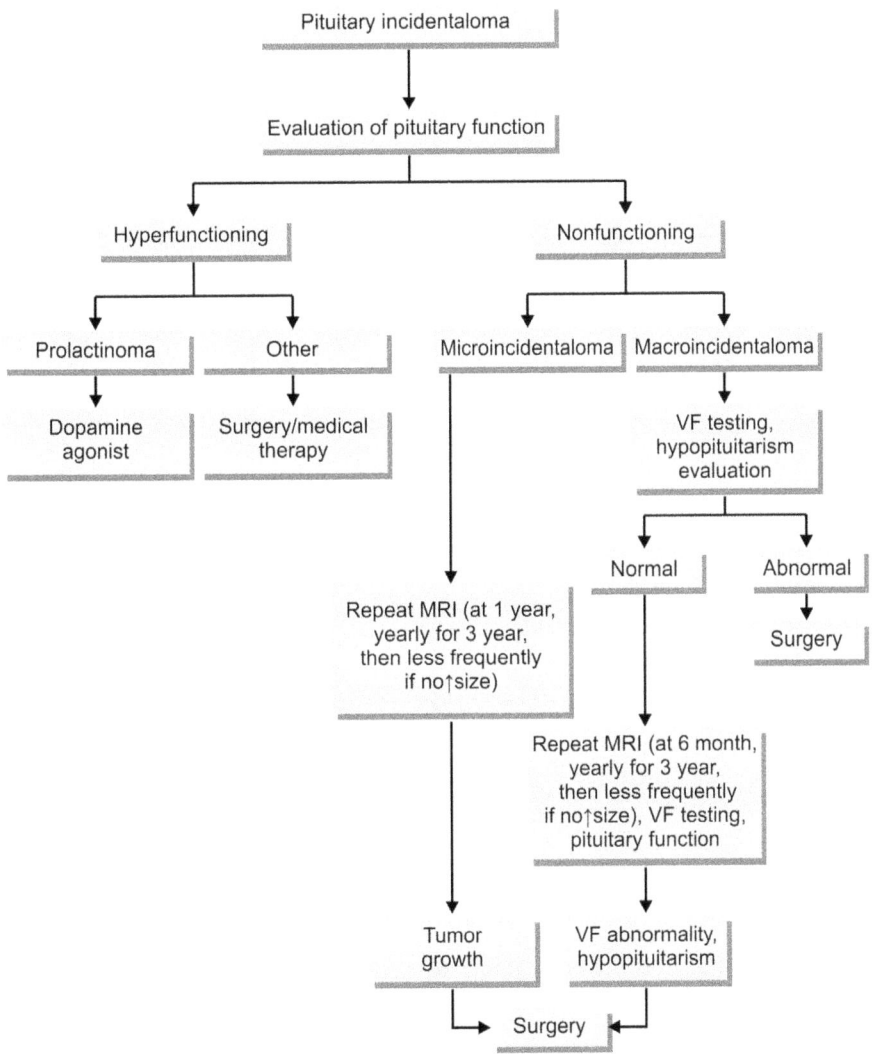

Q. What are the indications of surgery for pituitary incidentaloma?

Ans.

- Hyperfunctioning lesion other than prolactinoma
- Visual field defect due to lesion
- Hypopituitarism due to lesion
- Clinically significant growth in follow-up
- A lesion close to optic chiasma and plan to become pregnant
- Unremitting headache.

Q. What are the causes of intracranial calcification?

Ans.
- Craniopharyngioma
- Hypoparathyroidism
- Pseudohypoparathyroidism
- Hydatid cyst
- Neurocysticercosis
- Tuberous sclerosis
- Sturge-Weber syndrome (Tram track sign)
- Tuberculoma
- Physiological calcification may occur in pineal gland, choroid plexus and falx cerebri.

CHAPTER 23

Acromegaly

Q. Define acromegaly.

Ans.
- Acromegaly/hypersomatotropism is a clinical condition resulting from chronic growth hormone (GH) hypersecretion in adults from a pituitary adenoma, usually macroadenoma
- Age: At 40–60 years. Acromegaly in older people has milder disease with lower GH level and smaller tumor
- Sex distribution: Equal.

Q. Define gigantism/pituitary gigantism.

Ans.
- Gigantism/pituitary gigantism is a clinical condition resulting from chronic GH hypersecretion in children prior to fusion of epiphyses
- Most patients have associated hypogonadism, which delay epiphyseal closure. The combination of IGF-I excess and hypogonadism leads to striking acceleration of linear growth
- Increased growth velocity without premature pubertal onset should arouse suspicion of pituitary gigantism
- If GH hypersecretion persist into adulthood, patient of gigantism will also have features of acromegaly
- Differential diagnosis of gigantism:
  - Marfan syndrome
  - Homocystinuria
  - Precocious puberty
  - Cerebral gigantism (large at birth with accelerated linear growth and disproportionately large extremities, associated with normal GH, IGF-1).

Q. Define acromegaloidism.

Ans. Patients exhibit soft tissue and skin changes associated with acromegaly but normal baseline and dynamic GH and IGF-1 with no demonstrable pituitary or extrapituitary tumor.

Q. Discuss about physiology of growth hormone.

Ans.

1. **Diabetogenic effect of GH:**
   - Decreases glucose uptake in extrahepatic tissue
   - Increases hepatic glucose output
2. **Ketogenic effect of GH:**
   - Increases lipolysis leading to increased FFA
3. **Protein sparer effect of GH:**
   - Increases protein synthesis
   - Decreases protein catabolism
4. **Other causes of GH hypersecretion:**
   - Anxiety, stress, exercise
   - Pregnancy
   - Acute illness, CKD, CLD
   - Starvation, PEM, anorexia nervosa
   - Type 1 diabetes mellitus
   - Heroin addiction
   - These conditions may be associated with abnormal GH suppressibility by glucose
   - Patients with these conditions do not have clinical manifestations of GH excess and do not have elevation of IGF-I.

Q. Discuss about pathophysiology of acromegaly.

Ans.

- In acromegaly, GH secretion is increased in number, duration and amplitude of secretory episodes
- Secretion occurs randomly throughout a 24-h period
- Characteristic nocturnal surge (1–4 h after onset of sleep) is absent
- Glucose suppressibility is lost and GH stimulation by hypoglycemia is absent
- TRH may cause GH release (normally does not cause)
- Dopamine and dopamine agonist causes GH suppression in 70%–80% of patients with acromegaly (normally stimulate)
- The mediator of most of the effects of GH is by IGF-I except insulin resistance and carbohydrate intolerance (direct effect of GH).

Q. What are the causes of acromegaly?

Ans.

- Pituitary adenoma (>99% cases). Macroadenoma > microadenoma (10%)
- Fifteen percent tumor also contains lactotrophs releasing prolactin
- Ectopic GH or GHRH secretion: from lung carcinoma, carcinoid tumor and pancreatic islet cells tumor. Suspected in patients present with:

- Known extrapituitary tumor present with clinical and biochemical features of acromegaly
- Radiology show normal pituitary gland.

Q. Mention clinical features of acromegaly.

Ans.

1. **Symptoms**
   - Progressive increase in size of the body with enlargement of hands, feet and coarsening of facial features (increase in ring, glove and shoe sizes)
   - Headache
   - Increased sweating (hyperhidrosis), heat intolerance
   - Weight gain but weakness
   - Progressive visual field defect (H/o collision with doors due to defective temporal field of vision)
   - Convulsion
   - Arthralgia and arthritis
   - Disturbance of other endocrine functions:
     - Galactorrhea (15%)
     - Hypogonadism: Tumor growth impair gonadotropin secretion, associated hyperprolactinemia
     - Features of complications, for example, HTN, DM.

2. **Signs**
   - Comparison with old photograph, if available
   - Face:
     - Large coarse facies with prominent supraorbital ridge
     - Enlargement of lip, nose and tongue (macroglossia)
     - Malocclusion and widely spaced teeth
     - Skull is enlarged
     - Prognathism (protrusion of lower jaw forward, so lower teeth overbite the upper teeth)
   - Hand:
     - Large, bulky, doughy feeling with blunt spade like fingers
     - Warm and sweaty hand
     - Carpal tunnel syndrome: Median nerve compression at wrist detected by
       - Tinel sign: percussion over flexor retinaculum → paresthesia along nerve distribution (lateral three and half fingers)
       - Phalen sign: flexion/extension of wrist for 1 min → paresthesia along nerve distribution (lateral three and half fingers)
   - Eye: Visual field defect/bitemporal hemianopia, papilledema
   - Voice: Husky, cavernous voice due to enlargement of larynx

- Skin: Generalized thickening of skin with increased oiliness and sweating. Acanthosis nigricans in axilla and neck, skin tag (molluscum fibrosum), hypertrichosis in women
- Visceromegaly: Thyromegaly, enlargement of salivary gland, cardiomegaly
- Blood pressure: high
- Proximal myopathy.

3. **Complications:**
   - Cardiac:
     – HTN (25%)
     – Cardiomegaly (15%) due to HTN, CCF, acromegalic cardiomyopathy
     – CCF, IHD, cardiomyopathy
   - Insulin resistance and IGT (50%–70%), DM (20%)
   - Cerebrovascular disease
   - Sleep apnea: Central and obstructive (due to soft tissue swelling in nasopharyngeal region)
   - Increased risk of colonic carcinoma (2-4 times) as GH/IGF-1 stimulate colonic mucosal turnover
   - Renal calculi: Due to hypercalciuria induced by GH excess.

4. **Effects of tumor:**
   - Visual field defect
   - Hypopituitarism.

Q. What are the causes of death in acromegaly?

Ans.
- Cardiovascular disease: HTN, IHD, CCF, cardiomyopathy
- Cerebrovascular disease/stroke
- Colonic carcinoma
- Pituitary apoplexy.

Q. Mention differential diagnosis of symptomatology related to acromegaly.

Ans.
- **Heat intolerance:**
  – Thyrotoxicosis
  – Postmenopausal syndrome
  – Acromegaly
- **Warm and sweaty hand:**
  – Thyrotoxicosis
  – Acromegaly
- **Cold and sweaty hand:**
  – Anxiety neurosis
- **Weight gain but weakness:**
  – Hypothyroidism
  – Cushing syndrome
  – Acromegaly

- **Prominent supraorbital ridge:**
  - Acromegaly
  - Hereditary hemolytic anemia
  - Rickets
  - Hydrocephalus
  - Paget disease
  - Achondroplasia
- **Macroglossia (large tongue):**
  - Acromegaly
  - Hypothyroidism
  - Amyloidosis
  - Down syndrome
  - Tumor in tongue
- **Carpal tunnel syndrome:**
  - Pregnancy
  - Obesity
  - RA
  - Acromegaly
  - Hypothyroidism
  - CRF on long term dialysis
  - OCP
  - Idiopathic
- **Endocrine and metabolic cause of proximal myopathy:**
  - Hypothyroidism
  - Hyperthyroidism
  - Acromegaly
  - Cushing syndrome
  - Osteomalacia
  - Hypokalemia
- **Sleep apnea syndrome:**
  - Hypothyroidism
  - Acromegaly
  - Obesity
  - Nasal obstruction
  - Familial (more in male)
  - Alcohol.

Q. How will you investigate acromegaly?

Ans.
- **Glucose suppression:**
  - Most specific dynamic test for acromegaly
  - In healthy subject, oral 100 g glucose causes reduction of GH to <1 ng/mL at 60 min

- In acromegaly, GH levels paradoxically increase (50%), remain unchanged or fall modestly but never <1 ng/mL
- False positive: CKD, CLD, PEM, Type 1 DM, heroin addiction
- **Basal fasting GH level:**
  - Not useful in diagnosis of acromegaly
  - Normal 1–5, >10 ng/mL in >90% acromegaly patients
  - Single measurement is not reliable as GH secretion is episodic in acromegaly, and other conditions may increase GH
  - However, in untreated patient, random GH <1 ng/mL, possibility of acromegaly is less
- **IGF-I measurement:**
  - IGF-I level is elevated in virtually all patients with acromegaly
  - IGF-I has long half-life, so IGF-I levels fluctuate much less than GH levels
- **IGF-BP3**
- **MRI of brain:** Localize the tumor. Ninety percent have tumor size >10 mm
- **Radiology:**
  - **X-ray skull Towne view:** AP X-ray of skull with beam travel from 5 cm above nasion to foramen magnum
  - **X-ray skull lateral view:**
    - Skull is enlarged
    - Frontal and maxillary sinuses are enlarged
    - Sella turcica is enlarged
    - Erosion of anterior and posterior clinoid process
    - May be double floor (due to enlargement of tumor downwards)
  - **X-ray hand AP view:**
    - Hands are enlarged
    - Increased soft tissue shadow
    - All the bones of both hands are enlarged
    - Widening of joint spaces (increase width of intra-articular cartilage)
    - Arrowhead tufting of terminal phalanges
  - **X-ray foot to see heel pad thickness:** Normal in male up to 21.5 cm, in female 18 cm. In acromegaly >22 cm
  - **CXR P/A view:** Cardiomegaly
- **Others:**
  - Serum prolactin: Elevated (15%), also assessment of other anterior pituitary hormones if needed
  - OGTT: DM/IGT
  - Perimetry: Bitemporal hemianopia
  - ECG: LVH
  - USG abdomen: Organomegaly

- Serum calcium: May be high due to associated MEN-1. There is also hypercalciuria (risk of renal stone)
- Colonoscopy: All patients >40 years should have routine colonoscopy, and those with polyp should receive 3–5 years repeat colonoscopy.

Q. How will you treat a patient of acromegaly?

Ans.

- **Objectives of treatment:**
  - Removal of pituitary tumor
  - Reversal of GH hypersecretion
  - Maintenance of normal anterior and posterior pituitary function

1. **Surgical treatment:** Trans-sphenoidal selective removal of adenoma is first line treatment
   - Cure rate: 60%–80%
   - Cure rate is less (30%–60%) in
     - Those with large tumors (>2 cm)
     - Basal GH levels >50 ng/mL
     - Those with extrasellar extension
   - Recurrence rates: 5% at 5 years
   - Guidelines for remission:
     - Fasting GH of ≤1 ng/mL
     - Glucose suppressed GH ≤1 ng/mL
     - Normal level of IGF-I.

2. **Medical treatment:** Indicated in patient with persisting GH hypersecretion after surgery
   - Somatostatin analog:
     - Octreotide acetate or lanreotide
     - Adverse effects: GI symptoms, gallstones, IGT, pancreatitis
   - Cabergoline: Dopamine agonist, in patient with hyperprolactinemia
   - Pegvisomant:
     - GH receptor antagonist
     - Adverse effects: Elevated liver enzymes
     - Used limited in patients who have failed therapy with surgery and somatostatin analogs
   - Biological agent: Sunsumab.

3. **Radiotherapy:**
   - Indicated in those patients with inadequate response to surgery and medical therapy
   - Risk of hypopituitarism

Q. How can you measure response of treatment of acromegaly patients.
Ans.

1. **Clinical:**
   - Reduction of soft tissue bulk of the extremities (mark a line over wrist and submerge in a bowl of water and measure volume of water displaced in each month)
   - Decreased facial puffiness
   - Increased energy
   - Cessation of hyperhidrosis, heat intolerance
   - Headache, carpal tunnel syndrome, sleep apnea reversed

2. **Biochemical:**
   - Glucose intolerance reversed
   - Guidelines for remission achieved (bone changes typically do not regress).

Q. Discuss about follow-up of acromegaly patients after treatment.
Ans.
- Assessment of GH secretion, anterior pituitary function and tumor size
- Following surgery follow up after 4–8 weeks
  - If GH >1 ng/dL: Therapy with somatostatin analogs
  - If GH <1 ng/dL: Repeat GH, IGF-I at 6 month interval for 2 years and yearly thereafter to rule out recurrences
- Recurrent elevations in IGF-I: Repeat MRI of the sella.

CHAPTER 24

Prolactinoma

Q. Clinical information about prolactin.

Ans.
- Prolactin (PRL) is secreted by lactotrophs, account for 10%–25% of anterior pituitary cells
- Lactotrophs proliferate during pregnancy due to elevated estrogen and account for twofold increase in gland size
- Hypothalamic dopamine inhibits prolactin secretion. TRH increase prolactin secretion
- If patient not distressed by venepuncture, a random serum prolactin is sufficient to diagnose hyperprolactinemia
- Absence of galactorrhea despite markedly elevated prolactin level may be due to concomitant deficiency of gonadal hormones required to initiate lactation
- Patient with galactorrhea but normal menses may not have hyperprolactinemia and usually do not have prolactinoma. If prolactin level is normal, they may be reassured and followed with sequential prolactin measurement
- Patient with persistent hyperprolactinemia and hypogonadism but normal MRI managed by observation if hypogonadism is of short duration. In patient whose hypogonadism >6–12 months, dopamine agonist should be used to suppress prolactin secretion and restore normal gonadal function
- Normal serum prolactin: Male (54–340 mIU/mL), female (66–490 mIU/mL).

Q. What is hook effect?

Ans. Extremely high prolactin level may be falsely reported as normal or modestly elevated due to saturation of assay antibodies, known as hook effect. So in patient with macroadenoma with clear-cut clinical features of hyperprolactinemia with prolactin value not as high as expected, serum sample should be diluted $\geq$1:100 before assay to overcome the hook effect.

Q. What is macroprolactinemia/big prolactin?

Ans.
- In some patients, high molecular weight (>150 kDa, normal prolactin: 23 kDa) prolactin predominate consists of aggregates of monomeric PRL as well as PRL-immunoglobulin G complexes known as macroprolactin

- Macroprolactin have reduced biological activity. Many commercial assays do not distinguish prolactin from macroprolactin, so macroprolactinemia is a cause of spurious hyperprolactinemia. Screening for macroprolactinemia should be done in asymptomatic hyperprolactinemia patients.

Q. Mention causes of hyperprolactinemia.

Ans.
1. **Physiological:** Pregnancy, nipple stimulation, coitus, exercise, stress, sleep.
2. **Pituitary disorders:**
   - Prolactinoma
   - Acromegaly
   - Pituitary adenoma compressing stalk (disconnection hyperprolactinemia)
3. **Systemic disorders:**
   - Hypothyroidism
   - PCOS
   - CRF, CLD
   - Chest: Chest wall injury, herpes zoster
   - Seizure
4. **Drug induced:**
   - Dopamine antagonist:
     - Antipsychotic: Phenothiazine, haloperidol, risperidone
     - Antidepressants: TCA, SSRI, MAO inhibitor
     - Antiemetic: Domperidone, metoclopramide
   - Dopamine depleting drugs: Reserpine, methyldopa
   - Verapamil, opiates, cocaine
   - Omeprazole, H2 blocker, estrogen/OCP
5. **Idiopathic hyperprolactinemia:** No cause found.

Q. What are the indications for prolactin measurement?

Ans.
- Galactorrhea
- Enlarged sella turcica
- Suspected pituitary tumor
- Hypogonadotropic hypogonadism/unexplained gonadal dysfunction
  - Unexplained amenorrhea
  - Unexplained male hypogonadism/male infertility

Q. What is prolactinoma?

Ans.
- Prolactin secreting pituitary tumor
- Commonest functioning pituitary tumor

- Microprolactinoma is common than macroprolactinoma
- For microprolactinoma: F:M = 20:1 (due to earlier recognition of endocrine consequence of prolactin excess in female), for macroprolactinoma F:M = 1:1.

Q. Mention clinical features of prolactinoma.

Ans.

1. **Due to hyperprolactinemia (micro- and macroprolactinoma):**
   - **Galactorrhea:**
     - Lactation in absence of breastfeeding
     - Up to 50% of women and 35% of men with prolactinoma have galactorrhea
     - It may or may not be spontaneous, may be present only transiently or intermittently. It can be unilateral or bilateral, profuse or sparse and vary in thickness
   - **Gonadal dysfunction:**
     - In women:
       - Amenorrhea, oligomenorrhea with anovulation or infertility
       - Menstrual disorder usually presents concurrently with galactorrhea if it is present but may either precede or follow it. Amenorrhea is usually secondary and may follow pregnancy or oral contraceptive use
       - ↓ Vaginal lubrication, ↓ libido or other symptoms of estrogen deficiency
     - In men:
       - ↓ Libido, erectile dysfunction, oligospermia, infertility
       - ↓ Libido may not come to attention by both patient and physician due to psychological factors. So diagnosis of prolactinoma in men is frequently delayed and often present with marked hyperprolactinemia with mass effect
   - **Osteoporosis:** Hyperprolactinemia is associated with long-term risk of ↓ BMD.

2. **Mass effect (macroprolactinoma only):**
   - Headache
   - Visual field defect, ↓ visual acuity, optic atrophy, papilledema
   - Cavernous sinus: Diplopia, ophthalmoplegia, cranial nerve palsy
   - Seizure
   - Pituitary apoplexy
   - Hypopituitarism.

Q. Why gonadal dysfunction occurs in hyperprolactinemia?

Ans.

- Prolactin inhibits both normal pulsatile secretion of LH and FSH and midcycle LH surge, resulting in anovulation
- In men, prolactin excess leads to decreased testosterone synthesis and spermatogenesis
- High prolactin also directly inhibits ovarian and testicular function.

Q. How will you investigate a case of hyperprolactinemia?

Ans.
- Serum prolactin level:
  - Stress of venepuncture may cause mild hyperprolactinemia, sample best taken through an indwelling cannula after 30 min
  - Serum prolactin (500–1,000 mIU/mL): Induced by stress or drug and repeat measurement is indicated
  - Serum prolactin (1,000–5,000 mIU/mL): Drugs, microprolactinoma, disconnection hyperprolactinemia
  - Serum prolactin (>5,000 mIU/mL): Suggestive of macroprolactinoma. More than 10,000 mIU/mL is diagnostic of macroprolactinoma. There is relationship between prolactin level and tumor size. Higher the level, bigger the tumor
  - Prolactinoma can present with any level of prolactin elevation
- Exclude pregnancy at first in women of childbearing potential with amenorrhea
- Serum FSH, LH, FT_4, TSH
- Serum testosterone in men
- Liver and kidney function tests
- MRI of sella and perisellar region with contrast: If serum prolactin >1,000 mIU/mL.

Q. How will you treat a case of prolactinoma?

Ans.
- **Aims of treatment:**
  - **Microprolactinoma:** Lower prolactin level and restoration of gonadal function
  - **Macroprolactinoma:** Lower prolactin level, restoration of gonadal function, ↓ tumor size and ↓ risk of further tumor expansion, hypopituitarism and visual impairment
  - Most microprolactinoma do not progress (93%), but macroprolactinoma continue to expand and lead to mass effect

1. **Drug treatment (Dopamine agonists):**
   - Bromocriptine, cabergoline, quinagolide, pergolide. Dopamine agonists act by activation of D2 receptor in brain
   - Bromocriptine: Ergot derived dopamine agonist. Dose 1.25–15 mg/day.
   - Cabergoline: Ergot derived. .25–1 mg once or twice weekly. It has better side effect profile than bromocriptine. Cabergoline is more potent, much longer acting and better tolerated. Cabergoline has become the dopamine agonist of choice in prolactinoma unless pregnancy is desired. For fertility, bromocriptine is preferred as it is short acting and can be discontinued on pregnancy confirmation.

2. **Surgical treatment:**
   - Trans-sphenoidal surgery is indicated only for patients who are resistant to or intolerant of dopamine agonist treatment. The cure rate for macroprolactinoma treated with surgery is poor (30%) and therefore drug treatment is first line in tumors of all size.

3. **Radiotherapy:** Reserved for macroprolactinoma not responded to surgery or dopamine agonist.
4. **Chemotherapy:** Temozolomide for malignant prolactinoma.

Q. Mention adverse effects of dopamine agonists and how to minimize them?
Ans.
- **Adverse effects:**
  - Ergotamine-like side effects (nausea, headache, postural hypotension, constipation)
  - Nasal stuffiness, Raynaud-like phenomenon in hands, sudden onset of sleep, CSF rhinorrhea
  - Fibrotic reactions: Ergot derived dopamine agonist is associated with pulmonary, retroperitoneal and cardiac fibrotic reactions (e.g., tricuspid valve regurgitation) due to their affinity to serotonin receptors. Common in Parkinson disease where doses of dopamine agonists is 20–30 times higher than prolactinoma and administered daily rather than twice daily
- **How to minimize adverse effects?**
  - Start dopamine agonist at low dose (1.25 mg bromocriptine daily or .25 mg cabergoline weekly)
  - Increase dose gradually as tolerated
  - Taking drug with food before bedtime
  - Avoid activities that cause peripheral vasodilation, for example, hot bath to decrease risk of postural hypotension

Q. Mention duration of treatment of prolactinoma with dopamine agonist and follow-up.
Ans.
- **Duration of treatment:** Dopamine agonist may be tapered and perhaps discontinued after 2–3 years of treatment, provided there is normalization of prolactin level and no visible tumor remnant on MRI. 30%–40% patients with micro- or macroprolactinoma will remain in long-term remission. Patients who have recurrence of hyperprolactinemia after drug withdrawal may resume the drug or choose to have surgical excision
- **Follow-up:**
  - Measurement of serum prolactin every 3 months for first year and then annually thereafter
  - MRI, if prolactin increases above normal level.

Q. What is dopamine agonist resistance?
Ans.
- Failure to normalize prolactin and decrease tumor size to <50%
- Occurs in 24% treated with bromocriptine and 11% with cabergoline
- D_2 receptors are reduced in number but not efficacy
- **Treatment:** Increase dose of dopamine agonist to maximum tolerable dose, switch to another dopamine agonist, surgery.

Q. How will you select therapy for prolactinoma?

Ans. Depends on the wish of the patient, patient's plans for pregnancy, tolerance to medical therapy and availability of a skilled neurosurgeon.
- **Microadenoma:** Patients who respond to dopamine agonist should be treated for 2–3 years and then the drug should be withdrawn to determine if long-term remission will occur. Patients who have recurrence of hyperprolactinemia after drug withdrawal may resume the drug or choose to have surgical excision
- **Macroadenoma:** Medical therapy with dopamine agonist is primary therapy of choice. Therapeutic failure can result from drug intolerance, poor compliance or resistance and may need trans-sphenoidal surgery.

Q. How to manage a case of drug induced hyperprolactinemia?

Ans.
- A variety of medication cause minimal or moderate PRL elevation, but risperidone, metoclopramide or phenothiazine can lead to prolactin level >4,000 mIU/mL
- If patient taking antipsychotic medication, consult with patient's physician, whether drug can be discontinued or switch to drugs with little or no effect on prolactin, for example, olanzapine, clozapine, quetiapine, aripiprazole
- If drug can be discontinued, measure serum PRL after several weeks (≥3 days later). If prolactin level does not normalize, a pituitary MRI should be done
- If the drug cannot be discontinued, onset of hyperprolactinemia does not coincide with therapy initiation or patients have hypogonadal symptoms or low bone mass, a pituitary MRI should be done to exclude prolactinoma
- Whether to treat a patient with antipsychotic-induced hyperprolactinemia with dopamine agonist remain controversial due to increased risk of side effects (e.g., postural hypotension) and exacerbation of underlying psychosis. Some advocate cautious use of both drugs simultaneously.

Q. How will you manage prolactinoma in pregnancy?

Ans.
- **Effect of pregnancy on tumor size:** Risk of significant tumor enlargement resulting in visual field defect or headache in microprolactinoma (1%–2%) and macroprolactinoma (15%–35%)
- **Effect of dopamine agonist on fetus:**
  - Bromocriptine appears not to be teratogenic with no adverse fetal effects. Cabergoline also do not show adverse effects but the data are limited compared with large numbers for bromocriptine safety
  - It is recommended that for women with prolactinoma seeking fertility, bromocriptine is preferred to induce ovulation as there are more data on long-term safety of bromocriptine, and it is short acting and can be discontinued immediately on pregnancy confirmation, but cabergoline is being used increasingly as it is better tolerated. Both are category B drug

- **Microadenoma:**
  - Discontinue dopamine agonist when pregnancy test is positive
  - Periodic visual field examinations at each trimester during pregnancy
  - MRI is indicated in patient who become symptomatic, for example, visual field defect, headache
  - Serum prolactin measured after 6 weeks of delivery, if it is higher than prepregnancy level, pituitary MRI is indicated
- **Macroadenoma:**
  - Consider surgery before pregnancy
  - Bromocriptine should be continued throughout pregnancy to ↓ risk of tumor growth. Periodic visual field examinations at each trimester during pregnancy
  - Consider high dose steroid or surgery during pregnancy if vision is threatened or adenoma hemorrhage occurs
  - Postpartum MRI after 6 weeks of delivery.

CHAPTER 25

Diabetes Insipidus

Q. Define and classify diabetes insipidus (DI).

Ans. Excretion of large volume of urine (diabetes) that is dilute, hypotonic and tasteless (insipid).

1. **Classification:**
   - **Cranial DI:** Due to decreased synthesis or secretion of ADH (hypothalamic DI)
     - **Genetic:**
       - Familial hypothalamic DI
       - DIDMOAD (DI, DM, optic atrophy, nerve deafness)/Wolfram syndrome
     - **Acquired:**
       - Invasive: Pituitary adenoma, craniopharyngioma, meningioma, metastasis
       - Infiltrative: Sarcoidosis, hemochromatosis
       - Injury: Head injury, for example, RTA
       - Iatrogenic: Pituitary surgery
     (10% vasopressin cell sufficient to keep urine volume <4 L/day)
   - **Nephrogenic DI:** Renal tubules are unresponsive to ADH
     - **Genetic:** Aquaporin-2 mutation
     - **Acquired:**
       - Metabolic: Hypokalemia, hypercalcemia
       - Drug: Lithium, demeclocycline
       - CKD: PKD, sickle cell anemia
   - ↑ **Metabolism of ADH in pregnancy:** DI of pregnancy.

Q. What are the clinical features of diabetes insipidus?

Ans.
- Adult: Polyuria (5–20 L/day or more), nocturia and thirst
- Children: Polyuria, enuresis and failure to thrive
- Features of cranial DI may be masked by cortisol deficiency leading to failure to excrete a water load.

Q. How will you investigate diabetes insipidus?

Ans.
- Twenty-four-hour urinary output/voiding diary (time and volume of each voided urine)
- Blood sugar, urine R/M/E, serum creatinine (to exclude DM, RF)

- Serum electrolyte: Hypokalemia, hypercalcemia (nephrogenic DI)
- Plasma vasopressin level
- Water deprivation test
- Saline infusion test: Infuse hypertonic (5%) saline and measure ADH secretion in response to increasing plasma osmolality
- MRI brain: Tumor (hypothalamic, infiltration), loss of bright spot of posterior pituitary gland
- Serum ACE (sarcoidosis).

Q. **Discuss about water deprivation test.**

Ans.
- **Use:** To establish diagnosis of DI and differentiate cranial from nephrogenic causes
- **Protocol:**
  - No coffee, tea or smoking on the test day
  - Free fluids until 8 AM on the morning of the test but discourage patient from stocking up with extra fluid in anticipation of fluid deprivation
  - No fluid from 8 AM
  - Attend at 9 AM for body weight, plasma and urine osmolality
  - Record body weight, urine volume, urine and plasma osmolality and thirst score on visual analogue scale every 2 h for 8 h
  - Stop the test if the patient loses 3% of body weight
  - If plasma osmolality reaches >300 mOsm/kg and urine osmolality <600 mOsm/kg, administer DDAVP 2 μg IM and urine output and osmolality for additional 4 h
- **Interpretation:**
  - DI is confirmed by plasma osmolality >300 mOsm/kg with urine osmolality <600 mOsm/kg
  - Cranial DI is confirmed if urine osmolality rises ≥50% after DDAVP
  - Nephrogenic DI is confirmed if DDAVP does not concentrate the urine
  - Primary polydipsia is suggested by low plasma osmolality at the start of test

Diagnosis	Urine osmolality mOsm/kg	
	After fluid deprivation	After DDAVP
Cranial DI	<600	>600, ≥50% increase
Nephrogenic DI	<600	<600
Primary polydipsia	>600	>600
Partial central DI	300–600	>600

Q. **How will you treat diabetes insipidus?**

Ans.
- Maintenance of adequate fluid input: In patient with partial DI and intact thirst mechanism, drug therapy may not be necessary if polyuria is mild (<4 L/day)

- **Cranial diabetes insipidus:**
  - Desmopressin (DDAVP): Vasopressin analogue acting predominantly on V_2 receptor in kidney with little action on V_1 receptor at blood vessels. It thus has reduced pressor activity and ↑ antidiuretic efficacy
  - Desmopressin is available as tablet, solution for nasal spray and more potent parenteral solution. Satisfactory control is achieved with 1–2 intranasal spray/day
  - Desmopressin is only therapeutic agent recommended for pregnancy and has minimal oxytocic activity on uterus
  - Adverse effects: Water intoxication and hyponatremia (so monitor serum Na^+, osmolality)
  - If DI is associated with other anterior pituitary hormone deficiency, treatment with thyroid hormone and hydrocortisone needed to maintain normal renal response to vasopressin
- **Nephrogenic diabetes insipidus:**
  - Offending drug stopped and electrolyte abnormality corrected
  - Thiazide diuretic, for example, bendroflumethiazide 5–10 mg/day, amiloride 5–10 mg/day cause contraction of ECF volume, ↓ GFR and ↓ urine volume
  - NSAIDS, for example, indomethacin 15 mg 8 h (↓ action of PGs which locally inhibit the action of vasopressin)

Q. **How will you differentiate diabetes insipidus from primary polydipsia?**
Ans.

Points	Diabetes insipidus	Primary polydipsia
Etiology	Pituitary surgery or injury, hypokalemia, hypercalcemia	Psychiatric patient or hypothalamic lesion (organic)
Cause of excessive fluid intake	Thirst	Bizarre motives such as for body cleansing
Dehydration	May be present if fluid intake impaired	Never
Over hydration	Never	May occur if water excretion is impaired
Fluid deprivation	Causes weight loss	No weight loss
Plasma osmolality	High	Low
Treatment	Desmopressin (DDAVP), correction of electrolyte abnormality	Treatment of psychiatric disorder, propranolol (inhibit renin angiotensin system)

Q. **Discuss about SIADH (Syndrome of Inappropriate ADH Secretion).**
Ans.
- **Definition:** It is a condition where an endogenous source of ADH promotes renal water retention in absence of appropriate physiological stimulus

- **Causes:**
  - Tumors: Small cell lung cancer
  - CNS disorder: Stroke, trauma, infection
  - Pulmonary disorder: Pulmonary tuberculosis
  - Drugs: Carbamazepine, cyclophosphamide, haloperidol, amitriptyline, morphine
  - Idiopathic
- **Clinical features:**
  - Depends on rate of development and severity of hyponatremia
  - Fatigue, headache, nausea, anorexia
  - Confusion, seizure, coma
- **Clue of diagnosis:**
  - Patient is euvolemic
  - Low plasma Na$^+$ <130 mmol/L
  - Low plasma osmolality <270 mmol/kg
  - Urine osmolality >150 mmol/kg
  - Urine Na$^+$ concentration >30 mmol/L
  - Low-normal plasma urea, creatinine, uric acid
  - Exclusion of other causes of hyponatremia
  - Appropriate clinical context
  - Intact renal, adrenal, thyroid function with exclusion of CCF, CRF, CLD
- **Treatment:**
  - Treatment of cause, for example, stop offending drug
  - Fluid restriction: 600–1,000 mL/day
  - Demeclocycline 600–900 mg/day (↓ responsiveness to collecting duct to ADH)
  - Oral Urea: 30–45 g/day (provide solute load to promote water excretion)
  - Vaptans (oral vasopressin receptor antagonist)
  - In acutely symptomatic patient or serum Na$^+$ ↓ to dangerously low: Infusion of hypertonic saline, loop diuretic, for example, frusemide.

CHAPTER 26

Short Stature

Q. Define short stature.

Ans. Short stature can be defined as follows:
- Height >3.5 SD below the mean for chronologic age
- Growth rate >2 SD below the mean for chronologic age
- Height >2 SD below the target height when corrected for midparental height.

Q. Mention etiology of short stature.

Ans.

1. **Non-endocrine causes:**
   - Constitutional short stature (commonest cause)
   - Familial/genetic
   - Intrauterine growth retardation and SGA (small for gestational age)
   - Syndromes of short stature:
     – Turner syndrome
     – Noonan syndrome (Pseudo-turner syndrome)
     – Prader–Willi syndrome
     – Laurence–Moon–Bardet–Biedl syndrome
   - Chronic systemic illness:
     – Cardiac disorders: Left-to-right shunt, CCF
     – Pulmonary disorders: Cystic fibrosis, Bronchial asthma
     – Gastrointestinal disorders: Malabsorption, Celiac disease
     – Hepatic disorders
     – Hematological disorders: Sickle cell anemia, Thalassemia
     – Rheumatological disorders: Connective tissue disease, Juvenile idiopathic arthritis
     – Chronic infection, CRF
   - Malnutrition
   - Skeletal dysplasia:
     – Achondroplasia (short limb and normal trunk)
     – Hurler syndrome or mucopolysaccharidosis (short limb, short spine).

2. **Endocrine causes:**
   - GH deficiency and variants
     - Congenital GH deficiency (Isolated or with other pituitary hormone deficiency)
     - Acquired GH deficiency
     - Abnormalities of GH action: Laron dwarfism, Pygmies
   - Hypothyroidism
   - Cushing syndrome
   - Pseudohypoparathyroidism
   - Disorders of vitamin D metabolism
   - Diabetes mellitus, poorly controlled
   - Psychosocial dwarfism (Kasper Hauser syndrome).

Q. **What are the criteria of constitutional short stature?**

Ans.
- A variation of normal, and considered slowing down the pace of development
- Normal birth length and height
- Moderate short stature (not far below third percentile), thin habitus
- Delayed bone age; bone age (BA) = height age (HA) (CA > BA = HA)
- Family history of similarly affected members, e.g. delayed puberty
- Usually associated with delayed puberty for CA but normal for BA
- Healthy child with no signs or symptoms of disease
- Final height often less than predicted
- **Treatment:** Aromatase inhibitor for boys, inhibit conversion of androgen to estrogen so that bone age does not advance and growth continues longer.

Q. **What are the criteria for familial/genetic short stature?**

Ans.
- Family history present
- Bone age normal, i.e. CA = BA > HA
- Normal onset of puberty
- Final height short but appropriate for parental age.

Q. **Define idiopathic short stature.**

Ans. Height of an individual >2 SD below the corresponding mean height for a given age, sex, and population group without evidence of systemic, endocrine, nutritional, or chromosomal abnormalities.

Q. **How do you evaluate a case of short stature?**

Ans.
1. **History:**
   - Who is concerned, child or parents?
   - When did growth failure begin? Has the child always been small or is this a recent growth failure?

- Any previous measurements available, e.g. from parents, general physician, health visitor, school.
- Pregnancy events and records: Maternal illness in pregnancy, drug intake or substance abuse, H/o IUGR, gestational age at delivery, mode of delivery, birth trauma, or complications at labor including birth asphyxia, size at birth (weight, length, and head circumference), any congenital disease.
- Neonatal history: breech delivery, micropenis, hypothermia, hypoglycemia (GH deficiency or panhypopituitarism).
- Growth velocity and mile stones of development.
- School performance, intelligence/IQ.
- History or any evidence of chronic systemic illness (Respiratory, cardiac, GIT, renal or endocrinopathies).
- Any features of puberty and time of onset.
- Medication history, e.g. long-term steroid.
- Dietary history: Less intake, malabsorption.
- Psychosocial circumstances of the child and family.
- Family history:
    - Consanguinity of marriage
    - Parents' height
    - Family H/o short stature
    - Family H/o delayed puberty
    - Family H/o endocrinopathies or systemic illness that may affect growth.

2. **Examinations:**
    - Height
    - Weight
    - Height velocity over at least 6 months
    - Arm span
    - Upper segment
    - Lower segment
    - Upper/lower segment ratio
    - Signs of dysmorphic feature
    - Evidence of chronic systemic illness (respiratory, cardiac, GIT, renal) or endocrinopathies
    - Signs of syndromes
    - Nutritional status, e.g. skinfold thickness
    - Midline defects
    - Pubertal status
    - Measure parents heights and calculate mid-parental height (MPH)
    - Reduction of weight to height (malabsorption and systemic illness)
    - More weight but short height (hypothyroidism, Cushing syndrome, Prader-Willi syndrome, Laurence-Moon-Bardet-Biedl syndrome).

3. **Investigations:**
   - CBC with ESR
   - Urine R/E
   - Stool R/E
   - Renal function tests (urea, creatinine, electrolytes)
   - Liver function tests
   - FT_4, TSH
   - Serum calcium and phosphate
   - X-ray wrist and hand (bone age)
   - IGF-1 (do not misinterpret low values in constitutional delay or malnutrition)
   - IGFBP-3 to confirm low IGF-1 in GH deficiency
   - Serum prolactin to evaluate potential hypothalamic/pituitary disease
   - MRI brain with contrast (if CNS pathology suspected)
   - Celiac panel
   - Karyotype in any girl without other diagnosis
   - Growth hormone (GH) testing: GH stimulated test is last and only performed if no other diagnosis is found.

Q. Discuss about growth hormone deficiency.

Ans.

1. **Etiology:**
   - Congenital GH deficiency
   - Acquired GH deficiency resulting from CNS tumors, trauma, or infection.

2. **Findings that suggest GH deficiency.**
   - **In neonates:**
     - Hypoglycemia
     - Prolonged jaundice
     - Hypothermia
     - Microphallus (penis <2 cm in length at birth)
     - Traumatic delivery
     - Breech delivery
   - **In children with short stature or growth failure:**
     - Cranial irradiation
     - Head trauma or CNS infection
     - Consanguinity and/or an affected family member
     - Craniofacial midline abnormalities
     - Signs of multiple hormone deficiency
   - **Clinical features of GH deficiency:**
     - Short stature
     - Delayed bone age
     - Chubby or cherubic appearance (due to increased fat mass) with immature facial appearance

- Immature high-pitched voice
- Intelligence is normal unless repeated or severe hypoglycemia.

Q. How will you diagnose GH deficiency?

Ans.

1. **IGF-1:** Do not misinterpret low values in constitutional delay, starvation/malnutrition, and psychosocial dwarfism. In constitutional delay, IGF-1 value is low for chronological age but normal for skeletal age.

2. **IGFBP-3:** To confirm low IGF-1 in GH deficiency. Provide stronger evidence of GH deficiency than IGF-1 determination alone.

3. **Growth hormone testing:**
   - Never get basal serum GH unless you suspect gigantism.
   - **Stimulated tests:**
     - Levodopa
     - Clonidine
     - Post exercise
     - Insulin tolerance tests (ITT)
     - Arginine
     - Glucagon
     - Propanolol
     - 60–90 minutes after onset of sleep.
   - **Precaution about GH testing:**
     - GH testing should be done after an overnight fast. Carbohydrate or fat ingestion suppress GH response. Obesity suppresses GH secretion and an overweight or obese child may falsely appear to have GH deficiency.
     - Because 10% of healthy children do not have adequate rise in GH with one test of GH reserve, at least two methods of assessing GH reserve are necessary before diagnosis of classic GH deficiency is made. However, if GH rises >10 ng/mL in a single test, classic GH deficiency is eliminated.
   - **GH stimulation test with Levodopa:** Levodopa given orally according to body weight, <15 kg: 125 mg, 15–35 kg: 250 mg, >35 kg: 500 mg. Samples taken at 0, 60, and 90 minutes. Adverse effects are nausea and vomiting.
   - **GH stimulation test with Clonidine:** Clonidine given orally .1 mg/m². Samples taken at 0, 30, 60 and 90 minutes. Adverse effect is postural hypotension.
   - **Postexercise GH stimulation test:** Step climbing exercise cycle for 10 minutes. Samples taken at 0, 10 and 20 minutes.
   - **Insulin tolerance test (ITT)/Insulin-induced hypoglycemia test:**
     - Done for assessment of GH and ACTH reserve
     - **Procedure:**
       - NPO after midnight, water can be taken
       - Start IV low rate normal saline

- Regular insulin IV 0.05–0.1 U/kg
- Sample collection for glucose every 15 minutes. For GH and cortisol at 0, 30, 45, 60, 75 and 90 minutes.
– **Result:** Symptomatic hypoglycemia (tachycardia, sweating) with blood glucose <2.2 mmol/L (usually 20–35 minutes after insulin given) lead to GH >5 ng/mL and cortisol >550 nmol/L in normal subjects.
– **Contraindication:** Seizure, elderly, IHD, severe panhypopituitarism (cortisol <140 nmol/L).
– **Precaution:**
- IV 25% glucose and hydrocortisone ready
- A physician must be in attendance
- IV line before the test.

Q. Discuss about GH therapy.

Ans.
- **Indications:**
    – GH deficiency
    – Turner syndrome
    – Chronic renal disease
    – Small for gestational age
    – Idiopathic short stature
    – Prader-Willi syndrome
- **Dose of GH:** 25–35 µg/kg/day or 0.7–1 mg/m²/day subcutaneous every day in the evening during period of active growth before epiphyseal fusion.
- **Adverse effects of GH therapy:**
    – Glucose intolerance
    – Pseudotumor cerebri/benign intracranial hypertension: headache, visual disturbance
    – Worsening of scoliosis
    – Prepubertal gynecomastia
    – Slipped capital femoral epiphysis
    – Arthralgia and edema
    – Risk of leukemia, brain tumor recurrence
    – Adverse lipid profile (low HDL, high LDL).
- **Monitoring of patient on GH therapy:**
    – Close follow-up with a pediatric endocrinologist every 3–6 month
    – Determination of growth response
    – Evaluation of compliance
    – Screening for potential adverse effects
    – Interval measurements of serum IGF1 and IGFBP3 (increase with GH treatment)
    – Dose adjustment based on IGF-1 value (maintain IGF-1 to high normal range) and growth response

- Annual assessment of thyroid function to identify development of central hypothyroidism during treatment
- Periodic reevaluation of adrenal function.
- **Responses after GH therapy:**
  - One-third poor response
  - One-third response as expected (gain 5–10 cm)
  - One-third excellent responders.
- **Good predictor of GH response:**
  - Good baseline height
  - Younger age at onset of treatment
  - Longer treatment duration
  - Tall parents
  - Increase linear growth velocity in first six month of treatment.
- **When to stop GH therapy:**
  - Growth rate <2 cm/year
  - Bone age >16 (boys) or >14 (girls)
  - Decision of parents.

Part B: Thyroid Disorders

CHAPTER 27

Thyrotoxicosis

Q. Define thyrotoxicosis and hyperthyroidism.

Ans.
- **Thyrotoxicosis:** Clinical syndrome that results when tissues are exposed to high levels of circulating thyroid hormones. Thyrotoxicosis may be due to hyperthyroidism, also extrathyroidal source of thyroid hormones, for example, struma ovarii or excessive ingestion of thyroid hormone
- **Hyperthyroidism:** Hyperactivity of thyroid gland. Hyperthyroidism is a cause of thyrotoxicosis.

Q. What are the causes of thyrotoxicosis?

Ans.
- Graves' disease/diffuse toxic goiter/Von Basedow disease (76%)
- Toxic multinodular goiter/Plummer disease
- Toxic adenoma
- Thyroiditis:
  - Subacute/De Quervain thyroiditis
  - Postpartum/silent/painless thyroiditis
- Iodide-induced hyperthyroidism (Jod Basedow effect)
  - Drugs, for example, amiodarone
  - Radiographic contrast media
  - Iodine prophylaxis program
- Extrathyroidal source of thyroid hormone:
  - Thyrotoxicosis factitia
  - Struma ovarii
  - Hamburger thyrotoxicosis
- TSH induced:
  - TSH-secreting pituitary adenoma
  - Choriocarcinoma and hydatidiform mole
- Metastatic thyroid carcinoma (follicular).

Q. What are the causes of low radio iodine uptake thyrotoxicosis?

Ans.
- Thyroiditis:
  - Subacute/De Quervain thyroiditis
  - Postpartum/silent/painless thyroiditis
- Iodide induced hyperthyroidism (Jod Basedow effect)
  - Drugs, for example, amiodarone
  - Radiographic contrast media
  - Iodine prophylaxis program
- Extrathyroidal source of thyroid hormone:
  - Thyrotoxicosis factitia
  - Struma ovarii
  - Hamburger thyrotoxicosis.

Q. Define Graves' disease.

Ans. Graves' disease consists of one or more of the followings:
- Thyrotoxicosis
- Diffuse goiter
- Ophthalmopathy
- Pretibial myxedema
  - Age: 20–40 years, Sex: female:male = 5:1.

Q. Discuss the pathogenesis of Graves' disease.

Ans.
- In Graves' disease, T lymphocyte becomes sensitized to antigens within the thyroid gland and stimulate B lymphocyte to synthesize antibodies to these antigens
- There is production of IgG antibodies directed against TSH receptor on thyroid follicular cell membrane, which stimulates thyroid hormone production and proliferation of follicular cells leading to goiter in majority patients. These antibodies are termed thyroid stimulating immunoglobulin (TSI) or TSH receptor antibody (TRAb), detected in 80%–95% patients.

Q. What are the potential risk factors for Graves' disease?

Ans.
- **Genetic susceptibility:** Association of Graves' disease with HLA B8, DR3, and DR2
- **Viral or bacterial infection:** Certain gut organism *Escherichia coli*, *Yersinia enterocolitica* possess cell membrane TSH receptor. Antibody to these microbial antigens reacts with TSH receptor on host thyroid follicular cell
- **Stress**
- **Female gender**
- **Pregnancy:** Particularly the postpartum period
- **Iodide excess:** Particularly in geographic areas of iodide deficiency, where lack of iodide may hold latent Graves' disease in check.

Chapter 27: Thyrotoxicosis

Q. Discuss pathogenesis of Graves' ophthalmopathy and dermopathy.

Ans.
- Within the orbit (and the dermis) there is cytokine (e.g., IFN γ from local lymphocytes)-mediated proliferation of fibroblasts and preadipocyte resulting in increased amount of retro-orbital fat and hydrophilic glycosaminoglycans, secreted from fibroblast. The resulting increase in interstitial fluid content combined with chronic inflammatory cell infiltrate causes marked swelling and ultimate fibrosis of extraocular muscles and rise in retrobulbar pressure. The eye is displaced forward (exophthalmos) and in severe cases, there is optic nerve compression
- Smoking is a risk factor for ophthalmopathy by causing anoxia or simply by direct inflammation. Radio I_2 causes exacerbation of ophthalmopathy.

Q. Mention clinical features of thyrotoxicosis.

Ans.

1. **Symptoms:**
   - Weight loss despite normal or increased appetite (weight gain in 10% patients)
   - Heat intolerance
   - Palpitation
   - Increased sweating
   - Hyperdefecation
   - Tremor
   - Nervousness and irritability
   - Exertional dyspnea
   - Fatigue and muscle weakness
   - Periodic paralysis (predominantly in Chinese)
   - Amenorrhea/oligomenorrhea, infertility
   - Anxiety, psychosis
   - Sleep disturbances, for example, insomnia
   - Pruritus, ankle swelling.

2. **Signs:**
   - Patient is anxious, restless, frightened face with stare looks
   - Cachexia
   - Diffuse goiter with bruit (Graves' disease)
   - Hand:
     - Hand is warm and sweaty
     - Tremor of out stretched hands with fingers spread out
     - Tachycardia, atrial fibrillation
     - Palmar erythema
     - Thyroid acropachy/osteopathy (subperiosteal inflammation of the phalanges of hands and feet indistinguishable from finger clubbing)

- Onycholysis (separation of nails from bed—Plummer sign, due to rapid growth of nails)
  - Systolic hypertension, increase pulse pressure, cardiac failure
  - Proximal myopathy
  - Hyper-reflexia, ill-sustained clonus
  - Pretibial myxedema
  - Splenomegaly, gynecomastia

Q. Discuss eye signs of Graves' disease.

Ans.
- **Lid retraction:** Sclera above upper corneal margin is visible. Normally, upper one-third of cornea is covered by upper eyelid
- **Lid lag/Von Graefe sign:** Upper eyelid fail to follow finger down
- **Joffroy sign:** Absence of wrinkling of forehead on upward gaze
- **Mobius sign:** Impaired convergence of eyes
- **Stellwag sign:** Infrequent blinking
- **Jendrassik sign:** Paralysis of extraocular muscles
- **Ballet sign:** Weakness of at least one extraocular muscle
- **Chemosis/conjunctival edema**
- **Exophthalmos**
- **Corneal involvement/keratitis**

All causes of thyrotoxicosis can cause lid retraction and lid lag due to sympathetic over activity which supply levator palpebrae muscle, but other features of ophthalmopathy are present only in Graves' disease.

Q. Mention causes of weight loss despite normal or increased appetite.

Ans.
- Thyrotoxicosis
- Diabetes mellitus
- Kala azar.

Q. Mention endocrine causes of increased sweating.

Ans.
- Thyrotoxicosis
- Acromegaly
- Pheochromocytoma
- Hypoglycemia
- Carcinoid syndrome
- Postmenopausal syndrome.

Q. Mention features of thyrotoxicosis in children and elderly.

Ans.

1. **In children:**
   - Hyperactivity

- Behavioral abnormalities
- Rapid growth with accelerated bone maturation with reduced final height.

2. **In elderly:** Also known as apathetic/masked thyrotoxicosis
   - AF, tachycardia, CCF
   - Weight loss with anorexia
   - Muscle wasting and weakness
   - Depression, dementia
   - Osteoporosis, bone fracture.

Q. Discuss eye changes in Graves' disease (Werner classification).

Ans.

Class 0: No signs or symptoms
Class 1: Only signs, no symptoms (signs limited to lid retraction, lid lag, stare)
Class 2: Soft tissue involvement (symptoms and signs)
Class 3: Proptosis (measured with Hertel exophthalmometer)
Class 4: Extraocular muscle involvement
Class 5: Corneal involvement/keratitis
Class 6: Sight loss (optic nerve involvement)

- Easy to remember: NO SPECS
- This classification is useful in describing the extent of eye involvement, not helpful in following the progress of illness as one class does not necessarily progress into next
- Hertel exophthalmometer consists of two prisms with a scale. The prisms are placed on lateral orbital ridges, and the distance from orbital ridge to anterior cornea is measured on the scale. Upper limit of normal according to race: White Asian (20 mm), Black (22 mm). Increase in proptosis—mild involvement (3–4 mm), moderate involvement (5–7 mm), severe involvement (>8 mm)
- Inferior rectus muscle most commonly involved (upper gaze limitation). Next is medial rectus (impaired lateral gaze)
- Orbital muscle enlargement can be demonstrated by orbital ultrasound, orbital CT scan or MRI
- Although only one-third patients have eye involvement clinically, enlarged muscle is detected by imaging in >90% patients.

Q. How will you investigate thyrotoxicosis?

Ans.

- **FT_4, FT_3, TSH:** Elevated FT_4, FT_3, and suppressed TSH. In 5% patients, increased FT_3, normal FT_4 and suppressed TSH (T_3 thyrotoxicosis)
- **Thyroid autoantibodies:** TSH receptor antibody (TRAb)/thyroid stimulating immunoglobulin (TSI) present in 80%–95% of Graves' disease
- **Radioactive iodine uptake test:** Rapid uptake and rapid turnover. High uptake at 2 and 24 h and rapid washout at 48 h
- **Thyroid scan/thyroid scintigraphy:** Enlarged thyroid with intense diffuse homogenous uptake of isotope

- **Ultrasonography of neck:** To see single, multinodular or diffuse goiter, solid or cystic
- **Color flow Doppler (CFD) of thyroid:** Markedly increase signals (diffuse increase vascularity)
- **FNAC of thyroid:** If any nodule is present
- **ECG:** Sinus tachycardia, atrial fibrillation, left ventricular hypertrophy (due to HTN)
- **Chest X-ray:** Retrosternal extension of goiter, cardiomegaly
- **Urine R/M/E:** Lag storage glycosuria
- **RBS:** Secondary diabetes
- **Nonspecific:**
  - Increased ALT/SGPT, γ glutamyl transferase (GGT), ALP
  - Mild hypercalcemia
- **For thyroid ophthalmopathy:** Orbital USG, CT/MRI of orbit (extraocular muscle enlargement, compression of optic nerve, proptosis).

Q. Mention the prevalence of thyroid autoantibodies.

Ans.

	Antibodies to		
	Thyroid peroxidase (TPO)	*Thyroglobulin*	*TSH receptor*
Normal population	8–27	5–20	0
Graves' disease	50–80	50–70	80–95
Autoimmune hypothyroidism	90–100	80–90	10–20
Multinodular goiter	30–40	30–40	0
Transient thyroiditis	30–40	30–40	0

- TPO antibodies is principal component of what was previously measured as thyroid microsomal antibodies
- TRAb can be agonists/stimulatory causing Graves' disease or antagonists/blocking causing hypothyroidism.

Q. Discuss about radio iodine uptake test (RAIU) test.

Ans. Useful in determining the functional activity of thyroid gland and to differentiate among the causes of thyrotoxicosis
- **Procedure:**
  - I^{131}, 10 µCi given orally. Uptake seen by γ camera at 2, 24, and 48 h
  - Normal uptake: At 2 h (4%–10%), at 24 h (10%–25%)
- **Result:**
  - **Low uptake thyrotoxicosis:**
    - Thyroiditis
    - Iodide-induced hyperthyroidism: Drug, for example, amiodarone, radiographic contrast media, iodine prophylaxis program
    - Extra thyroidal source of thyroid hormone: Thyrotoxicosis factitia, struma ovarii

- **High uptake thyrotoxicosis:**
  - Graves' disease (rapid uptake and rapid turnover)
  - Toxic multinodular goiter
  - Toxic adenoma
- **In areas of iodine deficiency:** Rapid uptake and slow turnover.

Q. What is difference between ^{131}I, ^{123}I and ^{99m}technetium?

Ans.
- ^{131}I: Half-life: 8.1 days, has β (therapeutic) and ϒ (diagnostic) rays
- ^{123}I: Ideal but expensive. Half-life: 13 h, has ϒ ray. Absence of β-ray result is very low radiation dose to thyroid (approx. 1% of ^{131}I)
- ^{99m}technetium: Half-life: 6 h, has ϒ ray only.

Q. Discuss about thyroid scan.

Ans. Useful in determining morphology of thyroid gland and to differentiate among the causes of high uptake thyrotoxicosis.
- **Procedure:** ^{99m}technetium pertechnetate 2 mCi given IV, concentrated by thyroid gland but not organified. Image taken by gamma camera 30–60 min later
- **Results:**
  - Graves' disease: Enlarged gland with intense, diffuse, homogenous uptake of isotope
  - TMNG: Multiple discrete areas of increased uptake, especially corresponding to palpable nodules with suppression of extra nodular tissue
  - Toxic adenoma: Single area of intense uptake
- **Limitation:** Thyroid scan is not helpful in low uptake thyrotoxicosis
- **Types of nodule in thyroid scan:**
  - **Hot nodule/hyperfunctioning:** Areas of increased uptake with suppression of extra nodular thyroid tissue. Hot nodules are almost never malignant. FNAB not needed
  - **Cold nodule/hypofunctioning:** Areas of decreased uptake. A percentage of 5–10 cold nodule is malignant. FNAB is needed

Q. Discuss about sick thyroid syndrome/nonthyroidal illness/low T_3 syndrome.

Ans.
- This typically presents with low-serum TSH, low FT_3 and normal or low FT_4 in a patient with systemic illness who does not have any clinical evidence of thyroid disease
- Caused by ↓ secretion of TSH, ↓ peripheral conversion of T_4 to T_3, altered level of binding proteins and their affinity for thyroid hormones
- Thyroid function test should be repeated after recovery.

Q. Discuss about drug treatment of Graves' disease.

Ans.
- **Antithyroid drugs:** Thionamides (carbimazole, methimazole, propylthiouracil)
- **Choice of drug:** Propylthiouracil (PTU) preferred in

- First trimester of pregnancy (rare association of carbimazole with aplasia cutis)
- Breast feeding (lower concentration in breast milk)
- Thyroid storm (block peripheral T_4 to T_3 conversion)
- Mild allergic reactions to methimazole who refuses radioactive I_2 therapy or surgery

- **Mechanism of action of thionamides:**
  - Inhibit TPO mediated iodination of thyroglobulin to form T_4 and T_3 within the thyroid gland
  - PTU in large doses (600 mg) block peripheral T_4 to T_3 conversion by inhibiting deiodinase
  - Each of these drugs have immunosuppressive effect leading to reduction of TSH
  - Carbimazole metabolized to methimazole in liver (10 mg carbimazole metabolized to 6 mg methimazole)
  - Methimazole is 10 times more potent than PTU (5 mg of methimazole/carbimazole is equivalent to 50 mg PTU)
  - Serum half-life of methimazole (6 h), PTU (1.5 h). Both drugs accumulated by thyroid gland
  - Duration of action: Methimazole (>24 h), PTU (12-24 h)

- **Dose of antithyroid drugs:**
  - **Carbimazole** 40-60 mg/day once or divided doses until the patient is euthyroid followed by maintenance dose of 5-20 mg/day for 12-18 month, then taper and discontinued if TSH is normal at that time
  - **Methimazole** 10-20 mg/day once daily until the patient is euthyroid followed by maintenance dose of 5-10 mg/day
  - **PTU** 100-200 mg 8 hourly (depending on severity of hyperthyroidism) until the patient is euthyroid followed by maintenance dose of 50-100 mg two or three times daily

- **Follow-up of patients on antithyroid drugs:**
  - Subjective improvement within 10-14 days (decreased nervousness, palpitation, increased strength and weight gain)
  - Patient is clinically and biochemically euthyroid at 4-6 weeks. After 4 weeks of initiation of therapy, measurement of FT_4, FT_3, TSH done and dose of medication adjusted accordingly. TSH remain suppressed for several months after starting therapy, so not reliable index to monitor therapy early in the course of treatment
  - Appropriate monitoring intervals is every 4-8 weeks until the patient is euthyroid, then biochemical testing and clinical evaluation can be undertaken at intervals of 2-3 months
  - During treatment, size of thyroid gland is decreased in one-third to half of patients. In other patients, it may remain unchanged or even enlarge
  - If enlarged, it may be due to intensification of disease process (dose to be increased) or secondary to increased TSH due to excessive treatment/hypothyroidism (dose is to be decreased) or presence of neoplasm

- **Remission:** Normal thyroid function (FT$_4$, FT$_3$, TSH) for 1 year following discontinuation of antithyroid drug, occurs in 20%–50% of patients but may not be lifelong. Sustained remission is more likely if
  - Mild disease/disease controlled with small dose of antithyroid drug
  - Small goiter
  - Thyroid gland returns to normal size
  - Negative TRAb at the end of treatment course
- **Lower remission rate in**
  - Men
  - Older patients
  - Smokers
  - Large goiter ($\geq$80 g)
  - More active Graves' disease (high titers of TRAb and high thyroid blood flow identified by CFD).

Q. What is block and replace therapy?

Ans. Patient is treated with methimazole until euthyroid (about 3–6 months), but instead of tapering at this point, T$_4$ is added (100 µg/day). The patient then continues to receive the combination of antithyroid drug and T$_4$ for another 12–18 months. At the end of this time or when the size of the gland is returned to normal, the drugs are discontinued.
- **Advantages:** Fewer hospital visits for checks of thyroid function, decreased incidence of hypothyroidism
- This strategy is not recommended for most patients as relapse is the same as treatment with antithyroid drug alone, with more side effects.

Q. What are the adverse effects of drugs used in Graves' disease?

Ans.
- **Minor allergic reactions, for example, rash:** In 5% patients taking either methimazole or PTU. Managed with antihistamine unless it is severe. It is not an indication for discontinuing the medication. In the cases of serious allergic reaction, prescribing alternative drug is not recommended
- **Agranulocytosis:**
  - Occurs in .1%–.5% of patients. More common with PTU, usually within first few weeks or months of treatment. Older patients and patients taking higher doses are at risk. It is reversible on stopping antithyroid drug. All patients should have a baseline CBC with differential count and LFTs (SGPT, bilirubin, ALP)
  - Agranulocytosis require immediate cessation of antithyroid drug, institution of appropriate antibiotic therapy. Granulocyte colony stimulating factor may speed recovery and shifting to alternative therapy, usually Radio I$_2$. One drug should never be substituted by other due to risk of cross-reactivity between two drugs
  - Patient is instructed that if sore throat or fever develops, he should stop the drug and contact the physician and obtain a CBC with differential. Absolute neutrophil count <1,500/mL, drug should be withdrawn

- **Cholestatic jaundice:** Methimazole only
- **Fulminant hepatic necrosis:** PTU only. Liver transplantation may be necessary
- **ANCA positive vasculitis:** PTU is associated
- **Arthritis and lupus like syndrome:** Either methimazole or PTU
- **Aplasia cutis of scalp:** In babies born to mothers taking methimazole. Methimazole taken by mother in first trimester is associated with syndrome of methimazole embryopathy including choanal atresia and tracheoesophageal atresia.

Q. What are the other medical treatments used to treat Graves' disease?

Ans.
- **Beta-blocker:**
  - Useful in acute phase of thyrotoxicosis. Should be considered in all patients with symptomatic thyrotoxicosis (Resting HR >90/min)
  - Propranolol in high dose weakly block conversion of T_4 to T_3
  - Beta-blocker decreases heart rate, systolic BP, AF, many adrenergic symptoms, for example, tremulousness as well as improvement in degree of irritability, emotional lability and exercise intolerance
  - Propanol 10-40 mg 6-8 hourly (nonselective beta-blocker). In thyroid storm—40-80 mg orally 6 hourly or 0.5-1 mg IV over 10 min every 3 hourly
  - Relative β_1 selective blocker (metoprolol, esmolol)
  - Nadolol (nonselective beta-blocker once daily)
  - In patient with bronchial asthma: Nadolol or IV esmolol in thyroid storm
- **Cholecystographic agents:** Sodium ipodate or iopanoic acid (0.5 mg IV or orally twice daily in thyroid storm) inhibits thyroid hormone synthesis and release as well as peripheral conversion of T_4 to T_3
- **Cholestyramine or Colestipol:** Binds T_4 in gut. A quantity of 20-30 g/day in thyroid storm
- **Dexamethasone:** Has immunosuppressive effect and decreases peripheral conversion of T_4 to T_3. A quantity of 2 mg 6 hourly IV in thyroid storm
- **Iodide transport inhibitor:** Thiocyanate and perchlorate
- **Iodine and iodine-containing agents**
- **Lithium:** Inhibit thyroid hormone secretion.

Q. In which cases antithyroid drugs is therapy of choice?

Ans.
- Young patients (first episode in patients <40 years)
- Mild disease
- Small goiter
- Patient with previously operated or irradiated necks
- In pregnancy
- Premedication before radio I_2 therapy or surgery

Chapter 27: Thyrotoxicosis

- Afraid of radiation exposure
- Patients with moderate or severe active GO
- Individuals in nursing homes or other care facilities who have limited longevity and are unable to follow radiation safety regulations.

Q. What are the contraindication of antithyroid drugs.

Ans. Previously known major adverse effects with antithyroid drugs.

Q. Discuss about radioactive iodine therapy.

Ans.
- **Mechanism of action:** RAI is taken up and concentrated by thyroid gland causing cell damage and death, also long lasting inhibitory effect on survival and replication of follicular cells
- **Dose:** 10–15 mCi orally as a single capsule
- **Medical treatment before radio I_2:**
  - In elderly patients, those with underlying heart disease or other medical problems, severe thyrotoxicosis or large glands (>100 g), patients treated with methimazole until euthyroid before RAI due to occasional exacerbation of thyroid function following RAI
  - Methimazole stopped 3–7 days before RAI (methimazole decreases efficacy of RAI as it prevents organification of iodine in the gland), restarted 7 days later and tapered over 4–6 weeks as thyroid function normalizes
  - A pregnancy test should be obtained within 48 h prior to treatment with RAI in any female with childbearing potential
- **Follow-up following RAI:**
  - Within 1–2 months with FT_4, FT_3, TSH if patient remains thyrotoxic
  - Biochemical monitoring continued at 4–6 weeks interval
  - If hyperthyroidism persists 6 months following RAI, treatment is repeated with 1.5 times of the initial dose
  - When hypothyroidism develops, T_4 replacement with 50–200 µg daily instituted
- **Adverse effects of RAI:**
  - Hypothyroidism in >80% patients by 6 months
  - Radiation thyroiditis: Exacerbation of thyrotoxicosis 10–14 days after RAI
  - Thyroid storm
  - Exacerbation of moderate to severe GO. Common in smoker, prevented by prednisolone 30–60 mg/day for 1–2 months following RAI
  - No increased risk of thyroid or other cancer
- **RAI is therapy of choice in**
  - Most patients (patient >40 years)
  - Recurrence following surgery or antithyroid drugs
  - Comorbidities increasing surgical risk

- **Contraindications of RAI:**
  - Pregnancy or planned pregnancy within 6 months of RAI. Men are also advised against fathering children for 6 months
  - Lactation (RAI not given within 6 weeks after lactation stops)
  - Coexisting thyroid cancer or suspicion of thyroid cancer
  - Individuals unable to comply with radiation safety guidelines
  - Moderate to severe active GO.

Q. Write about surgical treatment of Graves' disease.

Ans.
- **Surgical treatment:** Total or near total thyroidectomy
- **Indication of surgical treatment of Graves' disease:**
  - Large goiter (≥ 80 g) or multinodular goiter
  - Local compressive symptoms
  - Coexisting thyroid cancer or suspicion of thyroid cancer
  - Patient who are allergic to or noncompliant with ATDs
  - Recurrence after course of ATDs
  - Patient who refuse RAI
  - Pregnant women with severe Graves' disease who are allergic or develop reactions to ATDs
  - Moderate to severe active GO
  - Large goiter and relatively low uptake of radioactive I_2
- **Preparation for surgery:**
  - Patient is prepared with ATDs until euthyroid (about 6 weeks). In addition, starting 2 weeks before the day of operation, patient is given saturated solution of potassium iodide (SSKI) five drops twice daily (50 mg iodide/drops) or Lugol iodine 5–7 drops twice daily (8 mg iodide/drops) mixed in water or juice. This regimen decreases vascularity of gland and intraoperative blood loss
  - Patient should be referred to high volume thyroid surgeon (>30 thyroid surgery/year)
- **Contraindications of surgery:**
  - Previous thyroid surgery
  - Dependent upon voice, for example, opera singer, lecturer
- **Complications of thyroid surgery:**
  - Hypothyroidism
  - Transient hypocalcaemia
  - Permanent hypoparathyroidism
  - Recurrent laryngeal nerve palsy
  - Thyroid storm in ill-prepared patient.

Chapter 27: Thyrotoxicosis

Q. Discuss about thyroid storm/thyrotoxic crisis/accelerated hyperthyroidism.

Ans.

- **Definition:** Acute life threatening exacerbation of thyrotoxicosis
- **Precipitating factors:**
  - Infection of unrecognized or inadequately treated thyrotoxic patient
  - Abrupt cessation of antithyroid drugs
  - Thyroid or nonthyroidal surgery in a unrecognized, inadequately treated or ill prepared patients
  - Following RAI therapy
  - Acute illness: MI, cerebrovascular accident, cardiac failure, parturition, trauma
- **Clinical features:**
  - Hyperpyrexia
  - Tachycardia, arrhythmia, atrial fibrillation, CCF
  - Vomiting, diarrhea, abdominal pain, jaundice
  - Agitation, delirium, psychosis, stupor, coma
- **Treatment of thyroid storm:**
  - Admitted in ICU for cardiac monitoring
  - Blood sample taken for FT_4, FT_3, TSH, CBC, blood and urine culture (leukocytosis may be present in absence of infection)
- **Supportive care:**
  - Fluid to correct dehydration
  - O_2
  - Cooling blanket, paracetamol
  - Broad spectrum antibiotic, if infection suspected
  - Management of AF or CCF
- **Specific measures:**
  - Propranolol 40–80 mg orally 6 hourly or 0.5–1 mg IV over 10 min every 3 h
  - Propylthiouracil 150 mg 6 hourly (preferred) or methimazole 20 mg 8 hourly or carbimazole 40–60 mg/day orally/NG tube or rectally
  - SSKI five drops orally twice daily or iopanoic acid 0.5 mg IV or orally twice daily
  - Dexamethasone 2 mg 6 hourly IV for 48 h followed by tapering
  - Cholestyramine or colestipol 20–30 g/day
  - If beta-blocker contraindicated, IV verapamil can be given
  - Extreme measures: Plasmapheresis or peritoneal dialysis
- **Causes of death and mortality rate of thyroid storm:** Cardiac arrhythmia and failure, mortality rate 20%–30%.

Q. Discuss about thyrotoxic periodic paralysis.

Ans.

- **Definition:** It is common in Asian male (M:F = 17:1) with thyrotoxicosis due to Graves' disease or toxic multinodular goiter

- **Pathogenesis:**

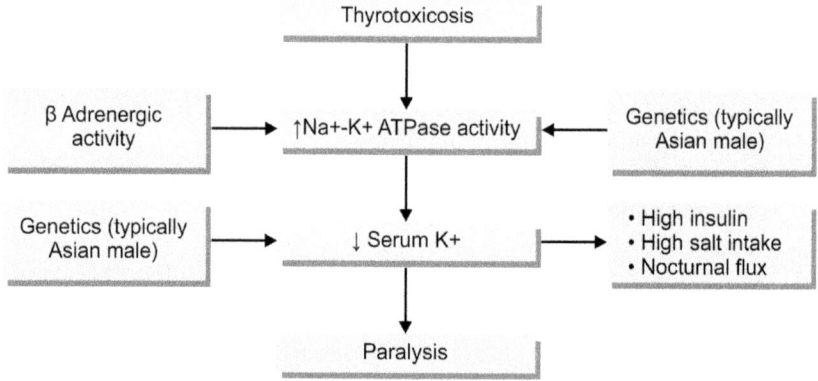

- **Clinical features:**
  - History of vigorous exercise or large high-carbohydrate meal before retiring
  - Recurrent episode of flaccid ascending paralysis, lasting minutes to days
  - Paralysis initially involves lower extremities but progress to girdle muscles followed by upper extremities. Proximal muscle groups are more affected than distal
  - Facial and respiratory muscles are not affected
  - Sensory function intact, tendon reflex depressed or absent
  - Bowel and bladder are not affected
  - No family H/o of periodic paralysis
  - Acute episode may be complicated by cardiac arrhythmia ($\downarrow K^+$)
- **Investigations:**
  - Serum K^+: Low during attack
  - ECG: Features of hypokalemia
  - FT_4, FT_3, TSH
- **Differential diagnosis:**
  - Familial periodic paralysis
  - GBS
  - Acute intermittent porphyria
- **Treatment:**
  - Oral K^+ supplement, monitor serum K^+
  - Oral propranolol 60 mg 6 hourly: block β adrenergic stimulation of Na^+-K^+ ATPase
  - Antithyroid drugs
- **Avoid:**
  - IV K^+
  - IV glucose →↑ Insulin →↓ K^+
  - β adrenergic agonist
- **Prognosis:**
  - With treatment, full recovery within 24–48 h and once thyrotoxicosis is controlled, the paralysis will not recur

Chapter 27: Thyrotoxicosis

- No role of K^+ supplement to prevent attack
- Acetazolamide decrease frequency of attack in familial periodic paralysis, but worsen attack of thyrotoxic periodic paralysis and should be avoided.

Q. Discuss about subclinical hyperthyroidism.

Ans.
- **Definition:** Serum TSH is subnormal despite normal/upper end of normal range of serum FT_4 and FT_3
- **Etiology:**
  - **Endogenous:** Toxic multinodular goiter, Graves' disease
  - **Exogenous:** Patient is on levothyroxine
- **Risks of subclinical hyperthyroidism:**
  - AF: 2.8 fold ↑ risk in persons over age 60
  - Accelerated bone loss/osteoporosis
  - Risk of progression to overt hyperthyroidism: 0.5 to 1% per year
- **Diagnosis:** TSH should be repeated over a 3-6 month period to confirm it as persistent, ruling out transient thyroiditis, nonthyroidal illness as etiology
- **Indication of treatment:**
  - **TSH (0.1–0.5 mU/L):** Insufficient data to conclude that patients will benefit from treatment
  - **TSH (<0.1 mU/L):**
    - All individuals ≥65 years of age
    - Postmenopausal osteoporosis
    - Cardiac risk factor: AF, recurrent cardiac arrhythmia, RHD with left atrial enlargement
    - Heart disease: CCF, angina pectoris
    - Infertility or menstrual disorder
    - Patient with hyperthyroid symptoms
- **Treatment option:**
  - Toxic multinodular goiter: RAI
  - Mild GD: Monitoring of thyroid function every 3 months (more chance of spontaneous remission)
- **Follow-up:** Annual follow-up is needed as risk of progression to overt hyperthyroidism.

Q. Discuss about thyrotoxicosis in pregnancy.

Ans.
- Thyrotoxicosis in pregnancy unusual as anovulatory cycles are common in thyrotoxic patients, and autoimmune disease tends to remit during pregnancy when the maternal immune response is suppressed
- Thyroid function test must be interpreted in caution as total T_4 and T_3 elevated in pregnancy due to ↑ TBG, so total T_4 and T_3 reference range adjusted at 1.5 times the nonpregnant reference range. The diagnosis of thyrotoxicosis in pregnancy should be made using serum FT_4, FT_3, and TSH with trimester specific normal reference ranges

- Serum TSH may be subnormal at the end of first trimester in 20% normal women due to ↑ hCG that activate TSH receptor. This is a transient and physiologic condition
- Hyperemesis gravidarum cause mild hyperthyroidism (gestational thyrotoxicosis) due to ↑↑ hCG. No treatment is indicated as hyperemesis is temporary
- Complications of thyrotoxicosis in pregnancy:

  Mother:
  - Increased and recurrent pregnancy loss
  - Pre-eclampsia
  - Preterm delivery
  - Increased maternal mortality

  Fetus:
  - IUGR
  - Fetal thyroid hyperfunction or hypofunction caused by TRAbs
  - Fetal goiter from excessive antithyroid drug treatment
  - Neonatal thyrotoxicosis
  - Increased perinatal mortality
  - Decrease IQ of offspring due to excessive antithyroid drug treatment
- **Treatment of thyrotoxicosis in pregnancy:**
  - ATDs used for thyrotoxicosis due to GD. PTU is preferred to methimazole in first trimester as methimazole has rare teratogenic effect (aplasia cutis and methimazole embryopathy), then switching to methimazole at the beginning of second trimester
  - The dose of ATDs kept to the minimal required to maintain FT_4 at or slightly above the upper limit of normal nonpregnant reference range. Thyroid function test done monthly, and ATDs dose are adjusted
  - Initial dose of PTU is 250 mg/day (in divided doses) or less and maintenance dose is 25–100 mg/day
  - TRAb measured in third trimester to predict possibility of neonatal thyrotoxicosis. If negative, indicated ATDs need to be reduced or stopped to avoid fetal hypothyroidism
  - RAI is contraindicated in pregnancy as it crosses placenta and induce fetal hypothyroidism
  - If subtotal thyroidectomy is necessary due to poor drug compliance or drug intolerance or increased dose of ATDs required, for example, >300 mg/day PTU. It should be done in late second trimester (first trimester—early pregnancy loss, third trimester—preterm labor)
  - Breast feeding is permitted with either ATDs but due to hepatic necrosis in either mother or child from maternal PTU use, methimazole is preferred in nursing mother

Q. Discuss about Graves' ophthalmopathy.

Ans.

1. **Activity of Graves' ophthalmopathy:** Best assessed by clinical activity score (CAS). Ten parameter with 1 point for each. GO is considered active in patients with CAS ≥3

- Pain in primary gaze
- Pain with eye movement
- Eyelid swelling
- Eyelid redness
- Conjunctival edema (chemosis)
- Conjunctival redness
- Caruncula swelling (fleshy body at medial angle of eye)
- Increased proptosis
- Decreased eye movement
- Decreased visual activity.

2. **Severity of Graves' ophthalmopathy:** 6 parameter—lid retraction, soft tissue involvement, proptosis, diplopia, corneal exposure, optic nerve compression
   - **Mild GO:** Patients whose eye disease have minor impact on daily life, generally insufficient to justify immunosuppressive or surgical treatment
   - **Moderate to severe GO:** Patient without sight threatening GO whose eye disease have sufficient impact on daily life to justify immunosuppressive (if active) or surgical treatment (if inactive)
   - **Sight threatening GO:** Patient with optic nerve compression and/or corneal breakdown, that warrants immediate intervention.

3. **Treatment of GO:**
   - **General measures:**
     - Stop smoking
     - Wearing dark glasses
     - Elevation of head of bed at night and diuretics (↓ periorbital edema)
     - Methylcellulose eye drop and gel, artificial tear (to counter gritty discomfort of dry eye)
     - Tinted glasses or side shields attached to spectacle frame decrease excessive lacrimation triggered by sun or wind
     - Antithyroid drugs to control thyrotoxicosis.
   - **Specific measures:**
     - **Glucocorticoid:**
       - For severe acute inflammatory episode, prednisolone 100 mg/day in divided doses for 7–14 days. If improvement occur, the dose is decreased over 6–12 weeks to lowest level at which improvement is maintained or IV methylprednisolone pulse therapy (500 mg initially, then 250 mg weekly for 6 weeks)
       - To prevent exacerbation of moderate to severe GO following RAI: Prednisolone 30–60 mg/day for 1–2 months
     - **External radiation:** If corticosteroid therapy is not effective or recurrence after the drug is tapered, external X-ray therapy to retrobulbar area. The lens and anterior chamber must be shielded. Adverse effects is retinal angiogenesis, and external radiation is contraindicated in DM

- **Orbital decompression:**
  - In sight threatening GO, orbital decompression that removes floor and lateral wall of orbit
  - Decrease exophthalmos by 5–7 mm
  - Diplopia and lid abnormalities can be corrected by eye muscle surgery or cosmetic lid surgery

Q. What is thyroid dermopathy/pretibial myxedema?

Ans.
- Thickening of skin particularly over the lower tibia with peau d' orange appearance and cannot be picked up between the fingers, occurs in 2%–3% of patients with Graves' disease
- Associated with significant GO and very high serum titer of TRAb
- Treated by topical high potency glucocorticoid with an occlusive dressing

Q. Discuss about thyrotoxicosis factitia.

Ans. Ingestion of thyroid hormone preparation usually for weight control. Usually woman connected with health-care field.

Clue for diagnosis:
- Clinical and biochemical features of thyrotoxicosis but goiter and eye sign absent
- Low RAIU
- Serum thyroglobulin low
- High $T_4:T_3$ ratio (70:1), in conventional thyrotoxicosis—30:1

Treatment: Stop thyroid hormone intake, psychotherapy.

Q. Discuss struma ovarii.

Ans.
- Ovarian teratoma containing thyroid tissue
- Clinical and biochemical features of thyrotoxicosis but goiter and eye sign absent
- Low RAIU
- Total body scan reveals uptake of radioiodine in pelvis rather than neck
- Treatment: surgical removal of tumor. Beta-blocker and ATDs used to restore euthyroidism before surgery.

CHAPTER 28

Hypothyroidism

Q. Define hypothyroidism.

Ans.

Definition: Clinical syndrome resulting from thyroid hormone deficiency causing generalized slowing down of metabolic process.

Pathology: Accumulation of hydrophilic glycosaminoglycans, mostly hyaluronic acid and chondroitin sulfate in interstitial tissues. The accumulation is not due to excessive synthesis but to decreased metabolism of glycosaminoglycans, producing in severe cases the clinical features of myxedema.

Q. Mention WHO recommended daily dietary iodine intake.

Ans. 150 µg/day.

Q. What are the causes of hypothyroidism?

Ans.

1. **Primary:**
   - Hashimoto thyroiditis
     - With goiter
     - Spontaneous atrophic hypothyroidism
   - RAI Therapy for Graves disease
   - Thyroidectomy for thyrotoxicosis, thyroid cancer
   - Iodine deficiency/endemic goiter
   - Drugs: Lithium, amiodarone, IFN-α, excessive iodide (radiocontrast dye), sunitinib
   - Transient hypothyroidism: Following subacute, postpartum thyroiditis
   - Infiltrative: amyloidosis, sarcoidosis, Riedel thyroiditis
   - Congenital: Inborn error of thyroid hormone synthesis/dyshormonogenesis
   - Goitrogen in food stuffs, for example, cabbage (contain thiocyanate).

2. **Secondary:** Hypopituitarism due to primary adenoma, pituitary surgery or radiotherapy.

3. **Tertiary:** Hypothalamic dysfunction.

4. **Peripheral resistance to thyroid hormone.**

Q. What are the causes of goitrous hypothyroidism?

Ans.
- Hashimoto thyroiditis
- Iodine deficiency/endemic goiter
- Infiltrative: Amyloidosis, sarcoidosis, Riedel thyroiditis
- Congenital: Inborn error of thyroid hormone synthesis/dyshormonogenesis.

Q. What are the causes of nongoitrous hypothyroidism?

Ans.
- Spontaneous atrophic hypothyroidism
- Thyroidectomy for thyrotoxicosis, thyroid cancer
- Secondary: Hypopituitarism due to primary adenoma, pituitary surgery or radiotherapy

Q. Mention difference between Hashimoto thyroiditis and spontaneous atrophic hypothyroidism.

Ans.

Hashimoto thyroiditis	Spontaneous atrophic hypothyroidism
Goiter	No goiter
Initially toxicosis (Hashitoxicosis)	No toxicosis
Thyroid peroxidase Ab positive	TSH receptor blocking Ab positive

Q. What is myxedema?

Ans. Myxedema is a severe form of hypothyroidism due to deposition of glycosaminoglycans, but all hypothyroidism may not be myxedematous.

Q. Discuss clinical features of hypothyroidism.

Ans. Female:Male = 6:1.

1. **Newborn infants/cretinism:**
    - Etiology:
        - Thyroid agenesis or ectopic thyroid (common in areas of iodine deficiency)
        - Placental transfer to embryo of blocking TRAb from mother with Hashimoto thyroiditis
        - Over treatment with ATDs to mother during pregnancy
    - **Symptoms:** Short stature, mental retardation, deaf mutism
    - **Signs:** Respiratory difficulty, cyanosis, jaundice, poor feeding, hoarse voice, umbilical hernia, marked retardation of bone maturation
    - **Newborn screening:** A drop of blood obtained by needle prick 24–48 h after birth. Serum T_4 <6 µg/dL or serum TSH >25 mIU/mL is suggestive of hypothyroidism
    - **Radiology:** Absence of proximal tibial epiphysis or distal femoral epiphysis (stippled epiphysis), delayed bone age.

Chapter 28: Hypothyroidism

2. **Children and adolescents:** Short stature, retarded growth, declining school performance, precocious puberty.
3. **Adults:**
   - **Symptoms:**
     - Weight gain
     - Cold intolerance (due to decreased cutaneous circulation)
     - Fatigue, somnolence
     - Constipation ($\downarrow$ peristaltic activity, $\downarrow$ food intake due to $\downarrow$ appetite)
     - Menorrhagia
     - Infertility
     - Aches and pains, muscle cramp, alopecia
     - Slowing of intellectual and motor activities, depression, psychosis (myxedema madness)
     - Deafness (Trotter syndrome)
     - Carpal Tunnel Syndrome
     - Sleep apnea syndrome.
   - **Signs:**
     - Face:
       - Puffy face with periorbital swelling and baggy eyelids
       - loss of lateral one third of eyebrows (Queen Anne sign)
       - Facial pallor (due to cutaneous vasoconstriction and anemia)
       - Lemon yellow tint (carotenemia)
       - Malar flush, purplish lip, macroglossia
     - Skin: Dry, rough, cold and thick, vitiligo, erythema ab igne (granny's tartan)
     - Hair: Dry and brittle, lusterless and tends to fall out
     - Voice: Low pitched, slurred, hoarse and croaky (diagnosis over telephone)
     - Non-pitting edema in legs, generalized swelling of whole body
     - CVS: Bradycardia, low voltage ECG, HTN, pericardial effusion, IHD, CCF
     - Ileus, Ascites
     - Neurological features:
       - Carpal Tunnel syndrome
       - Delayed relaxation of ankle reflexes (hung-up reflexes) due to $\downarrow$ muscle metabolism, best elicited by kneel down position on bed side
       - Peripheral neuropathy, proximal myopathy, dementia
       - Psychosis (myxedema madness), myxedema coma
       - Cerebellar ataxia
       - Myotonia due to interstitial myxedema with slowness of muscular activity (Hoffmann syndrome)
       - Deafness (Trotter syndrome)
       - Seizure due to $\downarrow$ Na^+.

Q. What is Pendred syndrome?

Ans. Inherited disorder (AR) associated with sensorineural deafness and goiter. It is due to inborn error of thyroid hormone synthesis.

Q. What are the types of anemia in hypothyroidism?

Ans.
- Normocytic normochromic (due to thyroxine deficiency)
- Microcytic hypochromic (menorrhagia, anorexia, decreased intestinal Fe absorption)
- Macrocytic (associated pernicious anemia).

Q. Mention indications of thyroid function tests.

Ans.
- Suspicion of hypothyroidism
- H/o thyroid surgery, RAI therapy for hyperthyroidism or external beam radiotherapy for head and neck malignancy
- Suspected hypopituitarism/following pituitary surgery
- Goiter/abnormal thyroid examination
- Those with autoimmune disease, for example, type 1 DM, pernicious anemia, Addison disease or first degree relative with autoimmune thyroid disease
- Unexplained edema/pericardial effusion/pleural effusion/pericarditis
- Short stature
- Cardiologist: Patient taking amiodarone, cardiac arrhythmia, unspecified HTN, hypercholesterolemia, low voltage ECG, prolonged QT interval
- Neurologist: Cerebellar ataxia, dementia, Carpal Tunnel syndrome
- Psychiatrist: Organic psychosis, depression, patient taking lithium
- ENT: Deafness
- Dermatologist: Dry skin, alopecia, vitiligo
- Gynecologist: Menorrhagia, infertility, pregnancy loss
- Geriatrician: Screening test or hypothermia
- Internist: Weight gain, proximal myopathy, malaise and fatigue, anemia, constipation
- Diabetologist: TSH in type 1 DM, dyslipidemia or women >50 years of age as routine test
- TSH Screening in asymptomatic adults:
  - **ATA:** Women and men >35 years age should be screened every 5 years
  - **AACE:** Older patient (age not specified), especially women.

Q. How will you investigate a case of hypothyroidism?

Ans.
- Serum FT_4 (low) and TSH (elevated). T_3 not done as it may be normal as it converted from T_4
  - In secondary hypothyroidism, FT_4 is low or low normal, TSH low, normal or even slightly elevated due to inactive TSH isoform in blood. In such case
    - MRI of brain
    - TRH stimulation test: ↑ TSH (hypothalamic cause), no or little rise (pituitary cause)

Chapter 28: Hypothyroidism

- Thyroid autoantibodies: Antibody to thyroid peroxidase (90%–100%), thyroglobulin (80%–90%) in autoimmune hypothyroidism
- ECG: Low voltage ECG, sinus bradycardia, prolonged QT interval, ST-T wave abnormalities
- Chest X-ray: Cardiomegaly due to HTN, HF, pericardial effusion, also pleural effusion
- Lipid profile: Increased total and LDL cholesterol
- Creatine kinase (CK), AST/SGOT, LDH: Elevated
- CBC: ↓ Hb% (anemia)
- Serum electrolyte: ↓ Na^+.

Q. How will you approach to suspected hypothyroidism?

Ans.

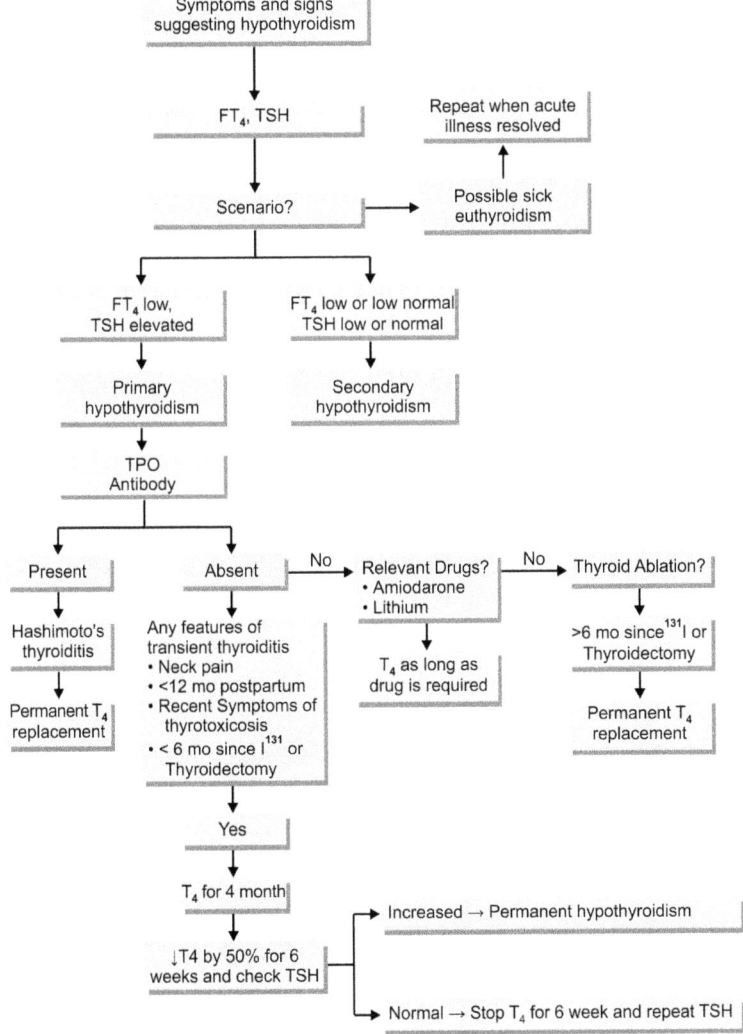

Q. How will you treat hypothyroidism?

Ans.
- Replacement dose of levothyroxine/T_4 depends on age, sex, body weight and certain clinical conditions
- In adult, replacement dose of T_4 is 1–2 µg/kg/day. Because of more rapid T_4 metabolism, infant and young children require high dose of T_4, for example, 0–6 months: 10–15 µg/kg/day. In elderly, replacement dose is usually lower. Females have higher dose requirement than male
- Levothyroxine should be taken once daily in empty stomach 30–60 min before breakfast (half-life of T_4: 7 days). 70% of oral dose is absorbed
- Malabsorptive state or drugs, for example, Al hydroxide antacid, bile acid binding resins, for example, cholestyramine, colestipol, Ca supplement, Fe compound decrease T_4 absorption. In these patients, T_4 given in empty stomach and others drugs taken 4 h later. PPI decrease T_4 absorption by ↓ gastric acid
- After 4–6 weeks, dose of T_4 adjusted. Monitor FT_4 and TSH every 4–6 weeks until dose of T_4 is stabilized (goal is to normalize serum TSH in primary hypothyroidism), then FT_4 and TSH monitored once every 6–12 months
- In some poorly compliant patients, T_4 is taken in excess for a few days prior to clinic visit, resulting high FT_4 and high TSH
- Patient feels better within 2–3 weeks. Reduction in weight and periorbital puffiness occur quickly, but restoration of skin and hair texture and resolution of any effusion may take 3–6 months.

Q. What are the adverse effects of T_4 overdose?

Ans.
- Symptoms and signs of hyperthyroidism
- Palpitation, insomnia, tremor
- Restlessness, excessive warmth
- Accelerated bone loss in postmenopausal patients

Managed by simply omitting the daily dose of T_4 for 3 days and then reducing the dosage will correct the problem.

Q. Discuss about thyroxine replacement in hypothyroidism and IHD.

Ans.
- Angina may remain unchanged, disappear or exacerbate to severe angina, MI or sudden death
- Thyroxine should be introduced at low dose (12.5–25 µg/day for 2–4 weeks) and increased very slowly (12.5–25 µg every 2–4 weeks) until a daily dose of 75 µg is reached
- The dose is continued for 6 weeks. Serum TSH is measured and the dosage adjusted accordingly
- It typically takes 2–4 months for a patient to reach full dosage

- If angina pectoris or cardiac arrhythmia develops, reduce the dose of T_4 immediately
- Beta-blocker and vasodilator should be added
- CABG or angioplasty is required in minority of patients with angina who cannot tolerate full thyroxine replacement therapy despite maximum antianginal therapy.

Q. Discuss about hypothyroidism in pregnancy.

Ans.

1. **Complications of hypothyroidism in pregnancy:**
   - **Mother:**
     - Increased and recurrent pregnancy loss
     - Pre-eclampsia
     - Preterm delivery
     - PPH
     - Increased maternal mortality
   - **Fetus:**
     - LBW
     - Still birth
     - Impaired intellectual and psychomotor development of fetus.

2. **Treatment of hypothyroidism in pregnancy:**
   - Overt hypothyroidism is uncommon in pregnancy as most women with untreated hypothyroidism are anovulatory
   - When a woman with hypothyroidism becomes pregnant, the dosage of levothyroxine should be increased by 25%–50% to keep serum TSH <2.5 mIU/mL in first trimester, <3 and <3.5 mIU/mL in second and third trimester, respectively, and FT_4 within trimester-specific normal reference ranges. This is due to increased TBG and increased thyroxine metabolism by placenta
   - When a patient with positive TPO antibody becomes pregnant, TSH measured, and if >2.5 mIU/mL, T_4 treatment should be initiated
   - Serum FT_4 and TSH is monitored every 4 weeks during first half of pregnancy and at least once between 26 and 32 weeks of pregnancy and thyroxine dose adjusted.

Q. Discuss about myxedema coma.

Ans.

- **Definition:** It is a medical emergency that is the end stage of untreated or inadequately treated hypothyroidism
- **Predisposing factors:**
  - Acute trauma
  - Infection, for example, UTI, pneumonia
  - Other illness, for example, MI, CVA
  - CNS depressants, for example, sedative, narcotic

- **Features:**
  - H/o thyroid surgery or RAI treatment or patient receiving thyroid hormone therapy that was discontinued
  - Stupor, coma
  - Hypothermia, hypoventilation, hypoglycemia, hyponatremia
  - Water intoxication
  - Seizure
  - Shock leading to death
  - On examination:
    - Bradycardia
    - Marked hypothermia as low as 24°C/75°F
    - Severe hypotension
    - Signs of severe myxedema
    - Fever may be masked by coexistent hypothermia
- **Investigations:**
  - Low FT_4 and markedly elevated TSH
  - RBS: Hypoglycemia
  - Electrolyte: Hyponatremia
  - ABG: ↓ PO_2, ↑ PCO_2
  - ECG: Sinus bradycardia, low voltage ECG, ST-T wave abnormality
  - Infection screen: CBC, urine R/M/E, blood and urine culture, portable chest X-ray
- **Treatment:**
  - Treated in ICU
  - Take blood sample for FT_4, TSH, cortisol before starting treatment
  - Identify and treat precipitating illness
  - Broad spectrum antibiotic after collection of blood for blood culture
  - Thyroxine 300–400 μg IV or by NG tube as loading dose followed by 50–100 μg IV or by NG tube daily. In addition, T_3 10 μg IV 8 h for first 48 h can be given
  - Hydrocortisone 50–100 mg IV 6 h initially and tapered over 1 week (necessary in hypopituitarism or polyglandular failure, not needed if initial serum cortisol >550 nmol/L)
  - Hypothermia: Blankets, gastric perfusion. Do not externally rewarm
  - Correct hyponatremia (water restriction), hypoglycemia (IV glucose), hypotension (cautious IV fluid, avoid fluid overload)
  - Intubation and mechanical ventilation if hypoventilating
  - Cardiac monitoring, ABG, pulse, BP, CVP, rectal temperature, urine output, O_2 saturation monitoring
- **Mortality rate of myxedema coma:** About 20%.

Q. Discuss about subclinical hypothyroidism/preclinical hypothyroidism/decreased thyroid reserve/early thyroid failure.

Ans.
- Serum FT_4 is normal or low normal and serum TSH is mildly elevated

- Repeat test 2-3 months apart needed to distinguish from non-thyroidal illness
- Most common cause is autoimmune thyroiditis/Hashimoto thyroiditis
- **Risk to patient:**
  - Progression to overt hypothyroidism (3%-20%). Risk greater in patients with goiter or thyroid antibodies or both
  - Cardiovascular effects
  - Dyslipidemia
  - Neuropsychiatric effects
- **Indications of treatment of Subclinical hypothyroidism:**
  - TSH >10 mIU/mL
  - TSH 5-10 mIU/mL in association with goiter or positive anti-TPO antibody or both
  - Typical features of hypothyroidism
  - Menstrual irregularity
  - Ovulatory dysfunction/infertility
  - Recurrent pregnancy loss
  - Relative: Obesity, dyslipidemia (↑ total or LDL cholesterol), non-pitting edema
- **Management of Subclinical hypothyroidism:**
  If treatment is indicated:
  - Levothyroxine 25-50 μg/day
  - TSH measured at 4-6 weeks later and levothyroxine dose adjusted
  - Target TSH: 0.3-3 mIU/mL
  - Once TSH level stable, annual thyroid function test is done

  If treatment not indicated: Annual follow-up both clinical and FT_4 and TSH.

Q. Define thyroiditis. What are the causes of thyroiditis?

Ans. Inflammation of thyroid gland leads to transient thyrotoxicosis followed by hypothyroidism.
- **Causes of thyroiditis:**
  - Autoimmune thyroiditis (Hashimoto thyroiditis, atrophic thyroiditis)
  - Subacute/De Quervain thyroiditis
  - Postpartum, silent or painless thyroiditis
  - Acute infectious/pyogenic thyroiditis
  - Riedel thyroiditis
  - Drug-induced thyroiditis: Lithium, amiodarone, IFN-α, excessive iodide, sunitinib
  - Postradiation thyroiditis
  - Sarcoidosis.

Q. Discuss subacute/De Quervain/granulomatous/giant cell thyroiditis.

Ans.

1. **Definition:** Acute inflammatory disorder of thyroid gland most likely due to viral infection (mumps, coxsackie virus, adenovirus). It is common in summer months and in women

2. **Pathophysiology:** Inflammation of thyroid gland leads to loss of follicular integrity associated with not only release of colloid and stored thyroid hormones but also damage to follicular cells and impaired synthesis of new thyroid hormones. As a result, thyroid hormones are raised until preformed colloid is depleted. Thereafter, there is usually a period of hypothyroidism of variable severity before the follicular cells recover and normal thyroid function is restored over weeks or months (thyrotoxic phase → hypothyroid → euthyroid phase).

3. **Clinical features:**
   - **Symptoms:**
     - Pain in the region of thyroid gland, radiates to the angle of jaw and ear and made worse by swallowing, coughing and movement of neck
     - Systemic upset: Fever, malaise
     - Symptoms of thyrotoxicosis: Palpitation, nervousness, sweating but no ophthalmopathy
   - **Signs:**
     - Thyroid gland is moderately enlarged, tender, firm and often nodular
     - No signs of local redness or heat suggestive of abscess formation
     - Signs of thyrotoxicosis: Tachycardia, tremor, hyperreflexia.

4. **Investigation:**
   - ESR: Raised, sometimes >100 mm in first hour
   - Thyroid autoantibodies: Not detectable
   - Thyroid function tests: Vary with the course of disease
     - Thyrotoxic phase: FT_4, FT_3 elevated with low serum TSH and ↓ RAIU
     - Hypothyroid phase: FT_4, FT_3 drop, TSH rises
     - Euthyroid phase: RAIU rises, reflecting recovery of the gland.

5. **Differential diagnosis:**
   - **Acute pyogenic thyroiditis:** Distinguished by presence of septic focus elsewhere, inflammatory reaction in the area of thyroid, greater febrile response and leukocytosis, RAIU and thyroid function usually preserved
   - **Graves' disease:** Distinguished by no thyroidal pain, presence of thyroid antibodies. High RAIU and elevated FT_4, FT_3 and suppressed TSH.

6. **Treatment:**
   - In mild cases: Aspirin or NSAIDs for symptom relief
   - In severe cases or patient not responding to NSAIDs: Prednisolone 20–40 mg/day for 7–10 days (For salvation of remaining thyroid gland)
   - Beta-blocker to control palpitation in thyrotoxic phase
   - Thyroxine 50–150 µg/day during hypothyroid phase if hypothyroid symptoms are present.

7. **Course and prognosis:**
   - 90% recover without any sequelae
   - 10% permanent hypothyroidism and require long term thyroxine therapy
   - Sometimes, patient begins to resolve and then suddenly become worse with involving first one lobe of thyroid gland and then the other (migrating or creeping thyroiditis).

Q. Discuss about Hashimoto thyroiditis/lymphocytic thyroiditis/chronic thyroiditis.

Ans.
- **Definition:** It is a common cause of hypothyroidism resulting from autoimmune destruction of thyroid gland. Occurs throughout adult life but increases with age. F:M = 4:1
- **Clinical features:**
  - Painless variable sized goiter, firm or rubbery in consistency. The surface is either smooth or irregular but well defined nodules are unusual
  - Patient may be euthyroid, mild or subclinical hypothyroid to overt hypothyroid
  - Thyroid gland may be painful due to more acute onset
  - There may be initial thyrotoxic phase (Hashitoxicosis)
  - Sometimes it may present as a part of syndrome—Schmidt syndrome, Addison disease, hypoparathyroidism, type 1 DM, Primary hypogonadism, chronic mucocutaneous candidiasis
  - Hashimoto thyroiditis is a risk factor for lymphoma of thyroid gland.
- **Investigations:**
  - Thyroid Function tests: Serum TSH high with low or normal FT_4, FT_3
  - RAIU: High, normal or low
  - Perchlorate discharge test: Positive
  - Thyroid auto antibodies: Thyroglobulin present in 80%–90% and TPO in 90%–100%
  - FNAB: Lymphocytic infiltration, varying degree of fibrosis, disruption of follicular architecture, enlarged follicular epithelial cell with eosinophilic cytoplasm laden with mitochondria (Hürthle cells), also done to exclude malignancy
- **Differential diagnosis:** Distinguished from other causes of nontoxic goiter by serum antibody and if necessary by FNAB
- **Treatment:** Indications of treatment of Hashimoto thyroiditis are goiter or hypothyroidism. Sufficient T_4 is given to normalize TSH and regression of goiter. Patient with positive antibody alone does not require therapy. Surgery is indicated if goiter does not regress and cause pressure symptoms.

CHAPTER 29

Thyroid Nodules

Q. Discuss about solitary thyroid nodules.

Ans.
- Prevalence: 3%–7% (palpation) and 20%–76% (USG) in general population
- A percentage of 20%–48% patient with one palpable nodule have additional nodule on USG
- Thyroid nodules are common in elderly, women (F:M = 4:1), iodine deficiency and history of radiation exposure
- Majority (95%) of thyroid nodules are benign.

Q. What are the differential diagnosis of solitary thyroid nodule?

Ans.
- Simple nodular goiter
- Palpable nodule of MNG
- Simple or hemorrhagic cysts
- Follicular adenoma
- Papillary carcinoma
- Follicular carcinoma including Hurthle cell carcinoma
- Poorly differentiated carcinoma
- Undifferentiated/anaplastic carcinoma
- Medullary carcinoma
- Lymphoma
- Sarcoma, teratoma, metastatic tumors.

Q. How will you evaluate a thyroid nodule?

Ans.

1. **History:**
   - Age of patient
   - Residence in endemic goiter area

- Rate of growth of mass
- Family H/o thyroid disease or cancer
- H/o head or neck irradiation
- Hoarseness/vocal cord paralysis, dysphagia or dyspnea
- Symptoms of hyperthyroidism or hypothyroidism
- Use of iodine containing drugs or supplements.

2. **Examination:**
   - Examination of thyroid gland (location, size, consistency, tenderness, mobility)
   - Cervical lymph nodes
   - Any metastasis.

3. **Features of malignant thyroid nodules:**
   - Age <14 or >70 years
   - Male sex
   - Size >1 cm (malignancy is not uncommon in nodules <1 cm in diameter. So diameter cut off for cancer risk is not justified)
   - Family H/o MTC, MEN 2, PTC
   - H/o head or neck irradiation
   - Hoarseness, dysphagia or dyspnea
   - Thyroid nodule: Rapidly growing, firm or hard, irregular, fixed to underlying structures
   - Cervical lymphadenopathy
   - Absence of carotid pulse (malignant infiltration of carotid sheath)
   - Metastasis.

4. **Investigation of thyroid nodule:**
   - **Serum factors:**
     - Serum TSH:
       - If TSH normal: No further blood test needed
       - If TSH ↓: Measure FT_4, FT_3
       - If TSH ↑: Measure FT_4, TPO antibody
     - Serum calcitonin: In patient with family H/o MTC or MEN 2
     - Serum thyroglobulin: H/o total thyroidectomy for PTC or FTC (to detect residual or metastatic disease)
     - Serum Ca^{++}, PTH or both: Intrathyroidal parathyroid adenoma on USG
   - **Thyroid USG:**
     - **Indication:**
       - Patient at risk of thyroid malignancy
       - Patient with palpable thyroid nodule or MNG
       - Patient with lymphadenopathy suggestive of malignancy

- **Role of USG:**
  - To confirm the cervical mass within thyroid
  - Measure the nodule size precisely
  - Detect other nonpalpable nodule elsewhere in the gland
  - Distinguish solid from cystic lesion
- **USG features suspicious of malignancy:**
  - Hypoechoic pattern
  - Irregular margin
  - More tall than wide shape
  - Microcalcification
  - Incomplete halo
  - Central vascularity/chaotic intranodular vascular spots (on Doppler)

(Comet tail artifact/colloid in nodule looks like Napoleon or puffy pastry favor benign nodule)

- **Thyroid scintigraphy:** In patient with low TSH, thyroid scintigraphy used to identify hot or cold nodule. Hot nodules are almost never malignant, and 5%–10% of cold nodules are malignant
  - **Indications:**
    - With a single thyroid nodule with suppressed TSH level
    - For MNG, without suppressed TSH to identify cold areas for FNAC
    - To diagnose ectopic thyroid tissue
    - To determine eligibility for RAI therapy
    - To distinguish among the causes of high uptake thyrotoxicosis
- **FNA biopsy:**
  - **Indications:**
    - Nodule >1 cm in diameter that is solid and hypoechoic on USG
    - Of any size with USG features suggesting of malignancy, extracapsular growth, metastatic cervical lymph nodes
    - Of any size with family H/o thyroid cancer, H/o head or neck irradiation or ↑ calcitonin level

(Hot nodule on scintigraphy should be excluded from FNA biopsy)

- **Cytologic diagnosis:**
  - Nondiagnostic (10%–15%): Inadequate sample or processing error
  - Benign (60%–80%): Colloid or hyperplastic nodules, Hashimoto's or granulomatous thyroiditis and cysts
  - Follicular lesion (10%–20%): Follicular neoplasm, Hurthle cell lesion and follicular variant of PTC
  - Suspicious (2.5%–10%): Suggest malignant but not fulfill criteria
  - Malignant (3.5%–10%): Malignant cytologic features
- **Follow-up of benign nonfunctioning nodule:**
  - Perform repeated clinical, USG and TSH measurement in 6–18 months
  - Repeated USG, FNA biopsy, if suspicious clinical, USG or ↑ >50% nodule size or >20% in two or three dimensions in 6–18 months

Chapter 29: Thyroid Nodules

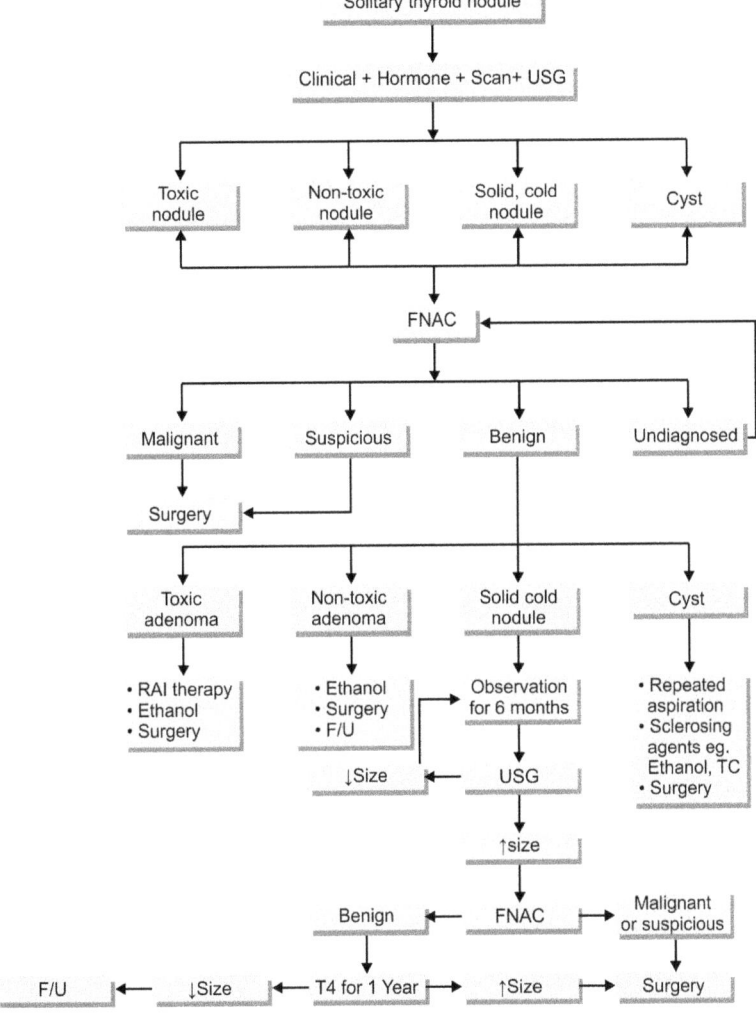

- **Levothyroxine therapy for benign nodule:** Levothyroxine may be considered in young patients who live in iodine deficient area and have small nodular non-functioning goiter
- **Percutaneous ethanol injection:** In benign thyroid cyst and complex nodules with a large fluid complement but recurrences are common
- **Fate of untreated thyroid nodule:**
  - May persist for a long time
  - Malignancy (5%–10%)
  - Spontaneous regression in 30%
  - Cystic changes due to hemorrhage within the nodule
  - Secondary infection

CHAPTER 30

Thyroid Neoplasm

Q. Classify thyroid tumors.

Ans.

Cell of origin	Tumor type	Frequency (%)	Age at presentation (years)	Spread	20 years survival (%)
Follicular cells	Benign: Follicular adenoma				
	Malignant: Papillary	80%	30–50 years	Lymphatic	95%
	Follicular (including Hurthle cell carcinoma)	10%	40–60 years	Hematogenous	60%
	Poorly differentiated				
	Undifferentiated (anaplastic)	3%	>60 years	Hematogenous	<1%
Parafollicular/ C cell	Medullary carcinoma	5%	>40	Local + Lymphatic + Hematogenous	50%
Others	Lymphoma, sarcoma, teratoma, metastatic (breast, lung, kidney)	1%			

*MTC associated with MEN 2B may present in childhood.

Q. Discuss about papillary carcinoma.

Ans.
- Common in female (3:1)
- Accounts for 90% of irradiation-induced thyroid cancer
- Spreads to regional lymph nodes. Ten percent of papillary carcinoma, especially in children presents with enlarged cervical lymph nodes
- It is confined to neck in over 95% cases, although 15%-20% have local extrathyroidal soft tissue invasion. Distant metastases, for example, lung in 1%-7% of patients only
- Multifocal in 30% cases

- Microscopically consist of papillae (fibrovascular core lined by a single layer of epithelial cells)
- About 40% of papillary carcinoma form calcified, laminated, stromal structure often at the tip of papillary projection called psammoma bodies
- Nuclear features: Larger nuclei, hypodense chromatin/ground glass appearance/ orphan Annie eye nucleus, deep nuclear grooves like coffee beans
- Most papillary carcinoma secrete thyroglobulin which can be used as a marker of recurrence or metastasis
- Prognostic factor: MACIS (metastasis, age, completeness of resection, invasion and size)
- Histological evidence of lymph node metastasis is present in two-thirds patients. Preoperative neck USG detect only half of involved lymph nodes.

Q. **How will you treat a case of papillary carcinoma?**

Ans.
- In low-risk group patients (age <45 years, size <1 cm, unifocal, intrathyroidal/do not extend beyond thyroid capsule, nonmetastatic or angioinvasive): Lobectomy or thyroidectomy done
- For all other patients, total or near total thyroidectomy (leaving 1 g of thyroid tissue contralateral to thyroid cancer site) with complete lymphadenectomy of involved lymph nodes done
- Postoperative RAI therapy (RRA—radioiodine remnant ablation) is advised for ablation of residual thyroid remnant (↓ recurrence rate), ↑ sensitivity of subsequent ^{131}I whole body scanning (WBS) and specificity of Tg measurement for detection of persistent or recurrent disease. Some thyrologist argue that RRA is not required in low-risk group patients if complete surgical resection is done
- To achieve maximum uptake of RAI into remnant, elevated serum TSH (>25 mIU/mL) is required
- Discontinuation of levothyroxine for at least 6 weeks before scanning. Liothyronine (T3) 25–50 µg/day can be given for 4 weeks, then discontinued for 2 weeks (half-life: 1 day) before WBS
- A low iodine diet is prescribed for 1–2 weeks to enhance uptake of RAI
- When TSH >25 mIU/mL, ^{131}I WBS done and Tg measured
- An undetectable serum thyroglobulin at the time of elevated serum TSH and negative scan indicate ablation of all functioning thyroid tissue
- If positive scan or rise of serum Tg to detectable level, radioactive ^{131}I 30–200 mCi administered depending on size and invasiveness of primary tumor. ^{131}I WBS is repeated 4–7 days later (post-therapy scan) to be sure no additional areas of radioiodine uptake is reveled. Nine to twelve months later, thyroid hormone therapy is withdrawn and WBS and serum Tg repeated to confirm ablation of all functioning thyroid tissue

- For the first year, patient is maintained on T_4 to suppress TSH <0.1 mIU/mL. Once it has been established that patient is free of disease, dose of T_4 is adjusted to keep TSH into low normal range (0.3–2 mIU/mL).

Q. Show a flowchart of treatment of PTC/FTC.

Ans.

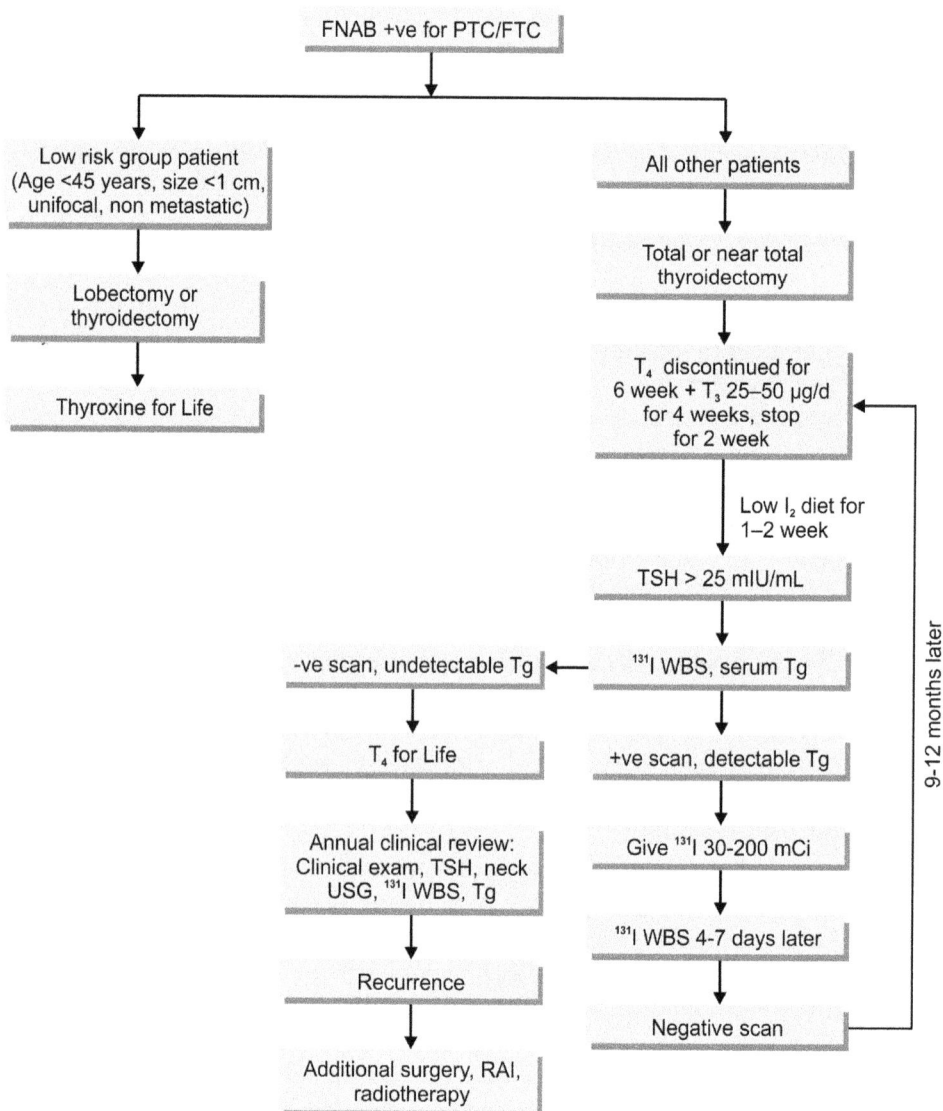

Chapter 30: Thyroid Neoplasm

Q. How will you follow-up a patient of papillary carcinoma?

Ans.
- F/U usually involves annual clinical review with clinical examination for presence of suspicious lymph node and measurement of serum TSH and Tg
- Serum Tg should be undetectable. A trend of increasing Tg requires investigation with WBS, neck USG, CT or MRI, bone scan, fluorodeoxyglucose PET scan
- WBS done annually for first 3 years. If negative, not repeated unless there is clinical indication of recurrence, for example, increased Tg level
- Recurrence is treated with additional surgery, RAI, radiotherapy.

Q. Discuss about follicular carcinoma.

Ans.
- Follicular carcinoma is characterized histologically by the presence of small follicles with poor colloid formation
- Common in areas of I_2 deficiency
- Spread to cervical lymph nodes is rare. Metastasis (5%–20%) is blood borne to lung, bone, brain
- These tumor often retain the ability to concentrate RAI from thyroglobulin and rarely synthesize T_3 and T_4
- A variant of follicular carcinoma is Hurthle cell/oxyphil cell/oncocytic carcinoma, characterized by enlarged follicular epithelial cells with pink staining/eosinophilic cytoplasm filled with mitochondria. They behave like follicular cancer except they rarely take up RAI.

Q. Discuss about medullary carcinoma.

Ans.
- Medullary carcinoma is capable of secreting calcitonin, CEA, serotonin, ACTH, prostaglandins, histaminase and other peptides (carcinoid syndrome and Cushing syndrome may occur) and variously responsible for flushing and watery diarrhea
- Calcitonin and CEA secreted by tumor is clinically useful marker for diagnosis and follow up. Despite high level of calcitonin, hypocalcaemia is extremely rare
- Microscopically consist of sheets of cells separated by pink staining substance that stains with congo red, typical of amyloid
- MTC is typically more aggressive than PTC and FTC, extending locally to cervical lymph nodes and into surrounding tissues. It may also invade lymphatics and blood vessels and metastasize to lungs, bone and liver
- Eighty percent of MTC is sporadic and remainder are familial fall into three patterns—MTC without associated endocrine disease, MEN 2A, MEN 2B

- RET proto-oncogene testing should be performed in all MTC patients. If positive, family members should be screened, if negative the tumor is sporadic
- Before surgery of MTC, hyperparathyroidism and pheochromocytoma should be evaluated
- Infusion of pentagastrin or Ca^{2+} increase calcitonin secretion, and the response may be exaggerated in patient with MTC
- **Prognostic factor:**
    - Age at diagnosis
    - Male gender
    - Initial extent of disease (e.g., nodal metastasis, distant metastasis)
    - Tumor size
    - Extrathyroidal invasion
    - Vascular invasion
    - Postoperative calcitonin level.

Q. Discuss management of medullary carcinoma with follow-up protocol.

Ans.
- **Treatment of medullary carcinoma:**
    - If FNAB is positive for medullary carcinoma, it should be confirmed with elevated serum calcitonin
    - Before surgery of MTC, HPTH and pheochromocytoma should be screened
    - RET proto-oncogene testing should be performed in all MTC patients. If positive, family members should be screened, if negative, the tumor is sporadic
    - Total thyroidectomy with complete lymphadenectomy of involved thyroid lymph nodes should be done
- **Follow-up:**
    - Follow-up postoperatively with clinical examination, calcitonin, CEA every 6 monthly. If normal, reevaluate every 6 months
    - If calcitonin is found to be elevated, neck USG, CT, MRI, PET, selective venous catheterization and sampling for serum calcitonin may reveal the lesion
    - If calcitonin >150 pg/mL, systemic metastasis localization with chest CT, PET, bone scan, indium-labeled somatostatin/octreotide scan are done
    - If the lesion is found but not operable, external X-ray therapy or chemotherapy with tyrosine kinase inhibitor—RET inhibitor (vandetanib) used
    - If the lesion is not found, patient should be followed-up until the metastatic lesion becomes evident by physical examination or imaging studies
    - As C cell do no concentrate I_2, there is no role of ^{131}I therapy and TSH suppressive doses of T_4 is not required.

Q. Show a flowchart of treatment of medullary carcinoma.

Ans.

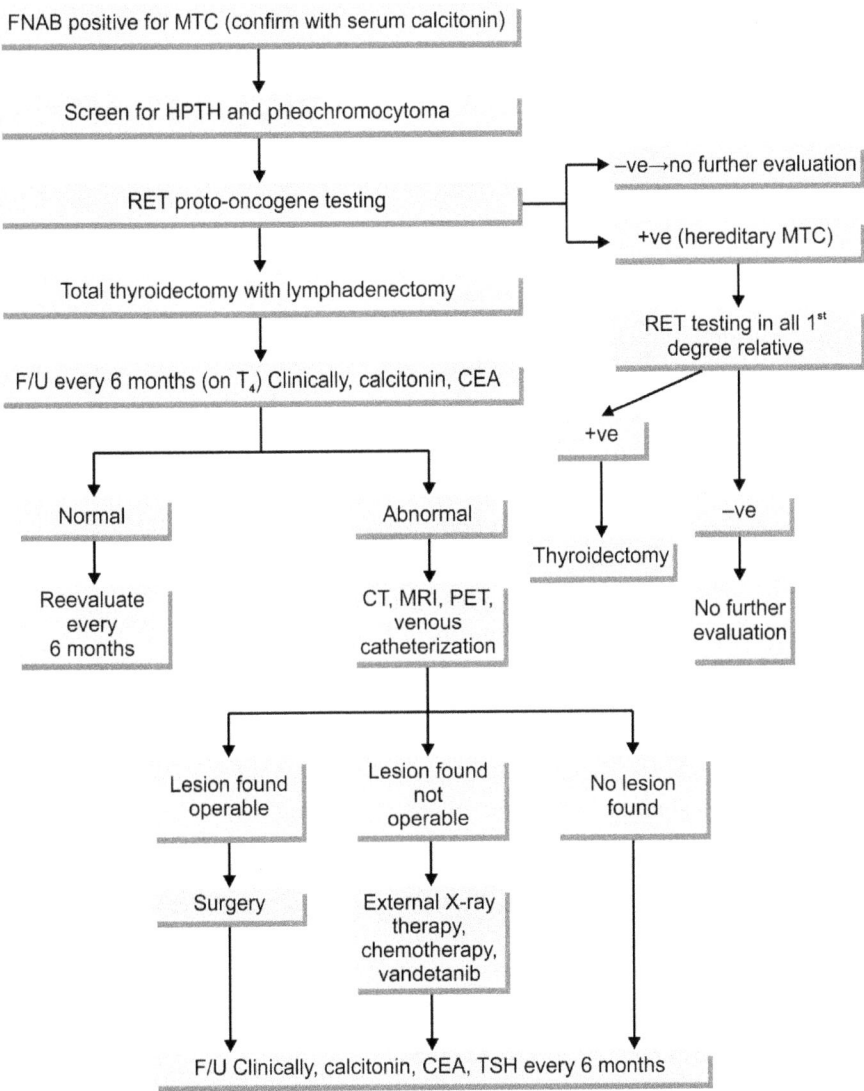

Part C: Bone and Mineral Disorders

CHAPTER 31

Hypercalcemia

Q. Mention the role of calcium in our body.

Ans. Calcium is called intracellular second messenger. Role of calcium is
- Excitation, contraction coupling in heart
- Synaptic transmission of nervous system
- Platelet aggregation and coagulation
- Secretion of hormones and other regulators by exocytosis.

Q. Mention calcium concentration in body fluid.

Ans.
- Total serum calcium: 8.5–10.5 mg/dL (2.1–2.6 mmol/L)
- Ionized calcium (50%): 4.4–5.2 mg/dL (1.1–1.3 mmol/L)
- 40%: Protein/albumin bound
- 10%: Complexed with citrate, phosphate
- Intracellular free calcium: 0.00018 mmol/L
- It is the ionized calcium which is biologically active and regulated by hormone
- 24-h urinary calcium: 50–300 mg (male), 50–250 mg (female).

Q. What is calcium/creatinine clearance ratio?

Ans. Calcium/creatinine clearance ratio: (Urine calcium ÷ serum calcium) × (serum creatinine/urine creatinine)
- Less than 0.01 in familial benign hypocalciuric hypercalcemia (FBHH)
- More than 0.02 in primary hyperparathyroidism (PHPT).

Q. How to calculate corrected serum calcium?

Ans.
- Hypoalbuminemia produces low total serum calcium because of reduction in albumin bound fraction of calcium, but the ionized Ca^{++} is normal
- Ionized Ca^{++} can be measured directly or the effect of hypoalbuminemia can be corrected by the following formula:
    - Corrected serum Ca^{++}: measured serum Ca^{++} + 0.8 (4 − measured serum albumin g/L/10)

    Or

Chapter 31: Hypercalcemia

- Adjust the value for calcium upwards by 0.1 mmol/L (0.4 mg/dL) for each 5 g/L reduction in albumin below 40 g/L.

Q. What are the causes of hypercalcemia?

Ans.

1. **Parathyroid dependent hypercalcemia:** With normal or elevated (inappropriately) PTH levels
   - Primary hyperparathyroidism (PHPT)
   - Tertiary hyperparathyroidism in CRF
   - Familial benign hypocalciuric hypercalcemia (FBHH)
   - Lithium therapy.

2. **Parathyroid independent hypercalcemia:** With low (suppressed) PTH levels
   - Malignancy:
     - Humoral hypercalcemia of malignancy:
       - Solid tumors: Squamous cell carcinoma of lung, breast, renal due to PTHrP
       - Lymphoma due to $1,25(OH)_2$ D
     - Local osteolytic hypercalcemia (multiple myeloma, breast, renal, leukemia, lymphoma)
   - Endocrinopathies: Thyrotoxicosis, adrenal insufficiency, pheochromocytoma
   - Drugs: Vitamin D intoxication, vitamin A intoxication, thiazide diuretics, milk alkali syndrome
   - Sarcoidosis
   - Immobilization.

Q. Discuss the following conditions related to hypercalcemia.

Ans.

- **Thyrotoxicosis:** Mild hypercalcemia found in 10% patient with thyrotoxicosis due to direct action of thyroid hormone to stimulate bone resorption
- **Adrenal insufficiency:** Hypercalcemia is due to hemoconcentration
- **Vitamin D intoxication:**
  - Due to ingestion of excess vitamin D or vitamin D analogs (>1 lac unit Vitamin D/day)
  - **Clinical feature:** Weakness, lethargy, polyuria, nausea, vomiting, headache, altered level of consciousness
  - **Diagnosis:** Very high serum levels of 25(OH) D
  - **Treatment:** Withdraw vitamin D, rehydration, reduce Ca^{++} intake, glucocorticoids
- **Thiazide diuretics:** Mild and transient hypercalcemia lasting for days or weeks but occasionally it persists
- **Milk alkali syndrome:** Ingestion of large amount of calcium with absorbable alkali produce milk alkali syndrome (triad of hypercalcemia, metabolic alkalosis and renal failure)

- **Sarcoidosis:** Hypercalcemia seen in 10% patients with sarcoidosis as lymphoid tissue and pulmonary macrophages of patients have 25(OH) D 1-hydroxylase activity, leading to overproduction of 1,25(OH)$_2$ D, treated with glucocorticoid
- **Lithium therapy:** Lithium used in bipolar affective disorder shift the set point for inhibition of PTH secretion to right causing mild hypercalcemia with normal or elevated PTH
- **Familial benign hypocalciuric hypercalcemia (FBHH):**
  - Autosomal dominant disorder
  - Asymptomatic, benign and mild hypercalcemia (10.5–12 mg/dL) with mild hypophosphatemia, hypermagnesemia with normal or slightly elevated PTH
  - 24 h urinary calcium <50 mg/24 h and calcium/creatinine ratio <.01
  - Importance of diagnosis: To distinguish it from PHPT and avoid unnecessary parathyroidectomy.

Q. **Mention clinical features of hypercalcemia.**

Ans.
- **CNS effects:** Lethargy, depression, ataxia, psychosis, impaired cognition, confusion, stupor, coma
- **Gastrointestinal:** Anorexia, nausea, vomiting, dyspepsia, peptic ulceration, constipation, pancreatitis
- **Neuromuscular:** Weakness, proximal myopathy, hypertonia
- **CVS:** HTN, bradycardia (even asystole), shortened QT interval
- **Renal:** Polyuria, polydipsia, renal stone, decreased GFR, hyperchloremic acidosis, nephrocalcinosis, uremia
- **Eye:** Band keratopathy
- **Systemic metastatic calcification.**

Q. **How will you investigate a case of hypercalcemia?**

Ans.
1. Repeat serum total or ionized Ca^{++}, preferably fasting and without venous occlusion (corrected for albumin)
2. **Serum PTH:**
   - If PTH is high → HPT → little further workup needed
     - RFTs
     - 24 h urinary Ca^{++}
     - Calcium/creatinine ratio
   - If serum PTH is low: Search for parathyroid independent hypercalcemia
     - CBC with ESR
     - Serum phosphate
     - CXR P/A view (sarcoidosis)
     - Thyroid function test
     - Plasma and urine protein electrophoresis (exclude MM)
     - 25(OH) D and 1,25(OH)$_2$ D

- Basal cortisol (9 AM) and rapid ACTH stimulation test (exclude adrenal insufficiency)
- Malignancy screening: Abdominal/chest CT, mammogram
- To determine end organ damage:
  - Renal USG (exclude calculi, nephrocalcinosis)
  - Skeletal radiographs, DEXA.

Q. Write down the treatment of hypercalcemia.

Ans.

1. **Asymptomatic/mild hypercalcemia:**
   - Maintain adequate hydration
   - Avoid thiazide diuretics and prolonged immobilization
   - Dietary calcium should not be restricted.
2. **Severe hypercalcemia/hypercalcemic crisis:** Serum calcium >14 mg/dL (3.5 mmol/L)
   - Commonly due to PHPT triggered by dehydration, for example, diarrhea, vomiting, diuretics, immobilization or parathyroid carcinoma, malignancy associated hypercalcemia
   - Indication for urgent treatment of hypercalcemia relates more to presence of clinical symptoms than to absolute level of serum Ca^{++}
   - Rehydration: 0.9% NS 2–4 L/day IV for 1–5 day
   - Frusemide: 20–40 mg IV (after rehydration) every 12–24 h
   - Zoledronic acid: 4 mg IV over 15–30 min—once—or pamidronate
   - Calcitonin: 4–8 IU/kg SC every 12–24 h
   - Glucocorticoid (for vitamin-D-dependent hypercalcemia, for example, lymphoma, sarcoidosis or MM)
     - HC 200–300 mg/day IV for 3–5 days
     - Prednisolone: 40–60 mg/day for 3–5 days
   - Cinacalcet: 30–60 mg BD or higher for parathyroid carcinoma
   - Dialysis.

Q. Discuss anatomy of parathyroid gland.

Ans.

- Weight 40–50 mg, usually four parathyroid glands. Supernumerary glands in 22%, fewer than 4 glands in 3–5%
- Location: As paired structures on posterior aspect of thyroid gland, 85% of parathyroid glands are found within 1 cm of point of intersection of recurrent laryngeal nerve and inferior thyroid artery. Superior parathyroid glands dorsal to the nerve and inferior glands ventral to it. Inferior glands more variable in position
- Common sites of ectopic glands: Paraesophageal (22%), mediastinal (26%), intrathymic (24%), carotid sheath, undescended/high cervical
- Histology: Chief cell secrete PTH, oxyphil cells—function unknown
- Blood supply: Inferior thyroid artery, also superior thyroid artery
- Development: Endodermal origin. Superior glands: fourth pharyngeal/branchial pouch, inferior glands: third pharyngeal/branchial pouch.

Q. What is primary hyperparathyroidism? Mention pathology and clinical features of primary hyperparathyroidism.

Ans.

- **Definition:** Autonomous secretion of PTH by parathyroid adenoma. Common in women over age 60, 2–3 times more common in women
- **Pathology:**
  - Single adenoma—85%
  - Multiple glands hyperplasia—11%
  - Double adenoma—3%
  - Parathyroid carcinoma—1% (short history, profound hypercalcemia, palpable parathyroid gland)
  - Often associated with other endocrine abnormalities particularly MEN 1 and 2
- **Clinical features:**
  - Majority of patients are asymptomatic (incidentally detected)
  - Pathological fracture
  - Features of hypercalcemia: Polyuria, polydipsia, renal colic, lethargy, anorexia, nausea, dyspepsia, peptic ulceration, constipation, depression, drowsiness, impaired cognition, dehydration (painful bones, renal stones, abdominal groans, psychic moans, fatigue overtones)
  - Hyperparathyroid bone disease:
    - Osteitis fibrosa cystica: Classic bone disease of hyperparathyroidism (<10%). ↑ Bone resorption by osteoclasts, marrow fibrosis, cystic lesion that may contain fibrosis tissue (brown tumors) manifested as bone pain, tenderness, fracture, deformity
    - Osteoporosis: Affect all sites but predominant loss of peripheral cortical bone
    - Joints (deposition of calcium pyrophosphate crystal within articular cartilage): Chondrocalcinosis, pseudogout
  - Hyperparathyroid kidney disease: Renal calculi (10–20%, usually Ca oxalate stones), nephrocalcinosis, gradual loss of renal function
  - Others: Pancreatitis, HTN (50% in primary hyperparathyroidism), pruritus (metastatic calcification of skin), conjunctival calcification.

Q. How will you investigate primary hyperparathyroidism?

Ans.

- Serum Ca^{++} level: ↑
- Serum phosphate level: Low normal (<3.5 mg/dL) or low (<2.5 mg/dL)
- Alkaline phosphatase level: Increased, suggest bone disease
- Intact PTH level: ↑
- Mild hyperchloremic metabolic acidosis
- Elevated 24-h urinary calcium
- Serum calcium/creatinine clearance ratio: >0.02 in PHPT
- RFTs
- DEXA: Osteoporosis

- **Radiological features:**
  - X-ray hand: Subperiosteal erosion, terminal resorption of phalanges (Hallmark of PHPT, particularly on radial side of middle phalange)
  - X-ray skull: Multiple small lytic lesion (pepper pot)
  - X-ray abdomen: Renal stone, nephrocalcinosis, pancreatic calcification
  - Dental film: Loss of lamina dura of teeth
- **Localization of abnormal parathyroid glands:**
  - ^{99m}Tc-sestamibi scan: ^{99m}Tc-sestamibi given IV. Early image at 10 min show tracer uptake in both thyroid and parathyroid gland. Delayed image at 2 h show persistence of tracer in abnormal parathyroid gland (isotope subtraction scan). Used in conjugation with SPECT to identify ectopic tumors
  - Neck ultrasound, MRI/CT scan
- **Invasive localizing studies:** Only in recurrent or persistent hyperparathyroidism
  - Highly selective venous catheterization for PTH
  - FNAC of suspected parathyroid mass
  - Arteriograms.

Q. How will you treat primary hyperparathyroidism?

Ans.

1. **Observation:** For asymptomatic patient with no evidence of end organ damage
   - Maintain adequate hydration
   - Avoid diuretics and prolonged immobilization
   - Dietary calcium should not be restricted
   - Follow-up:
     - 6 month–1 year: Plasma calcium, renal function, BP, symptoms
     - Every 1–2 years: DEXA, PTH, urine calcium, abdominal X-ray/renal USG
     - DEXA should be done at distal forearm that reflect cortical bone changes.

2. **Medical management:** Only indicated if patient not suitable for surgery
   - Hormone replacement therapy: Estrogen in high dose for postmenopausal female or selective estrogen receptor modulator (SERM)—Raloxifene
   - Bisphosphonate: Only transient effect on plasma and urine calcium, preserve bone mass
   - Calcium sensing receptor agonist/calcimimetic agents: Cinacalcet bind to parathyroid calcium sensing receptor and mimic the effect of ↑ extracellular Ca^{++} →↓ PTH. Indicated in tertiary hyperparathyroidism when parathyroidectomy is unsuccessful or not possible and parathyroid carcinoma. It is not licensed for use in 1° hyperparathyroidism.

3. **Surgical treatment:** Indications of surgery in primary hyperparathyroidism:
   - Serum calcium 1 g/dL above the upper limit of normal
   - eGFR <60 mL/min
   - Kidney stones or nephrocalcinosis

- BMD low (T score ≤ -2.5) at lumbar spine, hip or distal radius
- H/o fragility fracture or classic radiographic finding of osteitis fibrosa cystica
- Symptomatic or life threatening hypercalcemia
- Young age (<50 year)
- If long-term medical follow-up is not desired or possible.

In parathyroid adenoma, parathyroidectomy is done. If multiple enlarged glands/likely diagnosis is parathyroid hyperplasia either subtotal (resection of 3 and 1/2 glands) or total parathyroidectomy with primary parathyroid autotransplantation in forearm done.

Rapid intraoperative PTH assay is helpful to verify successful excision. As half-life of PTH in blood is <2 min, a decline of >50% within 10 min after surgery indicate successful surgery.

Q. Discuss postoperative care of patient undergoing parathyroidectomy.

Ans.
- Check Ca^{++}, PO_4, Mg^{++}, albumin on the evening of surgery and daily thereafter. Calcium begins to fall postoperatively after about 4–12 h and nadir is reached by 24–36 h
- Transient hypocalcemia that occurs 1–2 days postoperatively usually recovers spontaneously; however, one-third patients will require Ca^{++} support perioperatively, but half of the patients with postoperative tetany usually recovers so they do not require long-term replacement therapy
- Symptomatic hypocalcemia treated with IV Ca gluconate or oral calcium 1–3 g elemental calcium/day
- With the advent of minimally invasive parathyroidectomy and short hospital stays (<24 h), many centers advocate prophylactic calcium and vitamin D (calcitriol 0.5–1 µg/day) in all cases after surgery, which is continued until patient is reviewed 1–2 weeks later in outpatient clinic.

Q. What are the complications of parathyroidectomy?
- Recurrent laryngeal nerve injury
- Transient hypocalcaemia due to
    - Interruption of blood supply to parathyroid gland
    - Delayed recovery of other parathyroid glands due to long-term suppression
    - Parathyroid gland stunning due to intraoperative handling
- Hungry bones syndrome: In patient with severe hyperparathyroid bone disease, postoperative hypocalcaemia can occur following successful parathyroidectomy due to avid uptake of Ca^{++} and PO_4 by bones known as hungry bone syndrome. The syndrome is usually seen in patient with elevated preoperative ALP or severe uremic secondary hyperparathyroidism. Hungry bone syndrome distinguished from surgical hypoparathyroidism by serum PO_4 (low in hungry bone syndrome, high in surgical hypoparathyroidism)
- Permanent hypoparathyroidism: Rare (<2%). Check PTH level after day 3, level will be undetectable.

CHAPTER 32

Hypocalcemia

Q. What are the causes of hypocalcemia?

Ans.

1. **Parathyroid related disorder:**
   - Absence of parathyroid gland or PTH:
     - Postsurgical hypoparathyroidism
     - Congenital:
       - DiGeorge syndrome/Thymic aplasia
       - Autoimmune polyglandular syndrome type 1
   - Infiltrative disorder: Hemochromatosis, metastasis
   - Impaired secretion of PTH (functional hypoparathyroidism):
     - Hypomagnesemia
     - Chronic respiratory alkalosis
   - Resistance to PTH action: Hypomagnesemia, pseudohypoparathyroidism.

2. **Vitamin-D-related disorder:**
   - Vitamin D deficiency: Poor sunlight exposure, dietary absence, malabsorption
   - Accelerated loss: Anticonvulsant medication
   - Impaired 25 hydroxylation: Liver disease, INH
   - Impaired 1α hydroxylation:
     - RF
     - Vitamin D dependent rickets type 1 (Renal 25-OH vitamin D 1α hydroxylase deficiency)
   - Resistance to vitamin D action: Vitamin D dependent rickets type 2 (defective VDR).

3. **Acute complexion or deposition of calcium:**
   - Acute hyperphosphatemia: Crush injury with myonecrosis, tumor lysis syndrome
   - Acute pancreatitis (deposition of Ca soaps in fat necrosis)
   - Citrated BT.

4. **Critical illness/ICU patients:** Due to cytokine mediated inflammatory response, parathyroid gland suppression, failure to activate Vitamin D, Ca chelation, or hypomagnesemia.

Q. Mention clinical features of hypocalcemia.

Ans. Symptoms of hypocalcemia related to severity and rapidity of onset of hypocalcemia.
- Asymptomatic
- Neuromuscular manifestations: Due to increased neuromuscular excitability.
  - Tingling and paresthesia in fingers, toes and around mouth
  - Spontaneous or latent tetany
  - Hyper-reflexia
- CNS features:
  - Focal or generalized seizure
  - Psychosis
  - Pseudotumor cerebri
  - Papilledema, confusion, lassitude
  - Mental retardation in children
  - Calcification of basal ganglia with long-standing hypocalcemia associated with hyperphosphatemia (hypoparathyroidism or pseudohypoparathyroidism)
- Cardiac effect:
  - Prolong QT interval
  - Bradycardia
  - Impaired cardiac contractility and conduction
  - Ventricular arrhythmia including torsades de pointes
- Ophthalmological effects: Subcapsular cataract (chronic hypocalcemia)
- Skin: Skin is dry, flaky and the nails brittle
- Teeth: Enamel hypoplasia in children.

Q. Discuss about tetany.

Ans. State of painful spontaneous muscular contraction. Classic component is carpopedal spasm:
- Flexion of wrist and metacarpophalangeal joint
- Extension of interphalangeal joint
- Adduction of thumb (Main d'accoucheur posture)
- Life threatening spasm of laryngeal muscles
- In children triad of carpopedal spasm, stridor (spasm of glottis) and convulsion
- Tetany is not specific for hypocalcemia. It also occurs with hypomagnesemia and metabolic or respiratory alkalosis (e.g., hyperventilation)
- **Latent** (serum Ca^{++} 7.5–8.5 mg/dL) elicited by:
  - Chvostek sign: Tapping the facial nerve about 2 cm anterior to earlobe resulting in ipsilateral contraction of facial muscles. Specificity of the test is low. 25% normal individuals have mild Chvostek sign.

Chapter 32: Hypocalcemia

- Trousseau sign: Inflation of BP cuff midway between systolic and diastolic pressure for 3 min produce carpopedal spasm due to transient ischemia of hyperexcitable nerves innervating the hand. It is more specific than Chvostek sign (1%-4% normal individual have Trousseau sign).

Q. What is pseudohypoparathyroidism (PHP)/PTH resistance?

Ans. It is a genetic disorder of target organ unresponsiveness to PTH.
- **Clue to diagnosis:** ↓ Ca^{++}, ↑ PO_4, ↑ PTH, normal level of Vitamin D metabolites (with or without AHO), markedly blunted response to PTH.

Q. What is Albright hereditary osteodystrophy (AHO)?

Ans. A characteristic somatic phenotype of PHP type 1A and PPHP consists of short stature, rounded face, short neck, obesity, short fourth metacarpals and metatarsals, subcutaneous calcification, reduced intelligence. Due to short metacarpal, affected digits have a dimple instead of a knuckle when a fist is made.

Q. What are the causes of short fourth metacarpal?

Ans.
- Turner syndrome
- PHP
- PPHP
- Congenital or normal variant.

Q. What is pseudopseudohypoparathyroidism (PPHP)?

Ans. Certain individuals in family with PHP inherit the somatic phenotype of AHO without any disorder of calcium metabolism (Ca^{++}, PTH: normal). As the state mimic PHP, it is called PPHP.

The inheritance of the disorder is an example of genetic imprinting. Inheritance of the defective allele from a mother with PHP results in PHP in the offspring but inheritance from father results in PPHP.

Q. How will you differentiate pseudohypoparathyroidism from pseudopseudohypoparathyroidism?

Ans.

Points	PHP 1A	PHP 1B	PPHP
Hypocalcemia	Yes	Yes	No
Response to PTH	No	No	Yes
AHO	Yes	No	Yes
Other hormonal resistance	Yes	No	No
Urinary cAMP response to PTH (Ellsworth Howard test)	↓ed (resistance to PTH)	↓ed	Normal

Normally urinary cAMP increased after PTH administration.

Q. How will you investigate a case of hypocalcemia?

Ans.
- Serum total Ca^{++}, Mg^{++}, albumin, PO_4, ionized calcium
- Serum PTH
- Serum 25(OH) vitamin D, serum $1,25(OH)_2$ vitamin D.

Q. How you treat a patient of hypocalcemia?

Ans.

1. **Acute hypocalcemia:**
   - Patient with tetany or seizure requires urgent treatment with IV calcium until the sign and symptoms of hypocalcemia subside.
   - Approx. 100 mg of elemental calcium should be infused over 10–20 min
   - 10% Ca gluconate (90 mg elemental calcium/10 mL), less irritant than chloride
   - Ca gluceptate (90 mg elemental calcium/10 mL)
   - Ca chloride (272 mg elemental calcium/10 mL)
   - IV calcium is irritating to veins and best infused into large vein or CV catheter and should be diluted to minimize risk of phlebitis
   - Repeat if symptoms not resolved
   - If needed continuous calcium infusion can be given 400–1,000 mg/day with close monitoring of Ca^{++}
   - Failure to respond to infused calcium, check for hypomagnesemia and treat if needed.

2. **Chronic hypocalcemia:**
   - Aim is to keep patient free of symptoms and to maintain serum Ca^{++} 8.5–9.5 mg/dL
   - Oral calcium can be given in a dose of 1–3 g elemental calcium/day
   - Oral calcium preparation:
     - Calcium carbonate 1,250 mg (elemental Ca 500 mg/g)
     - Calcium acetate 667 mg (elemental Ca 167 mg/g)
     - Calcium lactate 300 mg (elemental Ca 84 mg/g)
   - Vitamin D preparation:
     - Ergocalciferol/Calciferol/Vitamin D_2
     - Cholecalciferol/Vitamin D_3
     - 1α-hydroxycholecalciferol/alfacalcidol/1α OH D_3
     - $1,25(OH)_2$ Cholecalciferol/calcitriol: .25–1 µg/day
     - Newer: Paricalcitol.

3. **Monitoring:**
   - Serum calcium should be monitored daily in profound hypocalcemia, weekly in moderate hypocalcemia
   - Measurement of PTH and 24 hour urinary Calcium done within 2–4 weeks of institution of therapy and repeat 1–3 monthly.

Q. Define rickets and osteomalacia.

Ans.
- **Rickets:** Disorder of mineralization of newly synthesized organic matrix of growing bone (in children), also occurring in growth plate and in mineralization of cartilage
- **Osteomalacia:** Disorder of mineralization of newly synthesized organic matrix of bone after the epiphyseal plates have closed (in adults).

Q. What are the causes of rickets and osteomalacia?

Ans.
1. **Disorder of vitamin D:**
   - Vitamin D deficiency: Poor sunlight exposure, dietary absence, malabsorption
   - Accelerated loss: Anticonvulsant medication
   - Impaired 25 hydroxylation: Liver disease, INH
   - Impaired 1α hydroxylation: RF, vitamin D dependent rickets type 1
   - Resistance to vitamin D action: Vitamin D dependent rickets type 2.
2. **Disorder of phosphate homeostasis/hypophosphatemia:**
   - Inadequate intake or absorption: Malnutrition, malabsorption/chronic diarrhea
   - Increased renal loss: Hyperparathyroidism, diuretics.
3. **Calcium deficiency.**

Q. Mention clinical features of rickets and osteomalacia.

Ans.
1. **Rickets:**
   - Growth failure/delayed development
   - Muscle hypotonia resulting potbelly and waddling gait
   - Craniotabes (small unossified area in membranous bones of skull with cracking feeling to finger pressure)
   - Frontal and parietal bossing (round eminence)
   - Delayed anterior fontanelle closure
   - Enlargement of epiphysis at lower end of radius
   - Deformities of shaft of long bones (knock knee or bowing of legs)
   - Swelling of rib at costochondral junction (rickety rosary)
   - Chest deformity: Pigeon chest
   - Bone pain and fracture
   - Eruption of teeth may be delayed and teeth may be pitted and poorly mineralized.
2. **Osteomalacia:**
   - Asymptomatic
   - Bone pain and fracture
   - Proximal muscle weakness (difficulty in climbing stairs or rising from chair/waddling gait).

Q. How will you investigate rickets and osteomalacia?

Ans.

1. **Biochemical features:** In vitamin D deficiency:
   - Serum calcium: Low/normal
   - Serum PO_4: ↓
   - Serum ALP, PTH: ↑
   - Serum 25(OH) D level: Low.

2. **Radiology:**
   - In growing bones:
     – Widening, splaying, cupping, and irregularity of metaphysis
     – Distance between epiphysis and metaphysis is ↑ed. (zone of provisional calcification is lost)
     – Bowing of long bones
   - X-ray spine: Generalized osteopenia with biconcave shape of body of vertebrae (fish mouth appearance)
   - Focal radiolucent area (pseudofractures/looser zones/milkman fractures): Uncommon but if present pathognomonic of rickets and osteomalacia. Commonly seen concave side of femoral neck, pubic rami, ribs, clavicles, lateral aspect of scapulae.

3. **Bone biopsy:** If diagnosis is in doubt. Site: rib, iliac crest.

Q. How will you treat rickets and osteomalacia?

Ans. Ergocalciferol which will restore the biochemistry to normal and heal the bony abnormalities. Although use of active metabolites of vitamin D will heal the bony abnormalities, it will not correct the underlying biochemical problem and is associated with ↑ed risk of hypercalcemia.

In adult: Ergocalciferol 20–25 µg/day in combination with calcium supplement.

CHAPTER 33

Osteoporosis

Q. Define osteoporosis.

Ans. A progressive systemic skeletal disorder characterized by low bone mass and microarchitectural deterioration of bone tissue with a consequent increase in bone fragility and susceptibility to fracture.

Q. Write down the pathophysiology of osteoporosis.

Ans.
- Peak bone mass achieved in late teenage years (early twenties in girls and by second decade in boys) that depend on
  - Genetic factors (approximately 70–80% of peak bone mass is genetically determined)
  - Nutrition: Calcium, protein, vitamin D
  - Physical activity
  - Circulating gonadal steroid
- Once peak bone mass is achieved, bone mass remains fairly stable until late third or early fourth decade. Thereafter, age-related bone loss starts with mean rate of bone loss 0.5–1% per year
- In 5 years after menopause, women lose as much as 5–8% of bone mass. Due to estrogen deficiency → increased IL-6 production → stimulate osteoclast, also with estrogen deficiency osteoprotegerin (OPG) secretion is low → stimulate osteoclast
- Osteoporosis may arise from
  - Failure to achieve optimal peak bone mass
  - Earlier than usual onset of bone loss
  - ↑ rate of bone loss caused by ↑ed bone resorption
  - Inadequate replacement of lost bone caused by ↓ed bone formation.

Q. Write down the classification of osteoporosis.

Ans.
- **Primary osteoporosis:** Osteoporosis in natural postmenopausal women or in older men and women due to age related factors
- **Secondary osteoporosis:** Osteoporosis due to specific clinical disorder. For example, Cushing syndrome. But patient may have a combination of primary and secondary causes

- **Localized osteoporosis:** Immobilization is the most common cause. For example, disuse osteoporosis of a limb.

Q. Discuss about glucocorticoid-induced osteoporosis.

Ans.
- Related to dose, route and duration of corticosteroid therapy
- Although there is no safe dose of corticosteroid, the risk increases when the dose >7.5 mg prednisolone or equivalent daily and continued for >3 months
- Corticosteroid inhibits renal tubular calcium reabsorption
- ↓ Intestinal calcium absorption →↓ plasma Ca^{++} → Compensatory hypersecretion of PTH →↑ bone resorption to maintain plasma Ca^{++}
- Inhibits osteoblastic maturation and activity
- High-dose glucocorticoid suppresses gonadotropin secretion and creates a hypogonadal state in men and women
- Associated with muscle weakness/myopathy →↑ risk of falling and fracture.

Q. What are the causes of secondary osteoporosis?

Ans.
- **Endocrine disorder:**
  - Cushing syndrome
  - Hyperparathyroidism
  - Hypopituitarism
  - Thyrotoxicosis
  - DM
- **Hypogonadal states:**
  - Premature menopause
  - Klinefelter and Turner syndrome
  - Anorexia nervosa
- **Drugs:**
  - Glucocorticoid
  - Heparin
  - Anticonvulsant
  - Thiazolidinediones
  - Chemotherapy, SSRI, PPI
- **Lifestyle factors:**
  - Low calcium intake
  - Vitamin D deficiency
  - Physical inactivity/immobilization
  - Low body weight
  - Smoking or alcoholism
- **GI disorder:** Malabsorption, coeliac disease, postgastrectomy
- **Hematological disorder:** MM, leukemia and lymphoma, sickle cell anemia

Chapter 33: Osteoporosis

- **Rheumatological disorder:** RA, ankylosing spondylitis
- **Miscellaneous:** Cystic fibrosis, CKD, COPD.

Q. What are the clinical features of osteoporosis?

Ans.
- Mostly asymptomatic until fracture
- Fragility fracture/low trauma fracture: Any fractures other than those affecting fingers, toes or face due to fall from standing height or less
- Osteoporotic fractures can affect any bone but commonly hip, vertebral fracture, distal forearm/Colles
- Vertebral fracture:
  - Two-third of vertebral fractures do not come to clinical attention
  - Patient may present with acute well localized back pain
  - May or may not be related to injury or exertion
  - Patient may also present with gradual onset of height loss and kyphosis with chronic pain
- In hip fracture, the affected leg is shortened and externally rotated
- Osteoporosis does not cause generalized skeletal pain
- Many patients present with incidental osteopenia on X-ray performed for other reasons.

Q. How will you investigate osteoporosis?

Ans.

1. **For diagnosis of osteoporosis:** Bone densitometry
2. **To find out secondary cause of osteoporosis:**
   - CBC with ESR
   - Serum Ca^{++}, PO_4, albumin, LFTs, RFTs
   - Serum 25(OH) D
   - Thyroid function test
   - Serum PTH
   - Tissue transglutaminase (tTG) assay, duodenal or jejunal biopsy: Coeliac disease
   - 24-h urinary free cortisol or other test: Cushing syndrome
   - Serum protein electrophoresis, BM study: MM
   - Undecalcified iliac crest bone biopsy with double tetracycline labeling: Suspected metabolic bone disease.
3. **Biochemical markers of bone turnover:**
   - Formation markers: Bone specific alkaline phosphatase, osteocalcin
   - Resorption markers: Collagen cross-links: For example, C terminal telopeptide (CTX) and N terminal telopeptide (NTX)
   - Utility:
     - Assessing overall risk of osteoporotic fracture

- To assess response of osteoporosis to treatment. Typically ↓ following treatment, can be detected at 3–6 months before changes in BMD measured by DEXA.

Q. Discuss about bone densitometry.

Ans. Bone densitometry used for measuring bone mass.
- Dual energy X-ray absorptiometry (DEXA)
- Quantitative computed tomography (QCT)
- Quantitative ultrasound (QUS)
- Quantitative radiography
- Single energy X-ray absorptiometry.

Q. What are the indications of bone densitometry?

Ans.
- Women aged 65 years or older and men aged 70 years or older regardless of clinical risk factors
- H/o fragility/low trauma fracture
- Clinical features of osteoporosis (height loss, kyphosis)
- Osteopenia on plain X-ray
- Use of long-term systemic glucocorticoid (≥7.5 mg prednisolone or equivalent daily for ≥3 months)
- Low body weight (BMI <20 kg/m^2)
- Early menopause (<46 years)
- Suspected secondary osteoporosis
- Assessing response of osteoporosis to treatment
- High fracture risk on FRAX analysis.

Q. Discuss about dual energy X-ray absorptiometry (DEXA).

Ans.
- For measurement of bone mineral density at lumbar spine, hip, periphery, also the whole body
- **Principle**: Calcium in bone attenuates passage of X-ray beams in proportion to amount of mineral present
- DEXA provides an image of the region studied. BMD measurement expressed as grams of hydroxyapatite/cm^2 and *T* score, *Z* score
- ***T* score:** How many standard deviation of patient's BMD value differ from that of young healthy adult of same sex?
- ***Z* score:** How many standard deviation of patient's BMD value differ from that of individual of same age and sex? Low *Z* score suggests secondary cause of osteoporosis but normal *Z* score does not rule out the possibility of underlying disorder
- **WHO criterion for postmenopausal women:**
  - Normal: *T* score at or above −1 SD
  - Osteopenia: *T* score between −1 and −2.5 SD

- Osteoporosis: *T* score at or below −2.5 SD
- Severe osteoporosis: *T* score at or below −2.5 SD with H/o fragility fracture

(WHO criterion is not applicable for premenopausal women and men but the same threshold is generally accepted).
- **Advantage of DEXA:**
  - Radiation exposure is minimum
  - Scanning time is short (5–20 min)
  - Variability of repeated measurement is <1%
- **Disadvantage of DEXA:**
  - PA measurement at lumbar spine in older patient are subject to error due to
    - Osteoarthritic change
    - Aortic calcification
    - Previous fracture
    - Radiodense material for example, surgical implant
    - Severe scoliosis
    - Extreme obesity
  - This can be overcome by performing lateral densitometry of lumbar spine but this measurement is less precise
  - Due to sources of error present in measurement of lumbar spine, ↑ reliance is placed on measurement derived from hip
- **Peripheral densitometry:** By DEXA or QCT done in obese patient at 1/3 (33%) radius site, fingers, heel/calcaneus. WHO criterion is not applicable to *T* score from peripheral densitometry.

Q. **What is FRAX (Fracture Risk Assessment Tool)?**

Ans.
- **Definition:** It is a diagnostic tool that integrates clinical risk factors and BMD at femoral neck to calculate 10-year probability of hip and major osteoporotic fracture (Spine, hip, forearm or proximal humerus)
- **FRAX risk factors:**
  - Age (40–90 years)
  - Sex
  - Weight (kg)
  - Height (cm)
  - Previous fracture
  - Previous fractured hip
  - Current smoking
  - Alcohol (≥3 units/day)
  - Glucocorticoid [≥5 mg/day of prednisolone for ≥3 months (ever)]
  - RA
  - Secondary osteoporosis
  - Femoral neck BMD (g/cm^2)

- **Application of FRAX:**
  - FRAX is intended for postmenopausal women and men age 40 years or older. It is not intended for use in younger adult (<40 years) or children
  - Not validated in patients currently or previously treated with pharmacotherapy for osteoporosis.

Q. How will you treat a patient of osteoporosis?
Ans.

1. **Goals of treatment:**
   - To prevent fracture by improving bone strength
   - Fall prevention
   - To relieve symptoms of fractures
   - To maximize physical function.

2. **Nonpharmacological treatment of osteoporosis:**
   - Adequate intake of dietary calcium (1,200 mg/day) and Vitamin D (800–1,000 IU/day)
   - Sunlight exposure [serum 25(OH) D should be ≥30 ng/mL/ ≥75 nmol/L]
   - Calcium rich food: Milk and milk products, liver, egg yolk, fish oil
   - Regular exercise. Both lack of exercise and excessive exercise cause osteoporosis
   - Avoid smoking and alcohol
   - Review of medication: Corticosteroid is truly needed or not, keep dosage and duration of administration to the minimum required for adequate treatment. If patient on thyroxine, TSH measured to avoid overdose.

3. **Fall prevention:**
   - Balance and exercise training
   - Rationalization of medication: Avoidance of unnecessary sedative, drugs causing postural hypotension, polypharmacy
   - Home environment hazard correction:
     - Grab bars in bath rooms
     - Hand rails on stair
     - Nonslippery tiles
     - Indoor and outdoor carpeting
     - ↑ lighting in high risk areas—bathrooms, stair
     - Walking aid
   - Correction of visual impairment, neurological problem.

4. **Pharmacological treatment:**
   - Indication: Postmenopausal women and men age 50 years or older presenting with
     - Hip or spine fracture (either clinical or radiological)
     - T score −2.5 or below at spine or femoral neck

- *T* score between −1 and −2.5 at spine or femoral neck and 10-year probability of hip fracture ≥3% or major osteoporosis related fracture ≥20% (humerus, forearm, hip, vertebral) based on FRAX tool
- Drugs used for osteoporosis:
  - Bisphosphonates: Alendronate, risedronate, ibandronate, zoledronic acid
  - Calcitonin
  - Estrogen/HRT
  - Selective estrogen receptor modulator (raloxifene)
  - Denosumab
  - Teriparatide/recombinant human PTH (1-34).

Q. Discuss about bisphosphonate.

Ans.

- **Bisphosphonates:** Alendronate, risedronate, ibandronate, zoledronic acid
- **Mechanism of action:** Bisphosphonates bind avidly to hydroxyapatite crystals in bone. When osteoclast attempt to reabsorb bone that contains bisphosphonates, the drug is released within the cell, interfere with protein prenylation in osteoclast causing impaired bone resorption and enhance osteoclast apoptosis resulting in gain in bone density partly due to increased mineralization of bone
- **Efficacy:** Bisphosphonate ↑ spine BMD 5-8% (0.5-2% per year) and hip BMD 2-4% during first 3 years of treatment and plateau thereafter
- **Use of bisphosphonate:**
  - Osteoporosis
  - Paget disease
  - Hypercalcemia of malignancy
  - Bone metastasis in breast cancer
  - MM
- **Swallowing of bisphosphonate:**
  - Bisphosphonate should be swallowed on empty stomach at morning with a full glass of plain water (≥8 oz/250 mL of water). Patient should remain upright (sitting or standing) for ≥30 min after talking tablet. Nothing other than plain water should be taken for 30 min (for alendronate and risedronate) or 60 min (for ibandronate)
  - The absorption of orally administered bisphosphonates is <1%. Taking with food substantially reduce the absorption of the drug
- **Adverse effect of bisphosphonates:**
  - Esophageal irritation: Esophagitis, esophageal erosion, ulcer, bleeding, perforation and association with esophageal cancer
  - IV bisphosphonate: Acute phase reactions in up to 30-40% of patient receiving their first dose, <2% in subsequent doses or patient who received previously oral bisphosphonate. Fever, myalgia, headache, arthralgia lasting several days

- Osteonecrosis of jaw: In patient receiving IV bisphosphonate (common in patient receiving higher dose for malignancy) and rarely with oral bisphosphonate. Characterized by presence of necrotic bone in mandible or maxilla typically occurring after tooth extraction when the socket fails to heal. Risk factors include poor dental hygiene, dental pathologic conditions, invasive dental procedure, infections, diabetes. Risk can be reduced by—maintain good oral hygiene, avoid invasive dental procedure. It is better to do a comprehensive dental checkup before therapy
- Atypical subtrochanteric fracture/chalk stick fracture
- Uveitis
- Atrial fibrillation (zoledronic acid)

- **Contraindications of bisphosphonate:**
  - Anatomic or functional esophageal abnormalities, for example, achalasia, stricture
  - Renal impairment (GFR <35 mL/min)
  - Hypocalcemia
  - Pregnancy and breastfeeding
  - Hypersensitivity to bisphosphonate

- **Precaution for zoledronic acid:**
  - Renal function (creatinine, CCR) and cardiac status (ECG) should be assessed before receiving zoledronic acid
  - Pre-existing hypocalcemia and other disturbances of mineral metabolism must be treated by adequate intake of calcium and Vitamin D
  - Patient must be appropriately hydrated prior to and following administration of zoledronic acid
  - Serum calcium and creatinine should be monitored.

Q. **Compare different drugs used for osteoporosis.**

Ans.

Drugs	Postmenopausal osteoporosis		Fracture risk reduction			Duration of treatment
	Prevention	Treatment	Vertebral	Nonvertebral	Hip	
Alendronate	5 mg PO daily 35 mg PO weekly	10 mg PO daily 70 mg PO weekly	Yes	Yes	Yes	4–5 years (1–2 years drug holiday)
Risedronate	5 mg PO daily 35 mg PO weekly	5 mg PO daily 35 mg PO weekly	Yes	Yes	Yes	7 years
Ibandronate	150 mg PO monthly	150 mg PO monthly	Yes	No effect demonstrated		3 years

(Contd...)

(Contd...)

Drugs	Postmenopausal osteoporosis		Fracture risk reduction			Duration of treatment
	Prevention	Treatment	Vertebral	Nonvertebral	Hip	
Zoledronic acid	5 mg IV every second year	5 mg IV yearly	Yes	Yes	Yes	3–6 years
Calcitonin (salmon calcitonin)	–	200 IU/1 spray on alternate nostril once daily	Yes	No effect demonstrated		5 years
Estrogen	Multiple formulations		Yes	Yes	Yes	
Raloxifene	60 mg PO daily	60 mg PO daily	Yes	No effect demonstrated		4 years
Denosumab	–	60 mg SC every 6 months	Yes	Yes	Yes	6 years
Teriparatide	–	20 µg SC daily	Yes	Yes	No	2 years

Q. Discuss other drugs used for osteoporosis.

Ans.

- **Calcitonin:** Inhibitor of osteoclastic bone resorption, also provide some analgesic effect. Adverse effects of nasal spray is rhinitis, epistaxis
- **Estrogen/HRT:** It may still be appropriate for treatment of menopausal symptoms. Prevention of osteoporosis no longer considered as primary indication. Used only when nonestrogen medication is not considered to be appropriate. When estrogen is prescribed for a patient who still has uterus, a progesterone also should be used to protect against endometrial proliferation
- **Selective estrogen receptor modulator/raloxifene:** Act as estrogen against on some tissues but antagonist on others. Adverse effects is venous thromboembolic disease
- **Denosumab:** Human monoclonal antibody to Rank-L. Adverse effects is serious infections including skin infection
- **Teriparatide/recombinant human PTH (1–34):**
  - Persistent elevation of PTH cause osteoporosis as in primary hyperparathyroidism but intermittent elevation of PTH causes net bone gain
  - Concomitant therapy with bisphosphonate blunt the anabolic effect of PTH but PTH therapy should be followed by bisphosphonate that maintain gain in BMD achieved with PTH
  - Measure serum Calcium, PTH, 25(OH) D before treatment with teriparatide
  - Adverse effects: Hypercalcemia (monitor Calcium), osteosarcoma

- Contraindications: Patient with ↑ed risk of osteosarcoma
  - Paget disease of bone
  - Unexplained elevation of ALP
- **Androgen:** ↑ Bone mass in hypogonadal men
  (Teriparatide, androgen are bone forming agents, others are antiresorptive agents)
- **Surgery for osteoporotic fracture:**
  - Femur neck: Partial or total hip replacement
  - Vertebral: Kyphoplasty and vertebroplasty

Q. How will you monitor and follow-up on a patient on treatment for osteoporosis?

Ans.
- Biochemical markers of bone turnover ↓ 3–6 months after therapy
- Monitor every 2 years until BMD is stable, then less frequently with evidence of persistent BMD stability
- DEXA of PA spine and hip (total hip or femoral neck) is gold standard
- As rich in trabecular bone, PA spine is more metabolically active and respond early to therapy and best site for monitoring than hip
- Monitoring should be done at same facility with use of same machine preferably by same technician and should involve the same region of interest
- To be sure that a change has occurred in a patient, about twice the precision (2% for spine, 5% for hip) is required
- ↓ BMD or new fragility fracture: Noncompliance, secondary cause of bone loss, new medication that may cause bone loss
- Fracture during drug therapy does not indicate treatment failure as most effective treatment only reduce fracture risk by 25–50%
- Screening for vertebral fracture in older patient, if height loss >4 cm in women and >6 cm in men.

Part D: Adrenal Disorders

CHAPTER **34**

Incidental Adrenal Mass

Q. Define incidental adrenal mass or adrenal incidentaloma.

Ans. Incidental adrenal mass or adrenal incidentaloma means incidentally detected adrenal mass. Adrenal incidentaloma detected in imaging studies in 2–4% patients, but in autopsy, the proportion is 1.5–7%.

Q. Mention differential diagnosis of adrenal incidentaloma.

Ans.
- Nonfunctioning benign adenoma (>85%)
- Functioning tumor:
  - Cortisol producing adenoma causing Cushing syndrome
  - Aldosterone producing adenoma
  - Androgen producing adenoma
  - Pheochromocytoma
- Adrenal carcinoma
- Metastatic deposit: From lung, GIT, kidney, breast
- Granulomatous infiltrations: TB, sarcoidosis
- Deep fungal infection: Histoplasmosis
- Adrenal cyst, Hamartoma, myelolipoma.

Q. How will you evaluate adrenal incidentaloma?

Ans.
- There are two questions to be resolved:
  - **Is the lesion secreting hormones (functional or not)?**
  - **Is it benign or malignant?**
- **Parameter to be assessed:** Clinical assessment for symptoms and signs of excess hormone secretion and signs of extra adrenal malignancy
  - **Size:** The larger the lesion, the greater the malignant potential. Around 90% of the adrenocortical carcinoma >4 cm in diameter but only 25% of such lesions are malignant
  - **Configuration:** Homogenous, round mass with regular margin likely to be benign. Non homogenous mass with irregular margin, vascular invasion is more likely to be malignant

- **Patient with known extra adrenal malignancy:** Presence of unilateral or bilateral adrenal mass in a patient with known malignancy probably represent metastatic disease and presence of metastatic lesions elsewhere increase the risk of malignancy but as much as two-third of adrenal incidentaloma in a patient with cancer are benign
- **Presence of lipid:** Adenomas are usually lipid rich. Lesions with low density (<10 HU—marker of radiodensity) on unenhanced CT scan is usually benign
- **Contrast washout:** Benign lesion demonstrate rapid washout of contrast (1–3 min, not >5 min), whereas malignant lesion tend to retain contrast (>10 min).

Q. How would you investigate adrenal incidentaloma?

Ans.
- CT/MRI of adrenal gland
- Endocrine evaluation:
  - 24-h urinary free cortisol
  - Midnight salivary cortisol
  - Overnight 1 mg dexamethasone suppression test
  - 24-h urinary fractionated metanephrines
  - Plasma metanephrine
  - Serum K^+
  - Plasma renin activity
  - Plasma aldosterone concentration
  - Measurement of DHEAS
- CT guided FNAC: Cannot distinguish adrenal adenoma from carcinoma, helpful to confirm metastatic lesion. Done once pheochromocytoma is excluded.

Q. How will you treat adrenal incidentaloma?

Ans.

1. **Surgical treatment:** Laparoscopic adrenalectomy if
   - Functional tumor
   - Tumor >4 cm—controversial (↑ likelihood of malignancy and definitely if >6 cm in diameter)
   - Imaging features suggestive of malignancy
   - Life-long follow-up after surgery as risk of recurrence (5–10%).

2. **Nonsurgical management:**
   - For radiologically benign, nonfunctioning lesions <4 cm in diameter
   - Repeat imaging at 6 and 12 months
   - Repeat biochemical screening annually
   - Up to 20% patients may develop hormone excess during follow up
   - If there is progressive tumor growth or hormonal excess, surgery should be done.

CHAPTER 35

Cushing Syndrome

Q. Define Cushing syndrome.
Ans. Symptoms and signs associated with prolonged exposure of tissue to inappropriately elevated levels of glucocorticoids.

Q. What are the causes of Cushing syndrome?
Ans.

1. **ACTH dependent:**
   - Pituitary adenoma secreting ACTH (Cushing disease)
   - Ectopic ACTH syndrome
   - Iatrogenic (ACTH therapy).

2. **ACTH independent:**
   - Adrenal adenoma and carcinoma
   - Iatrogenic/chronic glucocorticoid therapy: Most common cause
   - Primary pigmented nodular adrenal hyperplasia and Carney syndrome
   - Aberrant receptor expression: Food-dependent Cushing syndrome.

3. **Pseudo-Cushing syndrome:**
   - Depression
   - Alcoholism
   - Obesity
   - Eating disorder (anorexia, bulimia nervosa).

Q. Classify Cushing syndrome.
Ans. Two types of Cushing syndrome:
- Exogenous/iatrogenic
- Endogenous/spontaneous

Q. Discuss about iatrogenic Cushing syndrome.
Ans.
- Cushing syndrome due to prolonged administration of glucocorticoid

- Depends on dose, duration, route and potency of corticosteroid. Even topical or inhaled glucocorticoid in prolonged duration can produce Cushing syndrome
- Features more common than endogenous Cushing syndrome:
  - Cataract
  - Avascular necrosis of femoral head
  - Osteoporosis
  - Benign intracranial hypertension
  - Pancreatitis
- Features less common:
  - HTN
  - Hirsutism
  - Oligomenorrhea/amenorrhea
- Glucocorticoid components of skin creams (including bleaching agents), herbal medications, tonics and joint infections may be overlooked.

Q. What is Cushing disease?

Ans.

- Specific type of Cushing syndrome due to pituitary adenoma secreting ACTH
- Responsible for 80% of endogenous Cushing syndrome
- Age: 20–40 years, F:M = 5:1
- Usually benign microadenoma <10 mm in diameter. 10% may be larger and invasive or malignant
- ACTH secreting adenoma typically show Crooke changes (zone of perinuclear hyalinization due to chronic exposure of corticotroph cells to hypercortisolism)
- Endocrine abnormalities in Cushing disease:
  - Hypersecretion of ACTH with bilateral adrenocortical hyperplasia (ZF and ZR) and hypercortisolism
  - Absent circadian periodicity of ACTH and cortisol secretion
  - Absent responsiveness of ACTH and cortisol to stress (hypoglycemia or surgery)
  - ACTH-secreting pituitary adenoma functions at a higher than normal set point for cortisol feedback and typically maintains some responsiveness to usual feedback control factors, for example, high doses of glucocorticoid and CRH
- Characteristics:
  - Unlike patient of ectopic ACTH syndrome, patient of Cushing disease rarely have anemia, weight loss, hypokalemia, alkalosis, hyperpigmentation
  - Virilization occasionally seen in patient with adrenal carcinoma is unusual in Cushing disease
  - Symptoms due to tumor itself, for example, headache, visual impairment rare due to small size of adenoma
  - Insidious onset with slow progression over months or years.

Chapter 35: Cushing Syndrome

Q. Discuss about ectopic ACTH syndrome.

Ans.
- Arises when nonpituitary tumor synthesizes and hypersecretes biologically active ACTH
- Small cell lung carcinoma and bronchial carcinoid are responsible for 50% of cases, also pancreatic islet cell tumor, thymus, neuroendocrine tumor, gut, ovary or medullary carcinoma of thyroid
- Age: 40–60 years, M:F = 3:1
- Responsible for 10% of endogenous Cushing syndrome
- Typical features of Cushing syndrome may be absent due to acuteness of clinical course
- Hyperpigmentation common
- Anorexia, anemia, weight loss and other features of primary tumor may be apparent
- Features of mineralocorticoid excess (HTN, hypokalemia, alkalosis) is present due to increased secretion of deoxycorticosterone and mineralocorticoid effect of cortisol
- Tumor may be radiologically inapparent at the time of presentation
- Ectopic tumors have no residual negative feedback control and secretion of ACTH and cortisol is nonsuppressible with high doses of glucocorticoid
- Ectopic ACTH syndrome which is caused by benign tumor, for example, bronchial carcinoid, presents a more slowly progressive course with typical features of Cushing syndrome.

Q. Discuss about primary adrenal tumor.

Ans.
- Primary adrenal tumor (glucocorticoid producing adrenal adenoma and carcinoma) responsible for 10% of endogenous Cushing syndrome
- Both adrenal adenoma and carcinoma are common in women
- Adrenal adenoma: Gradual onset, clinical features of glucocorticoid excess alone
- Adrenal carcinoma: >4 cm size. Rapid onset with clinical features of excess glucocorticoid, androgen and mineralocorticoid and are rapidly progressive. Hypokalemia common, also abdominal pain, palpable mass, hepatic and pulmonary metastasis
- Subclinical Cushing syndrome reported in 10% of patients with adrenal incidentaloma.

Q. What is Carney syndrome?

Ans. Autosomal dominant disorder comprises atrial myxoma, spotty skin pigmentation, sexual precocity, acromegaly, peripheral nerve tumors.

Q. What is food-dependent Cushing syndrome?

Ans. Adrenal expression of glucose-dependent insulinotropic polypeptide (GIP) resulting in modulation of cortisol production after physiologic postprandial fluctuation of endogenous levels of GIP.

Q. Describe the clinical features of Cushing syndrome.

Ans.

1. **Symptoms:**
   - Obesity
   - Menstrual irregularity/gonadal dysfunction:
     - Amenorrhea in female due to ↑ androgen
     - Loss of libido in both sexes (cortisol inhibit GnRH pulsatility and LH/FSH secretion)
   - Hirsutism:
     - Due to hypersecretion of adrenal androgens
     - Facial hirsutism common
     - Also ↑ hair growth at abdomen, breast, chest, upper thighs
     - Acne and seborrhea usually accompany
     - Virilism is unusual except in adrenal carcinoma
   - Easy bruising
   - Fatigue
   - Proximal myopathy: Inability to climb stairs or get up from a chair
   - Psychiatric dysfunction: Emotional lability, depression, poor concentration, poor memory, insomnia, euphoria, psychosis
   - Backache:
     - Due to compressed vertebral fracture, loss of height due to osteoporotic vertebral collapse
     - Pathological fracture occurs spontaneously or after minor trauma, for example, in ribs (in X-ray: exuberant callus formation at the site of healing fracture)
     - Unexplained osteopenia in young and middle-aged adult need an evaluation for Cushing syndrome
     - Avascular necrosis of femoral head common in iatrogenic Cushing syndrome
   - Glucose intolerance, overt DM (in one-third patient), HTN, dyslipidemia (hepatic lipoprotein synthesis is stimulated →↑ cholesterol, TG), cardiovascular events
   - Peptic ulcer disease
   - Thirst and polyuria: Due to glucocorticoid inhibition of ADH secretion
   - Renal calculi: Due to glucocorticoid induced hypercalciuria
   - Infection:
     - Tendency to infection with poor wound healing
     - Fungal infection of skin and nails (onychomycosis) or mucosa (oral candidiasis)
     - Little inflammatory response (perforation of a viscus may be masked and patient may show no febrile response to an infection)
   - In children: Poor linear growth and weight gain

2. **Signs:**
   - Face:
     - Moon facies (accumulation of fat over cheeks and temporal region)
     - Facial plethora, acne, hirsutism
   - Obesity:
     - Centripetal obesity affecting mainly face, neck, trunk and abdomen with relative sparing of extremities (lemon on match stick appearance)
     - Generalized obesity in children. Fat depots over dorsocervical spine (buffalo hump) and supraclavicular region
   - Skin changes:
     - Skin thinning (atrophy of epidermis and its underlying connective tissue)
     - Wrinkling of skin on the dorsum of hand may be seen resulting in a cigarette paper appearance (Liddle sign)
     - Easy brushing following minor trauma
     - Striae in 50% patients but unusual in patients over 40 years age. Red to purple (increased vascularity), depressed below skin surface, wider (.5–2 cm), mostly horizontal or oblique in abdomen, also over breasts, buttocks, thighs
     - Striae must be differentiated from white vertical striae in abdominal wall below umbilicus in pregnancy (striae gravidarum) or rapid weight gain. Hyperpigmentation of skin common in ectopic ACTH syndrome
   - Hair thinning, psychosis, HTN, ankle edema
   - Cataract, mild exophthalmos (↑ed retro-orbital fat deposition).

Q. How will you investigate a case of Cushing syndrome?

Ans.
- **Diagnosis:** Does the patient have Cushing syndrome?
  At least two of the following three tests should be +ve to diagnose Cushing syndrome.
  - 24-h urinary free cortisol (≥2 tests)
  - Midnight salivary cortisol (≥2 tests)
  - Overnight 1 mg dexamethasone suppression test (DST)

1. **24-h urinary free cortisol (UFC):**
   - UFC is not affected by conditions and medications that alter corticosteroid binding globulin (CBG). For example, healthy women taking oral estrogen may have increased CBG and therefore high serum cortisol, but their UFC remains normal
   - Normal 24-h UFC: 14–135 nmol/24 h
   - Sample collection: The first morning void is discarded. All subsequent void collected, which is kept refrigerated (but not frozen) up to and including first morning void on second day
   - False +ve: Patient taking carbamazepine, fenofibrate

- False −ve: 8–15% patients of Cushing syndrome, moderate to severe renal impairment (CCR <60 mL/min)
- Simultaneous creatinine excretion (which differs by no >10% from day to day) may be used to ensure adequacy of collection
- Up to threefold elevation of UFC can occur in pseudo-Cushing syndrome but UFC >4 times normal indicate most likely diagnosis is Cushing syndrome.

2. **Midnight salivary cortisol:**
   - In healthy individual with stable sleep wake cycles, serum cortisol begin to rise at 3–4 AM and reaches peak at 7–9 AM, then falls for the rest of day to very low levels when the person is unstressed and asleep at midnight (serum cortisol <50 nmol/L at 11 PM to 2 AM)
   - Loss of circadian rhythm with absence of midnight cortisol nadir is consistent with Cushing syndrome
   - Circadian rhythm is blunted in many patients with depressive illness, in shift workers and may be absent in critically ill patients
   - Salivary cortisol concentration is not affected by serum CBG, salivary flow or composition and stable at room temperature for several weeks and can be mailed to a reference laboratory
   - Ask the patient to collect saliva sample on two separate days between 11 PM and 12 AM by passive drooling into a plastic pipette or by commercially available sampling device placed in mouth and chewing for 1–2 min
   - Normal midnight salivary cortisol <4 nmol/L
   - False +ve: Individuals using licorice, chewing tobacco, smoking, stress immediately before collection (so ideally collect sample at home)
   - Earliest and most sensitive markers for Cushing syndrome.

3. **Overnight 1 mg dexamethasone suppression test (DST):**
   - Patients take 1 mg dexamethasone (2 Tab. Oradexon .5 mg) at 11 PM and measure fasting plasma cortisol level at 8–9 AM the following day. Normal response is suppression of plasma cortisol level to <50 nmol/L.
   - Dexamethasone is used for testing as it does not cross-react with radioimmunoassays for cortisol
   - False −ve: Mild hypercortisolism, intermittent hypercortisolism
   - False +ve:
     - Drugs that increase dexamethasone metabolism, for example, phenytoin, phenobarbitone, rifampicin, carbamazepine, pioglitazone
     - Estrogen increased CBG → 50% chances of false +ve → so stop OCP for 6 weeks before testing

- RF, depression, alcoholism
- Patient undergoing stressful event or serious illness.

4. **Other initial tests:**
   - Done in patients with high clinical index of suspicion of Cushing syndrome but initial tests are not conclusive
   - **Diurnal rhythm of plasma cortisol:** Evening (5 PM) level >75% of morning (9 AM) level in Cushing syndrome
   - **48-hour low dose DST:** Plasma cortisol is measured at 9 AM at time 0 and again 48 h later after administration of dexamethasone 0.5 mg every 6 h for 48 h. Normal response is suppression of plasma cortisol level to <50 nmol/L
   - **Midnight serum cortisol:**
     - Sleeping midnight cortisol require impatient admission for 48 h or longer to avoid false +ve response due to stress of hospitalization. The blood should be collected within 5–10 min of waking patient or through indwelling line
     - Awake midnight serum cortisol far easier
     - Sleeping midnight serum cortisol >50 nmol/L or awake midnight serum cortisol >207 nmol/L: Cushing syndrome.

Q. **What is the cause of Cushing syndrome?**

Ans.

1. **Late afternoon (after 4 PM) ACTH:**
   - Late afternoon (after 4 PM) timing is important because ACTH level is normally low at that time
   - Normal plasma ACTH level: 9–52 pg/mL
   - ACTH >10 pg/mL: ACTH dependent Cushing syndrome (pituitary or ectopic ACTH secreting tumor). Plasma ACTH is higher in ectopic ACTH syndrome than Cushing disease
   - ACTH <5 pg/mL: ACTH independent
   - ACTH 5–10 pg/mL: Indeterminate. Do CRH stimulation test

2. **CRH stimulation test:** Administer CRH IV. ACTH and cortisol level measured before CRH injection and every 15 min for 2 h. Exaggerated response (ACTH >50% above basal, cortisol >20% above basal) suggest Cushing disease. Lesser or no response in ectopic ACTH syndrome. In normal subject, ACTH and cortisol >15–20% over basal

3. **Serum K^+, HCO_3^-:** Hypokalemic alkalosis present >95% patient with ectopic ACTH syndrome, also in <10% of patient with Cushing disease

4. **High-dose DST:**
   - Patient take dexamethasone 2 mg 6 hourly for 48 h. Collect 24 h urine sample before the test and during last 24 h of test
   - Urine cortisol suppression >50% basal suggest Cushing disease. In ectopic ACTH syndrome, no or minimal suppression
   - However, 10% of patient with Cushing disease do not suppress and 10% of ectopic ACTH syndrome mainly bronchial carcinoid show >50% suppression
   - For convenience 8 mg overnight DST done. 8 mg dexamethasone (Tab. Oradexon .5 mg, 16 tablets) given at 11 PM. Serum cortisol measured at 8 AM next morning. Serum cortisol suppression >50% basal suggest Cushing disease
5. **Inferior petrosal sinus sampling:**
   - For evaluation of patient with ACTH dependent Cushing syndrome when MRI does not reveal a definite adenoma
   - Catheters are advanced into inferior petrosal venous sinuses bilaterally via femoral vein
   - Simultaneous IPS and peripheral ACTH measurement before and after CRH stimulation
   - IPS to peripheral ACTH ratio >2:1 prior to CRH and >3:1 after CRH consistent with pituitary ACTH secreting tumor and <1.8:1 suggest ectopic ACTH syndrome
6. **MRI of pituitary with gadolinium enhancement:** Localize adenoma in upto 70% cases. However, 10% population of 20–40 years have pituitary incidentaloma. So some patient with ectopic ACTH syndrome may have radiographic pituitary lesion
7. **CT adrenals:** As adrenal incidentaloma present in 2%–4% of normal subjects. So adrenal imaging should not be performed unless biochemical investigation suggests primary adrenal cause, for example, undetectable ACTH
8. **Ectopic ACTH:**
   - CXR
   - HRCT of chest, abdomen and pelvis
   - Scintigraphy: Iodocholesterol scintigraphy (for diagnosis of adrenal adenoma), radiolabelled somatostatin analog scan (octreotide acetate scintigraphy)
9. **Other tests:** RBS, BMD, ECG, serum electrolyte.

Chapter 35: Cushing Syndrome

Q. Draw a flowchart about workup for Cushing syndrome.

Ans.

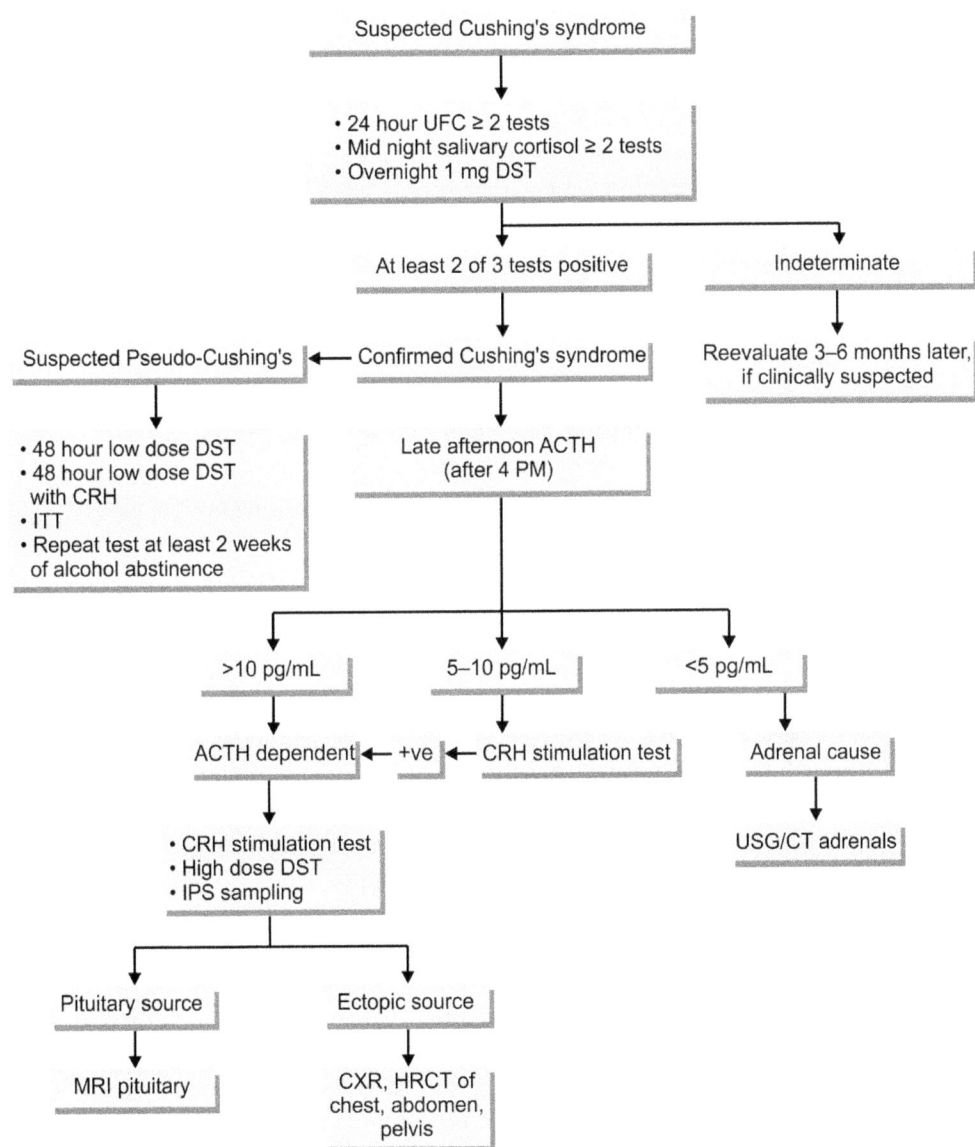

Q. How will you diagnose a case of Cushing syndrome in special populations?

Ans.
- **Pregnancy:** UFC, not DST in initial evaluation of pregnant woman
- **Epilepsy:** UFC, midnight salivary cortisol, not DST
- **Renal failure:** DST, not UFC in severe RF (CCR <60 mL/min)
- **Adrenal incidentaloma:** DST or midnight salivary cortisol rather than UFC in patient having mild Cushing syndrome
- **Cyclic Cushing syndrome:**
    - A small group of patients with Cushing syndrome there is episodic excessive secretion of cortisol in a cyclical pattern with peaks occurring at intervals of several days to many months
    - Screening tests for Cushing syndrome may be normal in between
    - Measurement of UFC or midnight salivary cortisol may best demonstrate cyclicity rather than DST
    - If clinical suspicion is high but initial tests are normal, follow-up should be done with repeat testing, best when clinical symptoms present
    - All causes of Cushing syndrome may be associated with cyclical secretion of cortisol but most patients thought to have pituitary dependent disease.

Q. Discuss about pseudo-Cushing syndrome.

Ans.
- In some conditions like depression, alcoholism, obesity, eating disorder (anorexia and bulimia nervosa), there is mild hypercortisolism (elevation of UFC, loss of diurnal rhythm, lack of low dose suppressibility) with presence of some clinical features of Cushing syndrome due to overactivation of HPA axis but without true Cushing syndrome (hypercortisolism is not autonomous) known as pseudo-Cushing syndrome
- 24-h UFC >4 times normal, pseudo-Cushing syndrome is unlikely
- 24-low dose DST: In pseudo-Cushing syndrome, plasma cortisol is suppressed to <50 nmol/L but in Cushing syndrome not suppressed
- 48-h low dose DST with CRH: Administration of dexamethasone 0.5 mg 6 hourly for 48 h followed by IV CRH 2 h after last dose of dexamethasone. As patients with pseudo-Cushing's are thought to be under chronic CRH stimulation thus showing a blunted response to CRH after dexamethasone suppression (cortisol 15 min after CRH >38.6 nmol/L in Cushing's and <38.6 in pseudo-Cushing's)
- Insulin tolerance test (ITT): Insulin induced hypoglycemia cause rise in ACTH and cortisol levels in pseudo-Cushing's but blunted rise in Cushing's. However, 20% Cushing's (especially cyclical Cushing's) show normal cortisol rise with hypoglycemia
- In alcoholic, repeat the initial tests after ≥2 weeks of abstinence
- No screening tests is 100% capable of distinguishing all cases of Cushing's from normal individual/pseudo-Cushing's.

Q. Write down the treatment of Cushing disease.

Ans.

1. **Surgical treatment:**
    - Selective transsphenoidal resection of ACTH secreting pituitary adenoma is treatment of choice (success rate 85%)
    - Complication: Transient or permanent DI, hypopituitarism
    - It is often useful to administer medical treatment for ≥6 weeks prior to surgery to allow improvement in wound healing and reduce anesthetic risk in those with severe metabolic problems.

2. **Radiotherapy:** For patient who have persistent or recurrent disease following pituitary surgery, who have undergone bilateral adrenalectomy or patients with established Nelson's syndrome. γ-Knife radiosurgery achieves remission in 65–75% cases.

3. **Medical treatment:**
    - Indicated during preoperative preparation of patient or while awaiting benefit from pituitary radiotherapy or if surgery or radiotherapy are contraindicated
    - They inhibit adrenal steroid biosynthesis
    - Ketoconazole: 600–1,200 mg/day. Adverse effects: Hepatotoxicity
    - Metyrapone
    - Trilostane
    - Aminoglutethimide
    - Mitotane/adrenolytic drug: Cause atrophy of ZF and ZR. Delayed response (weeks or months). Adverse effects: Nausea, vomiting, diarrhea, somnolence, skin rash
    - Etomidate
    - Thiazolidinediones: Rosiglitazone, doses up to 8 mg/day
    - Novel somatostatin analog: Pasireotide
    - Use of these drugs associated with ↑ ACTH (as cortisol concentration ↓) that overcome enzyme inhibition. So combined use of these drugs
    - Aim is to achieve mean plasma cortisol concentration 150–300 nmol/L during the day or normal UFC.

4. **Bilateral adrenalectomy:**
    - Indicated when pituitary surgery, radiotherapy and medical treatment failed to control the disease or in ectopic ACTH syndrome, when ectopic source cannot be found or inoperable
    - Risk of Nelson syndrome in <10% of patients that can be reduced with prophylactic pituitary radiotherapy
    - Correct hypercortisolism but produce permanent hypoadrenalism, require lifelong glucocorticoid and mineralocorticoid.

5. **Perioperative management following trans-sphenoidal surgery for Cushing syndrome:**
   - Most patients develop transient secondary adrenocortical insufficiency (as corticotrophs surrounding microadenoma are usually suppressed) requiring postoperative glucocorticoid support until HPA axis recovers (usually 2–18 months)
   - After 3–5 days postoperatively, 9 AM plasma cortisol measured with patient omitted hydrocortisone for 24 h (1 mg dexamethasone given at 10 PM day before testing)
     – <30 nmol/L considered cure
     – >300 nmol/L considered for radiotherapy.

6. **Follow-up:**
   - To detect recurrent Cushing disease
   - To assess recovery of HPA axis
   - If postoperative cortisol undetectable (<30 nmol/L) recurrence rate 2–20% and 50–75% if postoperative cortisol detectable
   - Physical features of Cushing syndrome disappear within 2–12 months. HTN and DM improve but may not resolve completely.

Q. What is Nelson syndrome?

Ans. If bilateral adrenalectomy is done in patients with Cushing disease, then there is risk (<10%) that pituitary tumor will grow in absence of negative feedback suppression previously provided by elevated cortisol level known as Nelson syndrome.
- Clinical features:
  – Hyperpigmentation with markedly elevated ACTH level (>1,000 pg/mL) with features of expanding intrasellar mass lesion
  – Usually within 2 years of adrenalectomy
  – Prevented by pituitary irradiation
- Treated by trans-sphenoidal surgery with postoperative radiotherapy
- MRI and ACTH monitoring initiated 6 months after adrenalectomy and continued annually for ≥6 years.

Q. Discuss about prognosis of Cushing syndrome.

Ans.
- Untreated Cushing syndrome is fatal with 50% mortality at 5 years
- Death is due to
  – Underlying tumor itself as in ectopic ACTH syndrome, adrenal carcinoma
  – Complication of sustained hypercortisolism: HTN, cardiovascular disease, stroke, thromboembolism, susceptibility to infection
- In Cushing disease: If postoperative cortisol undetectable (<30 nmol/L) then recurrence rate 2–20% and 50–75% in postoperative cortisol detectable
- Physical features of Cushing syndrome disappear within 2–12 months. HTN and DM improve but may not resolve completely.

Chapter 35: Cushing Syndrome

Q. How to treat adrenal adenoma?

Ans. Treated by unilateral adrenalectomy. As there is atrophy of contralateral adrenal gland, so it requires glucocorticoid support both during and following surgery until HPA axis recovered (6–18 months).

Q. How to treat adrenal carcinoma?

Ans.
- Surgery is useful to debulk tumor mass, also ↓ degree of steroid hypersecretion
- Medical treatment: Mitotane (Adrenolytic drug)
- Prognosis is poor. Median survival from onset of symptoms is 4 years.

Q. How you will treat Ectopic ACTH syndrome?

Ans.
- If tumor can be found and has not spread: Removal can lead to cure, for example, bronchial carcinoid
- Prognosis of small cell lung carcinoma with ectopic ACTH syndrome is poor. Mean survival <12 months. Treatment of tumor should be done. K^+ replacement to correct hypokalemia and spironolactone to block mineralocorticoid effect. Ketoconazole and metyrapone may be useful
- If ectopic source of ACTH cannot be found: Bilateral adrenalectomy and follow up the patient until primary tumor become apparent.

CHAPTER 36

Adrenocortical Insufficiency

Q. Define adrenocortical insufficiency.

Ans. Adrenocortical insufficiency results from inadequate adrenocortical function and may be primary (destruction or dysfunction of adrenal cortex in the setting of adrenal disease) or secondary (deficient ACTH secretion due to pituitary or hypothalamic disease). Exogenous glucocorticoid therapy is most common cause of secondary adrenocortical insufficiency.

Q. Discuss about pathophysiology of adrenocortical insufficiency.

Ans.
- In primary adrenocortical insufficiency, adrenal cortex destruction or dysfunction involves all three zones of adrenal cortex resulting in inadequate glucocorticoid, mineralocorticoid and androgen secretion
- Loss of >90% of both adrenal cortex results in clinical manifestations of adrenocortical insufficiency
- With gradual adrenocortical destruction, in initial phase basal cortisol, secretion is normal but secretion does not increase in response to stress (surgery, trauma, infection) leading to adrenal crisis
- Acute adrenocortical insufficiency may occur in context of septicemia or adrenal hemorrhage
- Mineralocorticoid deficiency leads to reduced Na^+ retention, hypotension with ↓ intravascular volume, also hyperkalemia due to ↓ renal K^+ and H^+ excretion
- Androgen deficiency presents in female with reduced axillary and pubic hair, ↓ libido (testicular production of androgen is more important in male)
- In secondary adrenocortical insufficiency, ACTH deficiency leads to ↓ cortisol and adrenal androgen secretion. Aldosterone secretion remains normal (as aldosterone secretion is not dependent on ACTH and renin–angiotensin–aldosterone axis is intact)
- 25% patients in crisis or impending crisis at the time of diagnosis.

Chapter 36: Adrenocortical Insufficiency

Q. What are the causes of adrenocortical insufficiency?

Ans.

1. **Primary/Addison disease:**
   - Autoimmune/autoimmune adrenalitis: Most common cause (>75%)
     - Sporadic
     - Polyglandular syndrome
   - Infection: TB, HIV, fungi (histoplasmosis, coccidioidomycosis), CMV
   - Metastatic malignancy (lung, GIT, breast, renal) or lymphoma
   - Bilateral adrenalectomy
   - Adrenal hemorrhage
   - Infiltration: Amyloidosis, hemochromatosis
   - CAH
   - Drugs: ketoconazole, metyrapone, aminoglutethimide, mitotane, etomidate.

2. **Secondary:**
   - Withdrawal of suppressive glucocorticoid therapy
   - Pituitary or hypothalamic disease.

Q. Discuss about different etiology of adrenocortical insufficiency.

Ans.

1. **Autoimmune adrenalitis:**
   - Pathologically adrenal glands are atrophic with loss of most cortical cells but medulla is usually intact
   - Adrenal autoantibodies detected in 75% cases
   - 50% of patients have an associated autoimmune disease, for example, Hashimoto thyroiditis, Grave disease, pernicious anemia, primary ovarian failure, hypoparathyroidism, IDDM, myasthenia gravis, celiac disease
   - Autoimmune adrenocortical insufficiency occur in autoimmune polyglandular syndrome type 1 (APS-1) and type 2 (APS-2)
   - APS-1/autoimmune polyendocrinopathy–candidiasis–ectodermal dystrophy syndrome (APCED): Triad of adrenal insufficiency, autoimmune hypoparathyroidism, chronic mucocutaneous candidiasis (only 2 is required for diagnosis)
   - APS-2/Schmidt syndrome: Triad of adrenal insufficiency, autoimmune thyroid disease, type 1 DM (≥ 2 is required for diagnosis).

2. **Infection:**
   - Tuberculous Addison disease results from hematogenous spread of infection from elsewhere in the body and only 5% of patients with disseminated TB

- Tuberculosis and fungal infections are associated with enlarged adrenals that may show calcification (50% of TB)
- Adrenal insufficiency may be precipitated by rifampicin (↑ cortisol metabolism) or ketoconazole (inhibit cortisol synthesis) and need ↑ replacement steroid dose

3. **Metastatic malignancy:** Bilateral adrenal involvement present in 50% patients but adrenal insufficiency does not occur with unilateral metastatic disease.

4. **Adrenal hemorrhage:** In septicemia (Waterhouse-Friderichsen syndrome following meningococcal septicemia), trauma, patient on anticoagulant for coagulopathy, heparin-induced thrombocytopenia, antiphospholipid antibody syndrome (lupus anticoagulant).

Q. Discuss clinical features of Addison disease.

Ans.
- **Common in females:** F:M = 2:1, Age: third to fifth decades
- **Triad of Addison disease:** Weakness or emaciation, pigmentation, hypotension
- **Due to glucocorticoid insufficiency:**
    - Weakness, fatigue, weight loss (up to 15 kg)
    - Anorexia, nausea, vomiting, diarrhea, abdominal pain
    - Postural symptoms
    - Hypoglycemia (loss of gluconeogenic effect of cortisol), more in secondary adrenal insufficiency
    - Hyponatremia (dilutional)
    - Hypercalcemia
- **Due to mineralocorticoid insufficiency:**
    - Salt craving (20%), dehydration, hypotension, shock
    - Hyponatremia (depletional), hyperkalemia
    - Acidosis
- **ACTH excess:**
    - Generalized hyperpigmentation of skin and mucosa at
        - Sun exposed areas
        - Pressure areas (elbow, knees, under bras and belts)
        - Palmar crease, knuckles, nail beds, axillae, nipples, areolae
        - Mucous membrane (buccal mucosa, gum, perivaginal and perianal mucosa)
        - Conjunctivae
        - Recent scars rather than old scars (scars that have formed after onset of ACTH access)
- **Adrenal androgen insufficiency:** Loss of axillary and pubic hair, loss of libido especially in female

- Vitiligo present in 10–20% patients with autoimmune Addison disease
- Low grade fever
- Amenorrhea may be due to weight loss, chronic illness or primary ovarian failure
- Adrenal insufficiency should be considered in differential diagnosis of unexplained weight loss and in patient with hypotension and fever.

Q. When to suspect acute adrenal hemorrhage as etiology of adrenocortical insufficiency?

Ans. Should be considered in deteriorating patient with unexplained abdominal or flank pain, vascular collapse, progressive hyperkalemia, rapidly falling Hb% particularly in the setting of septicemia or patient is on anticoagulant.

Q. Mention clinical features of secondary adrenocortical insufficiency.

Ans. Clinical features are same as primary adrenocortical insufficiency except
- Absence of pigmentation, skin is pale (low ACTH)
- Absence of mineralocorticoid insufficiency
- Associated features of underlying cause, for example, visual field defect in pituitary tumor
- Other endocrine deficiencies of hypopituitarism
    - LH/FSH (infertility, oligomenorrhea, amenorrhea, poor libido)
    - TSH (weight gain, cold intolerance)
- Acute onset may occur due to pituitary apoplexy.

Q. How will you investigate a case of adrenocortical insufficiency?

Ans.
- Serum electrolytes: Hyponatremia (90%), hyperkalemia (65%)
- CBC: Normocytic normochromic anemia, macrocytic (associated pernicious anemia)
- Hypercalcemia: In 6% patients, mild to moderate, marked in patient with coexisting thyrotoxicosis
- Blood glucose: Low
- ECG: ST-T wave abnormalities due to electrolyte imbalance
- CXR, MT, early morning urine culture (TB)
- X-ray abdomen: Adrenal calcification in infective (TB, fungus), malignant or hemorrhagic disorders
- CT adrenal/USG: Bilateral adrenal enlargement in infective (TB, fungus), malignant, hemorrhagic or infiltrative disorder, CAH. Adrenal gland small and atrophic in autoimmune adrenalitis
- CT-guided FNAC of adrenal gland: Suspected malignant deposit in adrenal

- Autoantibody to adrenal, thyroid, gastric parietal cell, pancreatic β cell
- Plasma renin activity: Elevated, plasma aldosterone: low or low normal (mineralocorticoid deficiency)
- Basal cortisol (9 AM): May be normal in partial adrenal insufficiency, so not used to confirm or exclude adrenocortical insufficiency. Basal cortisol <140 nmol/L suggest adrenocortical insufficiency and the lower the level the more likely the diagnosis. Adrenocortical insufficiency is unlikely if basal cortisol >550 nmol/L (μg/dL × 27 = nmol/L)
- Rapid ACTH stimulation test/tetracosactide/short synacthen test: Used for diagnosis of adrenocortical insufficiency
- Plasma ACTH level: Elevated in primary adrenocortical insufficiency, inappropriately normal or low in secondary adrenocortical insufficiency
- Long synacthen test:
  - Done if ACTH is equivocal to confirm secondary adrenocortical insufficiency
  - Prolonged ACTH stimulation ↑ cortisol secretion in ACTH deficiency but not in primary adrenal disease
  - 1 mg depot ACTH IM for 3 days → in secondary adrenal insufficiency, there is progressive rise of plasma cortisol with repeated ACTH administration but in Addison disease, cortisol <700 nmol/L at 8 h after last injection.

Q. Discuss about rapid ACTH stimulation test/tetracosactide/short synacthen test.

Ans. Low cortisol that does not rise following administration of ACTH indicates decreased adrenal reserve.
- **Procedure:**
  - 250 μg $ACTH_{1-24}$/synacthen/cosyntropin IM or IV at any time of day and plasma cortisol measured at 0, 30, 60 min. 0 min also for ACTH.
  - 1 μg ACTH: More physiological stimulus to adrenal cortex and more sensitive in detection of adrenocortical insufficiency. 500 mL NS + 1 amp synacthen (250 μg) → 2 mL IV. Priming of syringe mean washout of syringe that is used to mix synacthen and NS
- **Result:** Peak plasma cortisol
  - >550 nmol/L: Normal
  - 270–550 nmol/L: Partial adrenocortical insufficiency
  - <270 nmol/L: Adrenocortical insufficiency
- **Short synacthen test in patient on glucocorticoid:** If patient is already receiving glucocorticoid, rapid ACTH stimulation test can be done first thing in the morning >12 h after last dose of glucocorticoid or treatment changed to dexamethasone that does not cross-react with plasma cortisol radioimmunoassay
- **Limitation:** Normal response does not exclude partial secondary adrenocortical insufficiency/decreased ACTH reserve.

Q. Draw a flowchart to evaluate suspected primary or secondary adrenocortical insufficiency.

Ans.

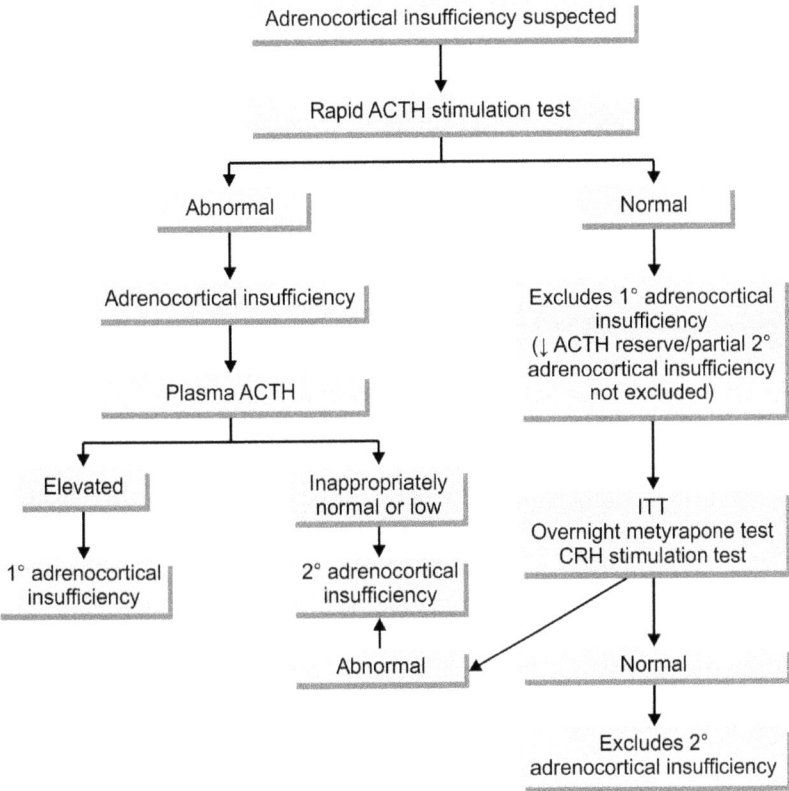

Q. Mention differences between primary and secondary adrenocortical insufficiency.

Ans.

Primary	Secondary
Primary involvement of adrenal gland	Pituitary or hypothalamic disease or exogenous glucocorticoid therapy
Autoimmune diseases are associated	Unlikely
Pigmentation present	Usually pallor
Secondary sex characters normal	Early loss of secondary sex characters, also associated with other pituitary hormone deficiency, e.g., secondary hypothyroidism
ACTH elevated	ACTH inappropriately normal or low
BP is low	BP is normal
Electrolytes ($\downarrow Na^+$, $\uparrow K^+$)	Usually normal electrolytes (absence of mineralocorticoid insufficiency)

Q. Discuss about acute adrenal crisis.

Ans.

- **Definition:** It is a medical emergency due to acute adrenocortical insufficiency
- **Causes:**
  - Following stress, for example, intercurrent disease, trauma, surgery, infection or dehydration due to vomiting or diarrhea
  - Sudden withdrawal of steroid in a patient on long term steroid
  - Following bilateral adrenalectomy or sudden destruction of pituitary gland (pituitary apoplexy)
  - Bilateral adrenal hemorrhage due to septicemia or patient on anticoagulant
  - When thyroid hormone or drugs which ↑ cortisol metabolism (rifampicin, phenytoin) or drugs which inhibit cortisol synthesis (ketoconazole, aminoglutethimide) given to patient of hypoadrenalism.
- **Clinical features:**
  - Acute onset of nausea, vomiting, abdominal pain, diarrhea
  - Unexplained fever (due to infection or hypoadrenalism per se)
  - Weakness, apathy, confusion
  - Circulatory shock with hypotension, dehydration, hyponatremia, hyperkalemia, hypoglycemia
  - Adrenal insufficiency should be considered in any patient with unexplained vascular collapse, not responding to pressor agents/inotropes.
- **Investigations:**
  - Infection screen: CBC with ESR, CXR, Urine R/M/E and culture, blood culture, CRP
  - Serum electrolytes
  - RBS
  - ECG
  - Random serum cortisol not helpful unless the level is very low (<140 nmol/L) during a period of great stress
  - Investigations to find etiology of adrenocortical insufficiency: According to suspicion.
- **Treatment:**
  - Establish IV access with a large gauze needle
  - Draw blood for serum electrolyte, glucose, CBC, Urine R/M/E and culture, blood culture and routine measurement of plasma cortisol and ACTH
  - Do not wait for laboratory results, start treatment as soon as diagnosis is suspected
  - Hydrocortisone 100 mg IV stat and 6 hourly for 24 h
  - When the patient is stable, reduce the dosage to 50 mg 6 hourly
  - When the patient can tolerate oral feeding, shift to oral replacement therapy, overlapping the first oral and last IV doses and gradual taper to maintenance therapy and add mineralocorticoid therapy as required
  - Correct volume depletion and hypoglycemia with IV fluid (NS) and glucose
  - Diagnose and treat infection and other precipitating factors

Chapter 36: Adrenocortical Insufficiency

Q. Discuss about maintenance therapy of primary adrenocortical insufficiency.

Ans.

1. **Glucocorticoid replacement:**
   - Cortisol/hydrocortisone is glucocorticoid of choice
   - Basal production rate of cortisol 8–12 mg/m^2/day, so maintenance dose of hydrocortisone is 15–25 mg/day in adults.
   - Hydrocortisone 10–15 mg on awakening and 5–10 mg in early afternoon (4–5 PM)
   - Some patients feel better with three doses daily, for example, 10-5-5 mg
   - Adverse effect: Insomnia, prevented by administering last dose in early afternoon

   Response to therapy:
   - Good appetite and sense of wellbeing guides adequacy of replacement
   - Replacement dose of glucocorticoid should be maintained at the lowest amount needed to provide the patient with a proper sense of wellbeing
   - Weakness, fatigue disappears. Anorexia and other GI symptoms resolve and weight return to normal
   - Hyperpigmentation invariably improves but may not entirely disappear
   - Signs of Cushing syndrome indicate over treatment
   - So use clinical assessment of patient wellbeing rather than biochemical criteria to assess adequacy of steroid replacement.

2. **Mineralocorticoid replacement:**
   - Fludrocortisone 0.05–0.2 mg/day orally in morning
   - Liberal salt intake
   - 10% patient can be managed with cortisol and adequate dietary Na$^+$ intake alone and do not require fludrocortisone

   Response to therapy:
   - Adequate mineralocorticoid replacement assessed by electrolyte, BP (supine and erect) and plasma renin activity
   - With adequate treatment BP is normal without orthostatic changes. Serum Na$^+$ and K$^+$ within normal range, PRA <5 ng/mL/h
   - HTN, edema, hypokalemia suggest excessive mineralocorticoid replacement.

3. **DHEA replacement:** 50 mg/day in female may improve mood and wellbeing.

Q. How will you prevent adrenal crisis in a patient with adrenocortical insufficiency?

Ans.

- **Patient education:** About the necessity of lifelong steroid therapy and need for increased dose during acute illness
- **Fever, diarrhea or intercurrent illness:**
  - ↑ Glucocorticoid dose 2–3 fold for the few days of illness
  - Do not change mineralocorticoid dose
  - Contact physician if symptoms worsen or persist for >3 days
- **Vomiting:** If unable to take drug by mouth, give parenteral hydrocortisone

- **Minor procedures under L/A (e.g., uncomplicated outpatient dental procedures) and most radiological studies:** No extra supplementation is needed
- **Moderately stressful procedures (e.g., endoscopy, angiography):** Hydrocortisone 100 mg IV just before the procedure
- **Minor surgery:** Hydrocortisone 100 mg IV/IM with premedication
- **Severe illness, for example, pneumonia:** Hydrocortisone 100 mg IV 8 hourly. Taper to maintenance level by decreasing by half every day. Adjust dose according to course of illness
- **Major surgery:**
  - Correct electrolyte, BP and hydration if necessary
  - Hydrocortisone 100 mg IV just before induction of anesthesia and 50 mg IV in recovery room and then 6 hourly for first 24 h
  - If progress is satisfactory, reduce dosage to 25 mg 6 hourly for 24 h and then taper to maintenance dosage over 3–5 day
  - Resume previous fludrocortisone dose when patient is taking oral medication
  - Maintain or ↑ hydrocortisone dosage to 200–400 mg/day if fever, hypotension or other complications occur
- **Pregnancy:**
  - Pregnancy proceeds normally in patient taking replacement therapy, but daily doses of hydrocortisone is usually increased modestly (5–10 mg/day) in last trimester
  - Fludrocortisone dose need to be increased (progesterone is a mineralocorticoid antagonist)
  - During labor, patient should be well hydrated with a saline drip and should receive hydrocortisone 50 mg IV 6 hourly until delivery, then doses can be rapidly tapered to prepregnancy level
- **Steroid card:** Patient should always carry this at all time. It should contain information regarding diagnosis, steroid dose.

Steroid card

Name of patient: _____

Address: _____

Phone: _____

Diagnosis: _____

Drug: _____

Dose: _____

Department/treating physician: _____

- I am on steroid regularly
- It is a life-saving medication
- It cannot be stopped without consultation of doctor
- In case of fever, diarrhea or other illness, dose of steroid may need to be increased 2–3 fold
- If you find me unconscious, please send me to a nearby hospital after the following treatment
  - Inj. Hydrocortisone (100 mg) 1 amp IV stat
  - Inj. NS 1,000 mL IV @30 drop/min
- **Steroid bracelet:** That has diagnosis and a reference number for central database.

CHAPTER 37

Judicious Use of Glucocorticoid

Q. Classify glucocorticoid.

Ans.
- Short to medium acting: Cortisol/hydrocortisone, cortisone, prednisolone, methylprednisolone
- Intermediate acting: Triamcinolone, fluprednisolone
- Long acting: Betamethasone, dexamethasone.

Q. Mention therapeutic use of glucocorticoid.

Ans.
- Endocrine: Replacement therapy (Addison disease, hypopituitarism, CAH), Graves ophthalmopathy
- Collagen disease: SLE, RA, polymyositis, dermatomyositis, giant cell arteritis
- Skin: Dermatitis, pemphigus
- Respiratory: Bronchial asthma, sarcoidosis, TB in special situation
- GIT: IBD, Chronic active hepatitis
- Renal: NS
- Hematological: Leukemia, lymphoma, AIHA, ITP
- CNS: Cerebral edema, MS
- Others: Septicemia, ARDS, fetal lung maturation, organ transplantation.

Q. What are the contraindications of steroid?

Ans.
- Cushing syndrome
- DM, HTN
- PUD
- CCF
- Infection
- Osteoporosis
- Psychosis
- Glaucoma.

Chapter 37: Judicious Use of Glucocorticoid

Q. Mention properties of glucocorticoids.

Ans.

Steroid	Anti-inflammatory effect	Salt retaining effect	Duration of action (h)	Equivalent oral dose
Hydrocortisone	1	1	8–12	20 mg
Prednisolone	5	0.3	12–36	5 mg
Methylprednisolone	5	0.25	12–36	4 mg
Triamcinolone	5	0	12–36	4 mg
Betamethasone	25–40	0	36–72	0.60 mg
Dexamethasone	30	0	36–72	0.75 mg

Q. What are the principles of judicious use of glucocorticoid?

Ans.

1. Do not administer glucocorticoid unless absolutely indicated or more conservative measures have failed.
2. Keep dosage and duration of administration to the minimum required for adequate treatment.
3. **Checklist prior to glucocorticoid treatment:**
   - Screen for tuberculosis with MT test or CXR
   - Screen for diabetes by blood sugar measurement
   - Evidence of HTN, cardiovascular disease or dyslipidemia (TG level)
   - Evidence of pre-existing or high risk for osteoporosis (DEXA scan)
   - Screen for cataract and glaucoma before treatment
   - H/o PUD, gastritis or esophagitis
   - H/o psychological disorders.
4. **Prophylactic measures to minimize undesirable metabolic effects of glucocorticoids:**
   - **Diet:**
     - Monitor calorie intake to prevent weight gain
     - Diabetic diet if glucose intolerant
     - Restrict sodium intake to prevent edema and minimize HTN
     - Provide supplementary potassium if necessary
   - Administer glucocorticoids with meal to prevent ulcer. Consider omeprazole 20-40 mg/day
   - **Minimize loss of bone mineral density:**
     - Adequate calcium intake 1,200 mg/day elemental calcium
     - Administer a minimum of 800–1,000 IU/day supplemental vitamin D

- Consider administering bisphosphonate prophylactically, for example, alendronate 10 mg daily or 70 mg weekly:
  - H/o low trauma fracture
  - At least 7.5 mg prednisolone or equivalent daily for ≥3 months
  - DEXA: *T* score <−1.5
- Treat hypogonadism
  ▪ Avoid prolonged bed rest that will accelerate muscle weakness and bone mineral loss
  ▪ Ambulate early after fractures
  ▪ Avoid elective surgery, if possible. Vitamin A 20,000 U daily for 1 week may improve wound healing
  ▪ Avoid activities that could cause fall or other trauma.

5. **Patient education:**
   ▪ Prepare the patient and family for possible adverse effect on mood, memory and cognitive function
   ▪ Inform the patient about side effects like weight gain, osteoporosis
   ▪ Avoid smoking and alcohol
   ▪ Dose to be increased during stress according to advice of doctor.

6. **Follow-up of patient receiving glucocorticoid:**
   ▪ **History:**
     - About mood, memory and cognitive function
     - Visual disturbance/cataract
     - Menstrual disturbance
     - Wasting and weakness of proximal thigh muscles
     - About urine test result at home weekly for glucose
   ▪ **Examination:**
     - Blood pressure
     - Body weight
     - Edema
     - Cataract and glaucoma screen: 3 months after treatment, then yearly
     - Height (serve to document degree of axial spine demineralization and compression)
   ▪ **Investigation:**
     - CBC
     - Blood sugar
     - Urine R/M/E
     - ECG
     - CXR
     - Serum electrolytes
     - Bone densitometry
     - Serum calcium

Chapter 37: Judicious Use of Glucocorticoid

Q. Discuss steroid withdrawal protocol.

Ans. Three issues exist with regard to withdrawal from steroid therapy:
- HPA axis suppression and resulting secondary adrenal insufficiency
- Possibility of worsening of underlying disease for which steroid therapy initiated.
- Steroid withdrawal syndrome: Patient encounter difficulty and even significant symptoms (lethargy, malaise, anorexia, myalgia, weight loss, postural dizziness, fever, skin desquamation) on discontinuing or decreasing steroid doses despite having demonstrably normal HPA axis.

Tapering of glucocorticoid indicated in:
- Glucocorticoid administered orally or systematically for >3 weeks.
- If patient receives frequent short course of corticosteroid (e.g. Asthma)
- If the dose is ≥7.5 mg/d prednisolone equivalent for a long period.
- If patient receives repeated doses in the evening.

Glucocorticoid must be withdrawn slowly at a rate dictated by dose, route and duration of treatment. If glucocorticoid therapy has been prolonged, it may take 6-9 months for HPA axis to recover.

Prednisolone withdrawal is done slowly in the following manner:

Prednisolone dose (mg/day)	≤3 Weeks	≥3 Weeks
≥7.5	Can stop	↓ 2.5 mg every 3–4 days ↓ Convert 5 mg prednisolone to 20 mg HC, then ↓ 2.5 mg/week to 10 mg/day ↓ After 2–3 months of HC 10 mg/day, do SST/ITT ↓ Pass (>550 nmol/L): Withdraw Fail (<550 nmol/L): Continue for another 2–3 months, then SST/ITT
5–7.5	Can stop	
<5	Can stop	

In patient receiving glucocorticoid, SST can be performed first thing in the morning with 12-24 h after last dose of glucocorticoid or treatment changed to dexamethasone that does not cross react in plasma cortisol rapid immunoassay.

Q. Write down the indication of immediate cessation (no tapering) of steroid.

Ans.
- Steroid induced psychosis
- Herpes virus induced corneal ulceration.

CHAPTER 38

Endocrine Hypertension

Q. Discuss about endocrine hypertension.

Ans. Hypertension is essential or idiopathic in most cases. 10% are secondary HTN.

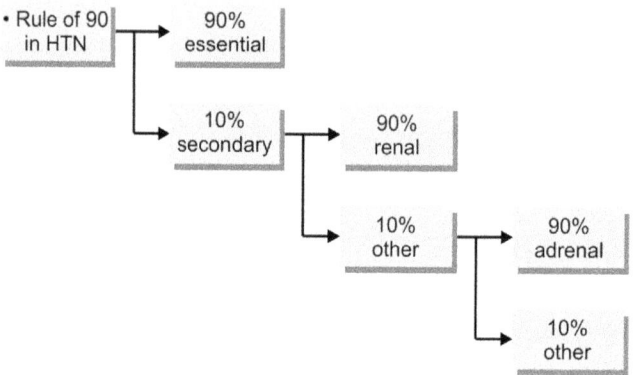

Endocrine causes of HTN: There are ≥14 endocrine disorders that cause HTN

1. **Adrenal dependent:**
   - Pheochromocytoma
   - Primary aldosteronism
   - Hyperdeoxycorticosteronism:
     - CAH (11β-hydroxylase deficiency, 17α-hydroxylase deficiency)
     - Deoxycorticosterone (DOC) producing tumor
   - Cushing syndrome
2. **Thyroid disorder:** Hypothyroidism, hyperthyroidism
3. **Parathyroid disorder:** Hyperparathyroidism
4. **Pituitary disorder:** Acromegaly, Cushing disease.

Q. What is juxtaglomerular apparatus?

Ans. Specialized tubular and vascular cells located at the vascular pole of renal corpuscle.
- Juxtaglomerular cell: Located in media of afferent arteriole. Synthesize, store and release renin

- Macula densa cell: Specialized group of distal convoluted tubular cells that act as chemoreceptors to monitor Na⁺ and Cl⁻ load in distal tubule
- Lacis cell: Function is unknown

Q. Discuss about renin angiotensin system.

Ans. Renin is an enzyme produced in juxtaglomerular apparatus of kidney secreted by
- Low renal perfusion pressure (e.g. hemorrhage, dehydration) or low Na⁺ and Cl⁻ delivery to distal tubule
- ↑ Sympathetic nervous system activity particularly in upright posture

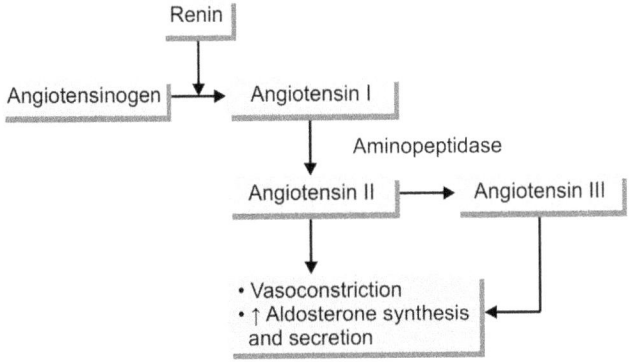

- Angiotensinogen is a globulin synthesized in liver
- Angiotensin I: Biologically inactive
- Angiotensin II: Biologically active, half-life in circulation <60 s
- ACE located in cell membrane of endothelium of lung vessels.

Q. Discuss about aldosterone.

Ans.
- Aldosterone secreted from zona glomerulosa of adrenal cortex
- Rapidly inactivated in liver and half-life is 15–20 min
- Aldosterone regulate extracellular volume and K⁺ homeostasis
- Aldosterone act on principal cells (P cells) of cortical collecting duct and cause Na⁺ reabsorption in exchange for K⁺ and H⁺, intercalated cells (I cells) concerned with acid secretion.

PRIMARY ALDOSTERONISM

Q. What is primary aldosteronism?

Ans. A group of disorders characterized by HTN, suppressed plasma renin activity, inappropriately high aldosterone production, relatively autonomous and nonsuppressible by sodium loading.
- **Causes:**
    - Aldosterone producing adenoma (APA)/Conn syndrome (35%)
    - Bilateral idiopathic hyperplasia (IHA, 60%)
    - Unilateral/primary adrenal hyperplasia (PAH)

- Aldosterone-producing adrenocortical carcinoma
- Ectopic aldosterone producing adenoma or carcinoma
- **Prevalence:** Primary aldosteronism present in 5%–10% of all patient with HTN.

Q. Mention clinical features of primary aldosteronism.

Ans.
- Age: Third to sixth decade of life
- Hypokalemia:
  - 30% patients with primary aldosteronism are not hypokalemic
  - Hypokalemia may be spontaneous or evident with addition of K^+ losing diuretic (e.g., hydrochlorothiazide, frusemide)
  - Muscle weakness, cramping or periodic paralysis
  - Polyuria, polydipsia, nocturia (hypokalemia-induced renal concentrating defect/nephrogenic DI)
- HTN: Moderate to severe, resistant to treatment, may present with hypertensive urgencies. More risk of target organ damage of heart (disproportionate LVH) and kidney
- Tetany due to $\downarrow$ in ionized Ca^{++} due to aldosterone-induced metabolic alkalosis
- Serum Na^+: High normal or slightly above upper limit of normal
- Edema is rare due to mineralocorticoid escape.

Q. When to consider testing for primary aldosteronism?

Ans.
- HTN and hypokalemia
- Resistant HTN ($\geq$3 drugs and poor BP control)
- Severe HTN (SBP $\geq$160 or DBP $\geq$100 mm Hg)
- Onset of HTN at young age (<30 years)
- Adrenal incidentaloma and HTN
- Whenever considering secondary HTN.

Q. How to detect primary aldosteronism?

Ans.

1. **Case detection testing:**

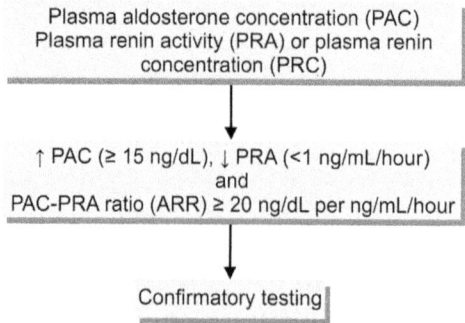

- **Protocols for measurement of aldosterone–renin ratio (ARR):**
  - Encourage the patient to liberalize (rather than restrict) sodium intake
  - Correct hypokalemia before testing
  - Withdraw drugs that markedly affect ARR for ≥6 weeks
    - Mineralocorticoid receptor antagonist, for example, spironolactone, eplerenone
    - K^+ wasting diuretics
  - Withdraw following drugs for ≥2 weeks
    - Beta-blocker, central α_2-agonist (clonidine, α-methyldopa), NSAIDs
    - ACEI, ARB, CCB
  - Control HTN with drugs that have minimal effect on ARR:
    - Non-dihydropyridine CCB, for example, verapamil, diltiazem
    - Vasodilator, for example, hydralazine
    - Alpha-blocker, for example, prazosin, doxazosin, terazosin
  - Collect blood at midmorning (8 AM–10 AM) after patient is out of bed for ≥2 h (sitting, standing or walking) and seated for 5–15 min
- PRA is suppressed (<1 ng/mL/h) in almost all patients with primary aldosteronism regardless of concurrent medication
- PRA level is undetectably low in patient taking ACEI, ARB: Primary aldosteronism is likely

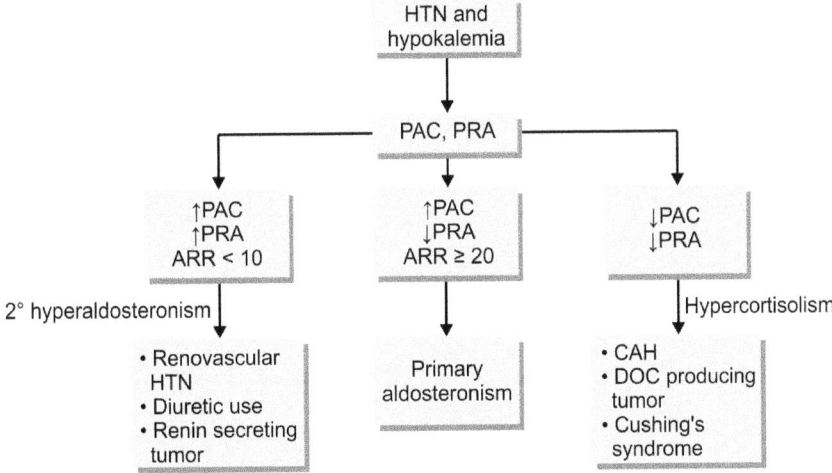

2. **Confirmatory testing:** Primary aldosteronism is confirmed by failure to suppress aldosterone level in face of sodium/volume loading.
    - **Oral sodium loading test:**
      - After HTN and hypokalemia are corrected, patient should ↑ Na^+ intake to >200 mmol/day for 3 days (supplemented with NaCl tablet if needed)
      - Serum K^+ monitored daily and K^+ supplementation given as needed
      - On the third day, 24 h urine collected for measurement of aldosterone, Na^+, creatinine (urinary Na^+ >200 meq/24 h verify adequate salt loading)

- Failure to suppress urinary aldosterone <12 μg/24 h consistent with primary hyperaldosteronism
- Sensitivity of the test 96%, specificity 93%
■ **Saline infusion test:** Patient stay in recumbent position for ≥1 before and during infusion of 2L NS IV over 4 h starting at 8 AM with BP and HR monitored throughout the test. Failure to suppress postinfusion PAC <10 ng/dL in primary aldosteronism. PAC level is <5 (normally), 5–10 ng/dL (bilateral idiopathic hyperplasia).

3. **Subtype studies and lateralization:**
    ■ **Adrenal CT:**
    - APA: Solitary unilateral hypodense (hounsfield units <10), nodule (>1 cm and <2 cm)
    - IHA: Normal on CT or nodular changes
    - Aldosterone producing adrenocortical carcinoma: >4 cm in diameter
    - Adrenal CT is not accurate in distinguishing between APA and UAH (apparent APA may represent area of hyperplasia)
    - High probability of APA: More severe HTN, more frequent hypokalemia, higher PAC (>25 ng/dL) and urinary aldosterone (>30 μg/24 h)

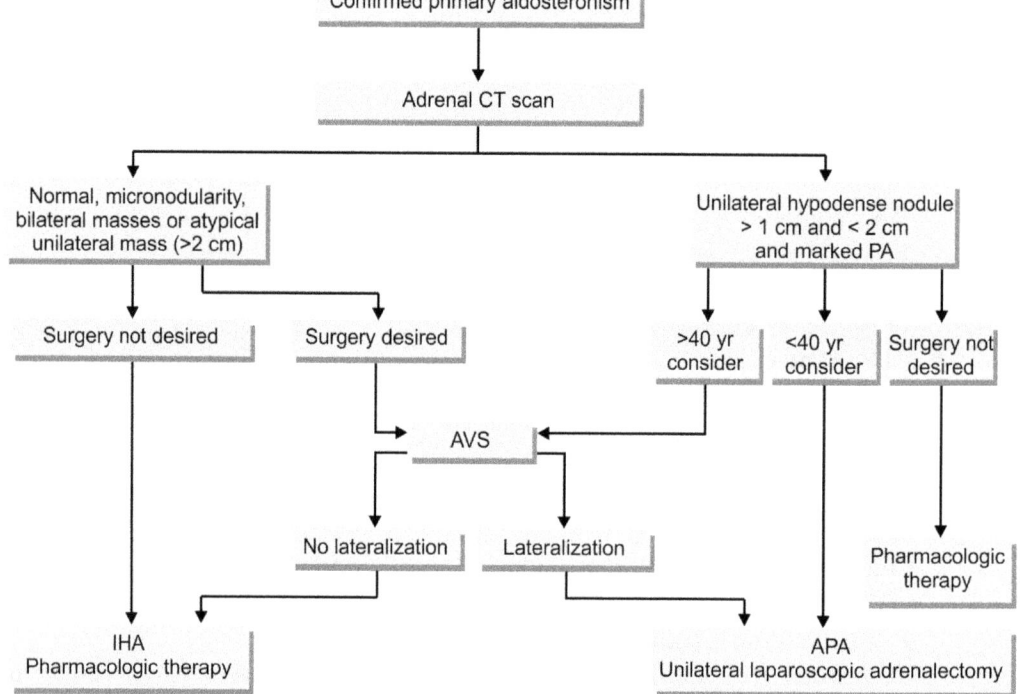

■ **Adrenal venous sampling:**
    - To distinguish between unilateral and bilateral disease in patients with PA who want surgical management for HTN

- Adrenal veins are catheterized through percutaneous femoral vein approach. Right adrenal vein is difficult to catheterize as it is short and enter IVC rather than renal vein
- Adrenal vein/IVC cortisol ratio >10:1 indicates successful adrenal vein catheterization
- Cortisol corrected aldosterone ratio >4:1 indicates unilateral aldosterone excess.

Q. **How will you treat primary aldosteronism?**

Ans.
- **Goal:** To prevent mortality and morbidity associated with HTN, hypokalemia and cardiovascular damage as excess aldosterone is associated with ↑ risk of cardiovascular disease
- **Surgical treatment of APA:**
  - Unilateral laparoscopic adrenalectomy causes normalization of hypokalemia in all, HTN is improved in all and cured in 30%–60% patients
  - HTN resolves 1–3 months postoperatively
  - Hypokalemia should be corrected with K^+ supplement or mineralocorticoid receptor antagonist preoperatively
  - PAC measured 1–2 days after surgery to ensure biochemical cure
  - Serum K^+ monitored weekly for 4 weeks as hyperkalemia may develop, often need short-term fludrocortisone
- **Pharmacological treatment:** If patient is unable or unwilling to undergo surgery
  - Na^+ restricted diet (<100 mmol Na^+/day)
  - Maintain ideal body weight
  - No smoking
  - Regular physical exercise
  - Spironolactone
    - Mineralocorticoid receptor antagonist
    - Start with 12.5–25 mg/day and ↑ to 400 mg/day as necessary to maintain serum K^+ in high-normal range. Hypokalemia respond promptly, but HTN may take 4–8 weeks to correct
    - Serum K^+ and creatinine monitored frequently in first 4–6 weeks
    - Adverse effects: Painful gynecomastia, ED, ↓ libido in men (antagonism at testosterone receptor), menstrual irregularities in women (progesterone agonist)
  - Eplerenone:
    - Competitive and selective mineralocorticoid receptor antagonist
    - Start with 25-mg BD and ↑ dose to achieve high-normal K^+ level
    - Minimal antiandrogen and progesterone agonist effect compared with spironolactone.

CHAPTER 39

Pheochromocytoma

Q. Outline the steps of biosynthesis of catecholamine.

Ans. PNMT: Phenylethanolamine N-methyltransferase. Cortisol serves as a cofactor for PNMT, that explains why epinephrine secreting tumor almost exclusively localized to adrenal medulla.

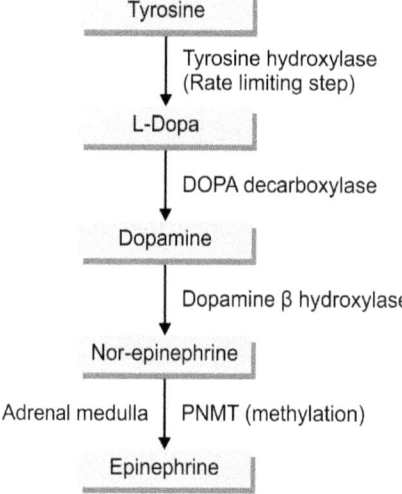

Q. Outline steps of catecholamine metabolism.

Ans.

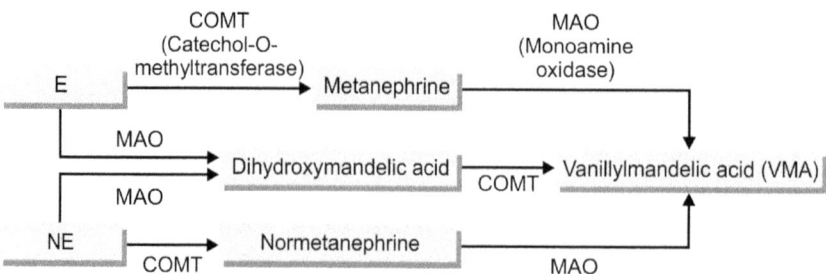

Chapter 39: Pheochromocytoma

- Epinephrine → β adrenoceptor → paroxysmal β adrenergic manifestation (anxiety, tremor, diaphoresis, tachycardia, palpitation, hyperglycemia)
- NE → α adrenoceptor → vasoconstriction → HTN
- Epinephrine and dopamine secreting tumor associated with orthostatic hypotension
- Circulating → epinephrine (100% from adrenal medulla), NE (90% from peripheral sympathetic synapse).

Q. Discuss about pheochromocytoma.

Ans.
- Catecholamine secreting tumor that arise from chromaffin cells of adrenal medulla is known as pheochromocytoma
- Account for <0.1% of all causes of hypertension
- Account for 90% of all pheochromocytoma/paraganglioma tumor in adults and 70% in children
- Equal sex distribution, common in third to fifth decade
- Rule of 10: To describe characteristics of catecholamine secreting tumor. 10% malignant, 10% extra-adrenal, 10% in children, 10% familial, 10% multiple or bilateral, 10% recur after surgical removal
- Bilateral pheochromocytoma common in genetic syndrome
- Diagnosis of pheochromocytoma is important as
  - HTN is curable with surgical removal of tumor
  - Risk of fatal hypertensive crisis
  - 10% of tumors are malignant
  - 10% familial, so diagnosis in proband results early diagnosis in other family members
- Differentiating benign and malignant tumor is difficult and mainly based on presence of metastasis
- Secretory products: Epinephrine, NE, dopamine, PTHrP (hypercalcemia), ACTH (Cushing syndrome), chromogranin A (tumor marker)
- Genetic syndrome associated with pheochromocytoma: Multiple endocrine neoplasia type-2, Von Hippel-Lindau disease, neurofibromatosis type-1, familial paraganglioma.

Q. Discuss about paraganglioma.

Ans.
- Catecholamine secreting tumor that arise from chromaffin cells of sympathetic ganglia is known as paraganglioma
- Located in abdomen along para-aortic sympathetic chain (organ of Zuckerkandl), perinephric, urinary bladder, along sympathetic chain in mediastinum and heart

- Paragangliomas are more likely to be malignant and metastasize to liver, lungs, lymph nodes and bone
- 36–60% of paragangliomas are secretory.

Q. Write down the clinical features of pheochromocytoma.

Ans.

1. **HTN:** Severe/hypertensive crisis, resistant, paroxysmal or sustained, orthostatic hypotension, shock, normotension (10%, due to adrenergic receptor desensitization called tolerance, tachyphylaxis).

2. **Spell-related signs and symptoms:**
   - Episodic anxiety and fear of impending death (angor animi)
   - Headache, diaphoresis, palpitation, HTN
   - Epigastric and chest pain, dyspnea, nausea and vomiting, pallor, tremor
   - Episodic paroxysms may occur multiple times daily or may not recur for months (due to episodic release of catecholamines)
   - Each spell lasts minutes to hours (typical: 15–20 min), symptoms usually begin abruptly and subside slowly
   - Most patients with spell usually do not have pheochromocytoma
   - Hypotension is due to chronic volume depletion due to pressure natriuresis, loss of vascular tone due to impaired sympathetic reflexes, arrhythmia or cardiac damage
   - Triggers for paroxysm:
     - Spontaneously
     - Anxiety, straining, exercise
     - Bladder catheterization, surgery
     - Drugs: Anesthetics, MAO inhibitor, TCA, sympathomimetics, decongestants
     - Pressure on abdomen: Posture change, lifting, bending, defecation, abdominal palpation
     - Foods containing tyramine (precursor of catecholamine): Tea, coffee, chocolate, Coca-Cola, milk, egg, banana, red meat, alcohol.

3. **Chronic signs and symptoms:**
   - Cold hands and feet, facial pallor (peripheral vasoconstriction)
   - Constipation
   - Weight loss
   - CCF, hypertensive retinopathy, CVA
   - Ectopic hormone secretion, for example, PTHrP, ACTH
   - Hyperglycemia, DM (α-adrenergic inhibition of insulin release).

4. **Not typical of pheochromocytoma: Flushing.**

Q. What are the complications of pheochromocytoma?

Ans.
- Cardiovascular: MI, acute LVF, DCM, arrhythmia, CCF, dissecting aortic aneurysm
- Metabolic: DM
- Neurological: Hypertensive encephalopathy, CVA.

Q. Mention differential diagnosis of pheochromocytoma type spells.

Ans.
- **Endocrine:**
  - Hypoglycemia, insulinoma
  - Postmenopausal syndrome
  - Thyrotoxicosis
- **Cardiovascular:**
  - Paroxysmal cardiac arrhythmia
  - Angina
- **Psychological:**
  - Severe anxiety and panic disorder
  - Somatoform disorder
  - Factitious
- **Pharmacological:**
  - Combination of MAOI and decongestant
  - Sympathomimetic drug ingestion
  - Illegal drug for example, cocaine
- **Others:**
  - Autonomic seizures
  - Carcinoid syndrome.

Q. Who should be screened for pheochromocytoma?

Ans.
- Hyperadrenergic spells
- Resistant HTN
- Marked lability of BP
- Onset of HTN at young age (<30 years)
- Family H/o pheochromocytoma MEN2, VHL, neurofibromatosis
- Patient develop hypertensive crisis during anesthesia, surgery
- Patient with adrenal incidentaloma.

Q. How will you investigate a case of pheochromocytoma?

Ans.

1. **Diagnosis:**
   - **24 h urinary fractionated metanephrines (metanephrine, normetanephrine):**
     – Fractionated mean free/unconjugated form
     – Most patients with elevated fractionated metanephrines do not harbor a pheochromocytoma unless it is >3 times × ULN (metanephrine >600 μg/day, normetanephrine >1,500 μg/day)
     – In patients with pheochromocytoma, catecholamine secretion is episodic but metanephrines are produced continuously, eliminates the need to catch a paroxysm
   - **24 h urinary fractionated catecholamines (E, NE) and dopamine**
   - **24 h urinary VMA (vanillylmandelic acid):**
     – Sensitivity only 63%
     – Collection of urine with acid preservative/6N HCL is needed for 24 h urinary fractionated catecholamines and dopamine assay and for 24 h urinary VMA assay only if urine stored for >5 days before analysis but not needed for 24 h urinary fractionated metanephrines assay
     – Measurements of urinary creatinine verify adequate collection
     – TCA and other drugs should be tapered and discontinued ≥2 weeks before hormonal assessment
     – Avoidance of foods containing tyramine for ≥3 days
   - **Plasma fractionated metanephrines:**
     – Most sensitive test for pheochromocytoma
     – Smoking, exercise, stressful illness (e.g., stroke, MI) may cause misleading elevation in free metanephrines
     – Diagnosis is likely if plasma metanephrine >3 times × ULN (plasma metanephrine >236 pg/mL or normetanephrine >400 pg/mL)
     – Best way for collection of blood sample: Indwelling heparin blocked IV cannula for 20 min after an overnight fast and resting supine
   - **Plasma fractionated catecholamines:**
     – Normal levels drawn during an episode strongly against the diagnosis
     – Poor overall accuracy
   - **Serum chromogranin A:** Tumor marker, increased in 80% patients with pheochromocytoma

- **Clonidine suppression test:**
  - Confirmatory test help to distinguish pheochromocytoma from false +ve increase in normetanephrine level
  - Clonidine is a central α_2 adrenergic blocker that suppress release of NE at sympathetic nerve synapses, thereby reducing circulating normetanephrine but does not affect normetanephrine secretion from pheochromocytoma
  - The patient must be fasting overnight and avoid smoking
  - An indwelling venous catheter is inserted and patient should remain recumbent
  - 30 min later blood is drawn for baseline plasma free normetanephrine
  - Clonidine .3 mg given orally, 3 h later blood is again drawn for plasma free normetanephrine
  - In normal individual, clonidine suppress plasma normetanephrine level >40% or <112 pg/mL but fail to suppress in patients with pheochromocytoma.

2. **Localization studies for pheochromocytoma:**
   - **CT/MRI of abdomen and pelvis:**
     - Hypertensive crisis may be provoked with ionic IV contrast in CT scan but less threat with nonionic contrast
     - IV gadolinium contrast in MRI does not cause hypertensive crisis
     - MRI is choice in children and pregnancy (no radiation exposure) but not suitable for claustrophobic patient and if metallic prosthesis present
     - Hounsfield unit: Marker of radiodensity in unenhanced CT scan. More fat content of a mass → less HU → more chance of benign
   - **^{123}I-MIBG (metaiodobenzylguanidine) scintigraphy:**
     Indication:
     - If abdominal imaging is negative
     - To confirm whether an extra-adrenal mass is paraganglioma or not
     - Adrenal mass >10 cm (↑ risk of malignant disease) → to screen metastasis
     - Paraganglioma → to screen additional paraganglioma
     (MIBG is a radiopharmaceutical agent, accumulate preferentially in catecholamine producing tumor.)
   - **PET scan with 18F-flurodeoxyglucose (FDG).**

3. **Genetic testing:** In bilateral or extra-adrenal paraganglioma or positive family history of pheochromocytoma/paraganglioma.

Q. Draw a flowchart to evaluate a case of suspected pheochromocytoma.
Ans.

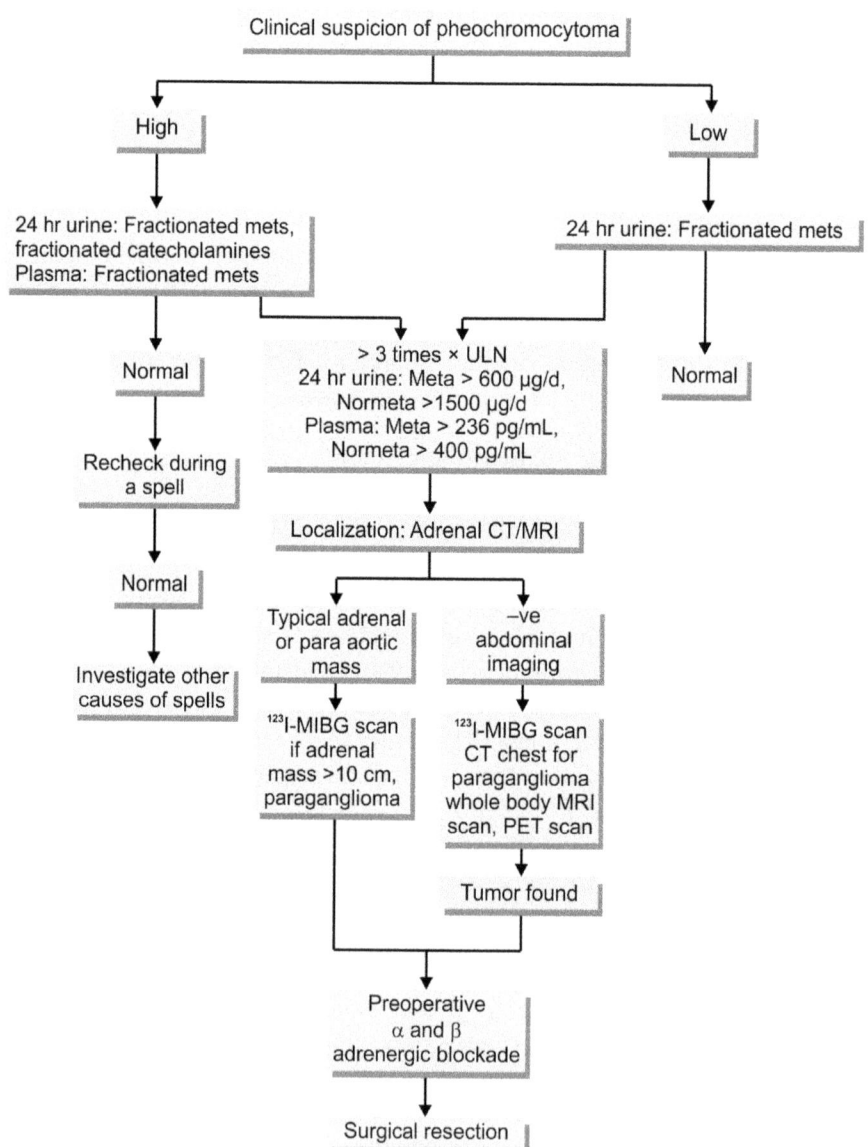

Chapter 39: Pheochromocytoma

Q. How will you differentiate different types of adrenal mass?

Ans.

Tumor type	Size	Shape	Texture	Laterality	Contrast enhancement	Unenhanced CT and % of contrast at 10 min	MRI (intensity compared with liver)	Necrosis, Hge or calcification
Cortical adenoma	≤3 cm	Round to oval with smooth margins	Homogenous	Usually unilateral	Limited	<10 HU, >50% washout	Isointense	Rare
Cortical carcinoma	>4 cm	Irregular with unclear margins	Inhomogeneous	Unilateral	Marked	>10 HU, <50% washout	Hyperintense	Common
Pheochromocytoma	>3 cm	Round to oval with smooth margins	Inhomogeneous with area of cystic degeneration	Unilateral and solitary	Marked	>10 HU, <50% washout	Hyperintense	Common
Metastasis	Variable	Irregular with unclear margins	Inhomogeneous	Often bilateral	Marked	>10 HU, <50% washout	Hyperintense	Common

Q. How will you manage a case of pheochromocytoma?

Ans.

1. **Preoperative medical management:**
   - Patient should be treated with oral antihypertensive 1–3 weeks prior to surgery to prevent intraoperative hypertensive crisis
   - Daily measurement of pulse and BP in lying, sitting and standing positions
   - Target BP: 130/80 mm Hg or less prior to surgery while avoiding symptomatic orthostasis
   - Phenoxybenzamine, long acting ($t_{1/2}$: 24 h) irreversible nonselective alpha-blocker, start with 10–20 mg daily, increase every 2–3 days (max. dose 100 mg/day) until patient become normotensive or intolerable side effects develop (orthostatic hypotension, tachycardia)
   - After adequate alpha-blocker, beta-blocker can be added to control tachycardia. Propranolol 10–40 mg 6–8 hourly
   - Beta-blocker should never be started before alpha-blocker due to risk of hypertensive crisis due to unopposed α-mediated vasoconstriction
   - Other alpha-blocker: Prazosin (max. dose 20 mg), doxazosin, terazosin (max. dose 20 mg) or CCB, for example, nicardipine can be used
   - Activities to avoid: Vigorous exercise, particularly involving bending or heavy lifting, emotional stress
   - Food containing tyramine should be avoided.

2. **Intraoperative management:**
   - Severe HTN can occur during catheterization, intubation, anesthesia or during surgery. Catecholamine release is stimulated by tumor manipulation
   - Acute hypertensive crisis before or during surgery managed with Na-nitroprusside (.3–1 µg/kg/min), phentolamine (nonselective alpha-blocker), nicardipine or GTN .6–1.2 mg/h
   - An arterial line is used to monitor BP continuously. A CV line used to monitor intravascular volume status
   - Tachyarrhythmia is treated with IV Esmolol (beta-blocker) and ventricular arrhythmia treated with lidocaine.

3. **Postoperative management:**
   - After tumor devascularization, hypotension can occur treated with volume replacement and occasional presser agent, for example, noradrenaline
   - Blood glucose should be monitored and hypoglycemia treated with IV dextrose.

4. **Follow-up:**
   - Biochemical testing repeated 2 weeks after surgery and repeated annually for life
   - BP is usually normal by the time of hospital discharge

Chapter 39: Pheochromocytoma

- Sustained HTN (25%) may be due to
  - Recurrence at surgical site
  - Multiple/bilateral tumor
  - Occult metastasis
  - Structural changes of blood vessels
  - Functional or structural renal changes.

Q. **How will you treat pheochromocytoma in pregnancy?**

Ans.
- Pheochromocytoma in pregnancy can cause death of both fetus and mother
- MRI (without gadolinium enhancement) is preferred imaging modality and ^{123}I-MIBG is contraindicated
- Treatment of hypertensive crisis is same as for nonpregnant patient except use of Na-nitroprusside
- Diagnosis in first and second trimester—surgery done
- Diagnosis in third trimester—single operation (C/S with tumor surgery)
- Spontaneous labor and delivery should be avoided.

CHAPTER 40

Congenital Adrenal Hyperplasia

Q. Define congenital adrenal hyperplasia (CAH).

Ans. A group of autosomal recessive disorders characterized by deficiency of enzymes necessary for adrenal corticosteroid biosynthesis.

Q. Mention enzyme deficiency in CAH.

Ans. There are six major types of enzyme deficiencies in CAH.
- 21α-hydroxylase: >90% of CAH
- 11β-hydroxylase: HTN (due to ↑ mineralocorticoid deoxycorticosterone, virilization)
- 17α-hydroxylase: HTN (due to ↑ mineralocorticoid deoxycorticosterone, pseudohermaphroditism in male, primary amenorrhea in female).

Q. Mention features of 21α-hydroxylase enzyme deficiency in CAH.

Ans.
- More than 90% of CAH is due to 21α-hydroxylase deficiency
- The gene that encodes 21α-hydroxylase is located on the short arm of chromosome 6
- 21α-hydroxylase deficiency results in cortisol and aldosterone deficiency. There is ACTH oversecretion due to loss of normal negative feedback inhibition that causes adrenocortical hyperplasia and accumulation of 17 hydroxyprogesterone and other steroid precursors proximal to enzymatic block that is shunted to androgen synthesis pathway
- The net result is cortisol deficiency, variable mineralocorticoid deficiency and excessive secretion of adrenal androgen
- There is correlation between severity of enzymatic detect and clinical severity of the disorder.

Chapter 40: Congenital Adrenal Hyperplasia

Q. Classify CAH.

Ans.

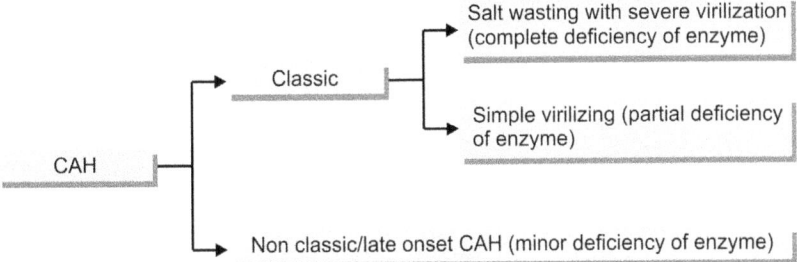

Q. Draw a flowchart of steroid biosynthesis.

Ans.

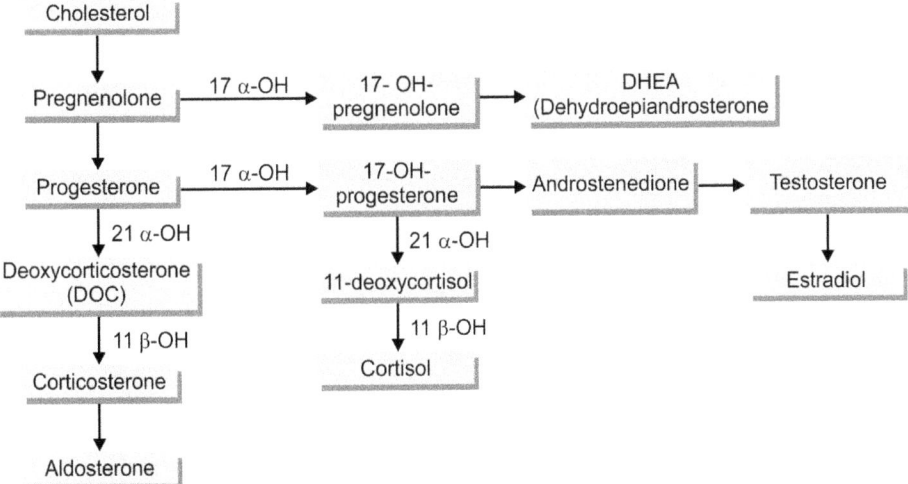

Q. Discuss features of different types of CAH.

Ans.
- **Salt wasting with severe virilization:**
  - Accounts for 80% of patients with classic CAH with complete deficiency of 21α-hydroxylase leading to impaired synthesis of both cortisol and aldosterone
  - Neonate commonly present after fifth day of life (may occur as late as 6–12 weeks) with poor feeding, vomiting, failure to thrive, hyponatremia, hyperkalemia, acidosis, dehydration, hypovolemia and shock
  - Masculinization of external genitalia of affected female fetus is more severe than simple virilizing form
- **Simple virilizing CAH:**
  - Accounts for 20% of patients with classic CAH with partial deficiency of 21α-hydroxylase leading to impaired synthesis of cortisol but retains enzymatic activity

to produce sufficient aldosterone to prevent hyponatremia/hyperkalemia under normal circumstances

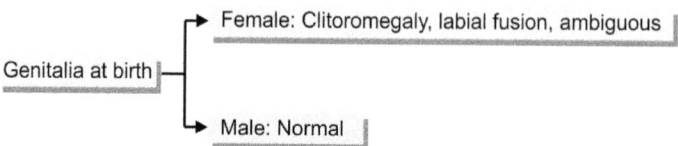

- If untreated, both sexes present in early childhood with signs of precocious pseudopuberty (sexual precocity, pubic hair, rapid height velocity, advanced bone maturation) due to androgen excess that stimulate premature epiphyseal closure leading to short final height
- **Late onset CAH:**
  - Due to minor deficiency of 21α-hydroxylase, glucocorticoid and aldosterone production is normal, but there is overproduction of androgen and 17-OH progesterone
  - Present in childhood or early adulthood with premature pubarche or a phenotype similar to PCOS (hirsutism, acne, primary/secondary amenorrhea or anovulatory infertility)
  - Some male becomes symptomatic in childhood with premature pubarche, advanced bone age with short final height.

Q. Mention differences among different types of CAH.
Ans.

Phenotype	Classic salt wasting CAH	Simple virilizing CAH	Non classic/late onset CAH
Age at diagnosis	Newborn–6 months	F: Newborn–2 years M: 2–4 years	Child to adult
Genitalia at birth	F: ambiguous M: normal	F: ambiguous M: normal	F: virilized M: normal
Aldosterone	↓	↔	↔
Renin	↑	↔/↑	↔
Cortisol	↓	↓	↔
Testosterone	↑	↑	Variably ↑
17 OHP	>5,000 ng/dL	2,500–5,000 ng/dL	500–2,500 ng/dL (ACTH stimulation)
Growth	−2 to −3 SD	−1 to −2 SD	Probably ↔

Q. How do you diagnose CAH?
Ans. CAH should be suspected by
- Patient with ambiguous genitalia who have 46, XX karyotype with uterus, ovaries on USG
- Apparent cryptorchid males

- Infant present with shock, hypoglycemia and serum chemistries compatible with adrenal insufficiency
- Males or females with signs of virilization before puberty including premature pubarche
- Investigations: Serum 17-hydroxyprogesterone (8 AM)
  - More than 800 ng/dL: Diagnostic
  - 200–800 ng/dL → 17 OHP after IV ACTH (250 μg) → >1,000 ng/dL: Diagnostic
  - Less than 200 ng/dL: Excluded
- 17 OHP measured in follicular phase of menstrual cycle as 17 OHP produced by corpus luteum can lead false positive result if measured in luteal phase. So simultaneous measurement of progesterone should be done to exclude ovulation
- Newborn screening should be done after 48 h of age
- Other investigations:
  - Basal cortisol (9 AM)
  - Serum electrolytes
  - Plasma renin
  - Serum testosterone, DHEAS
  - Serum ACTH: Grossly elevated in classic, normal in late onset CAH.

Q. Discuss the management of CAH.

Ans.

- **Goal of treatment:**
  - To replace glucocorticoid and mineralocorticoid and prevent adrenal crisis
  - To normalize adrenal androgen secretion to permit normal growth, development, bone maturation and to restore regular menses and fertility in female
  - To avoid glucocorticoid over replacement
  - ↑ Dose of glucocorticoid during stress
- **Newborn to adolescence:** Hydrocortisone 10–15 mg/m²/day orally in three divided doses
- **In postpubertal patients who have reached their final height:** Prednisolone 5–7.5 mg/day divided into two doses. One-third of total dose given on awaking (7 AM) and two third on retiring/just before going to bed (reverse treatment to suppress early morning ACTH peak and thus androgen secretion)
- **Salt loser:** Need fludrocortisone 0.05–0.2 mg/day and added dietary salts (1–3 g/day)
- **Reconstructive surgery:** Clitoral recession or clitoroplasty for markedly enlarged clitoris, vaginoplasty
- Education of patient about need for ↑ steroid during stress
- **Monitoring of hormonal therapy:**
  - Height velocity and bone age: If hydrocortisone therapy is insufficient, initial accelerated linear growth with advanced bone age and ultimate short stature due to premature epiphyseal closure. If HC therapy is excessive, growth will be suppressed

- 17 OHP, androstenedione and testosterone at 8 AM before morning dose of HC. Target concentration of 17 OHP 400–1,200 ng/dL with androstenedione and testosterone level in normal range
- Mineralocorticoid dose adjusted to keep electrolytes, BP, plasma renin activity in normal range

- **Genetic counseling:** Parents should be informed of 25% risk of recurrence in future offspring
- **Treatment of late onset CAH:**
    - Similar to PCOS
    - Hirsutism: Antiandrogen therapy
    - Ovulation induction rates with gonadotropin therapy improved after suppression of ACTH with dexamethasone 0.25–0.5 mg/day.

Q. How to manage a case of CAH in pregnancy?

Ans.
- Indication of prenatal treatment:
    - Maternal classic CAH
    - Previous child from same partner with CAH
- Aim: Prevention of virilization of affected female fetus

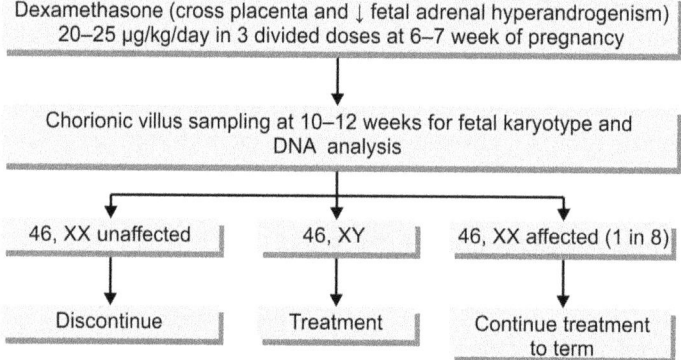

Part E: Reproductive Endocrinology

CHAPTER 41

Puberty

Q. Define puberty.

Ans. Puberty is the sequence of physical and physiological changes first developed to the point where reproduction is possible. Average age at onset of puberty is 8–13 years (female), 9–14 years (male).

Q. Mention factors that influence puberty.

Ans.
- **Historical:** Age at onset of puberty is declining at the rate of 1–3 months per decade for last several hundred years due to improved childhood nutrition and general state of health (now more due to obesity epidemic)
- **Genetic:** Age at onset of puberty is partly familial (similar in mother and daughter)
- **Ethnicity:** Black girl has earlier puberty than white due to different pattern of weight gain
- **Weight gain:** Obese girl has earlier puberty. Chronic illness and malnutrition delay puberty. Excessive exercises delay puberty, often have combination of exercise-induced amenorrhea, premature osteoporosis and disordered eating (female athletic triad).

Q. Describe endocrine changes from fetal life to puberty.

Ans.
- Pituitary gonadotropin secretion is controlled by pulses of GnRH from hypothalamus
- Control of GnRH secretion is exerted by hypothalamic pulse generator in arcuate nucleus and sensitive to feedback control from sex steroid and inhibin
- **In males:**
  - FSH → stimulates Sertoli cell to produce inhibin which feedbacks to inhibit FSH
  - LH → stimulates Leydig cell to secrete testosterone
- **In females:**
  - FSH → stimulates granulosa cell to produce estrogen and follicles to secret inhibin
  - LH → plays minor role until menarche when it triggers ovulation and later stimulate theca cells to secret androgens

- **Fetal life:** Pituitary content of gonadotropin rises at midgestation leading to increased serum concentration of FSH and LH and then gradually declines until term
- **Changes at birth:** Postnatal episodic peaks of serum gonadotropin may occur until 2 years of age (mini-puberty of infancy) followed by low serum gonadotropin in later years
- **Juvenile pause:** Serum gonadotropin concentration is low in childhood known as juvenile pause
- **Peripubertal gonadotropin increase:**
  - Within 1 year before development of physical change, GnRH secretion increases in amplitude and frequency during early hours of sleep
  - Later, peak serums FSH and LH occur more during waking hours, and in late puberty, the peaks occur at all times, eliminating diurnal variation
  - During peripubertal period, gonadotropin secretion is less sensitive to negative feedback inhibition
  - Trigger for onset of puberty is unknown, but several neurotransmitters are involved—N-Methyl-D-aspartate, GABA, metastin coded by *KISS1* gene
  - The response to GnRH administration reverses from the prepubertal FSH predominance to a higher response in LH level in peripubertal period.

Q. What is leptin?

Ans.
- Leptin is a hormone produced in adipose cells that suppress appetite through interaction with its receptor in hypothalamus.
- Leptin plays a major role in pubertal development in mice and rats.
- Genetically leptin-deficient mice do not initiate puberty.
- Leptin is a necessary component of pubertal development in human being but not a major stimulant to this development.

Q. What is adrenarche?

Ans. Secretion of adrenal androgen dehydroepiandrosterone (DHEA), dehydroepiandrosterone sulfate (DHEAS), androstenedione rises 2 years before puberty starts and persists until late puberty. This usually causes no physical changes but occasionally results in early pubic hair and acne (premature adrenarche).

Q. Mention role of hormones in pubertal growth spurt.

Ans.
- Pubertal growth spurt is due to combined effect of thyroid hormone, growth hormone, and estrogen.
- Estrogen indirectly stimulates IGF-1 production by ↑ secretion of GH.

- Estrogen also directly stimulates IGF-1 production in cartilage and stimulates maturation of chondrocytes and osteoblasts leading to epiphyseal fusion.
- In girls, pubertal growth spurt begin in early puberty and is mostly completed by menarche.
- In boys, the pubertal growth spurt occur toward the end of puberty 2 years later than girls.
- Total height attained during puberty is 28 cm in boys and 25 cm in girls.

Q. What are the physical changes associated with puberty?

Ans.

1. **Male changes:**
   - First sign of puberty: ↑ Size of testis (4 mL or more)
   - Spermarche: Appearance of spermatozoa in early morning urinary specimen at mean 13.4 years (gonadal stage 3-4 and pubic hair stage 2-4)
   - Boys achieve reproductive maturity prior to physical maturity and certainly prior to psychologic maturity
   - Secondary sexual characteristics:
     - Internal genitalia: ↑ Size of testis, seminal vesicles enlarge, secrete and begin to form fructose (main nutritional supply for spermatozoa), prostate and bulbourethral glands enlarge and secrete
     - External genitalia: Penis increases in length and width. Scrotum become pigmented and rugose
     - Voice: Larynx enlarges, vocal cord increase in length and thickness, voice breaks and becomes deeper
     - Hair growth: Beard appears, hairline on scalp recedes anterolaterally, pubic hair grows with male pattern. Hair appears in axilla, on chest and around anus. General body hair increases
     - Mental: More aggressive, active attitude, interest in opposite sex develops
     - Body conformation: Shoulders broaden and muscles enlarge
     - Skin: Sebaceous gland secretion thickens and increases (predisposing to acne).

2. **Female changes:**
   - First sign of puberty: Breast development (thelarche) followed by pubarche (development of axillary and pubic hair), then menarche (first menstrual period)
   - Breast developed by ovarian estrogen. The size and shape of the breast may be determined by genetic and nutritional factors
   - Pubic hair developed by adrenal and ovarian androgen
   - Girls acquire reproductive maturity prior to physical maturity and certainly prior to psychologic maturity.

Q. What are the stages of puberty (Marshall and Tanner stages)?

Ans.

1. **Boys:**

Stages	Genitalia	Pubic hair	Other events
G1	Prepubertal: Testes, scrotum and penis are about same size and proportion	P1: Vellus not thicker than that over abdomen (no pubic hair)	TV <4 mL
G2	Enlargement of scrotum and testes	P2: Sparse long slightly pigmented hair at the base of penis	TV: 4–8 mL Voice starts to change
G3	Lengthening of penis	P3: Darker, coarser, curlier and spread over pubes	TV: 8–10 mL Axillary hair
G4	Penis increase in length and breadth and development of glans	P4: Adult type hair but covering a smaller area	TV: 10–15 mL Upper lip hair Peak height velocity
G5	Genitalia adult in size and shape	P5: Adult type hair distributed as inverse triangle, spread to medial surface of thigh	TV: 15–25 mL Facial hair spread to checks Adult voice

2. **Girls:**

Stages	Breast	Pubic Hair	Others
G1	B1: Elevation of papilla only	P1: Vellus not thicker than that over abdomen (no pubic hair)	
G2	B2: Breast bud stage, elevation of breast and papilla	P2: Sparse long slightly pigmented hair along labia	Peak height velocity
G3	B3: Further enlargement of breast and areola	P3: Darker, coarser, curlier and spread over pubes	
G4	B4: Projection of areola and papilla to form a secondary mound on top of breast	P4: Adult type hair but covering a smaller area	Menarche
G5	B5: Mature stage—projection of papilla only and recession of areola	P5: Adult in quantity and type with inverse triangle of classic feminine distribution	

Q. Define delayed puberty.

Ans.

- Any boy of 14 years or girl of 13 years of chronological age without signs of pubertal development, that is, 2.5 SD above the mean is considered to have delayed puberty.
- By this definition .6% of healthy population have delayed puberty.
- Clinically boys are more likely to present with delayed puberty than girls.
- Some children present with delay in progression from one pubertal stage to the next for >2 years.

Q. What are the causes of delayed puberty?

Ans.

1. **Constitutional delay in growth and puberty.**

2. **Hypogonadotropic hypogonadism:** Gonadal hormone low with low level of FSH and LH.
   - **CNS disorders:** Pathology in pituitary and hypothalamus
     - Invasive: Pituitary adenoma, craniopharyngioma, meningioma
     - Infiltrative: Sarcoidosis, hemochromatosis, Langerhans histiocytosis
     - Infarction: Pituitary apoplexy
     - Infection: TB, syphilis, mycotic infections
     - Injury: Head injury, for example, RTA, battered children
     - Iatrogenic: Pituitary surgery, radiotherapy
     - Immunologic: Lymphocytic hypophysitis
     - Idiopathic
     - Isolated, for example, isolated GH deficiency
   - **Isolated gonadotropin deficiency:**
     - Kallmann syndrome
     - Gonadotropin deficiency with normal sense of smell
   - **Miscellaneous disorders:**
     - Prader-Willi syndrome
     - Laurence-Moon-Bardet-Biedl syndrome
     - Functional gonadotropin deficiency:
       - Chronic systemic disorder (respiratory, cardiac, GIT, renal)
       - Weight loss/malnutrition
       - Anorexia nervosa
       - Increased physical activity in female athletes
       - Stress (physical and psychological)
       - Hypothyroidism.

3. **Hypergonadotropic hypogonadism:** Gonadal hormone low with high level of FSH and LH.
   - **Male phenotype:**
     - Klinefelter syndrome
     - Other causes of primary testicular failure:
       - Trauma
       - Surgery
       - Chemotherapy/radiotherapy to gonads
       - Tuberculosis
       - Mumps orchitis
     - Bilateral anorchia (vanishing testes syndrome), cryptorchidism

- **Female phenotype:**
  - Turner syndrome
  - Other causes of primary ovarian failure:
    - Trauma
    - Surgery
    - Chemotherapy/radiotherapy to gonads
  - Pseudo-Turner syndrome
  - Noonan syndrome.

Q. Mention the criteria and management of constitutional delay in growth and puberty.

Ans. It is the most common cause of delayed puberty.
- **Criteria:**
  - A variation of normal
  - Males more often seek assistance
  - Patient usually has short stature but appropriate height and growth rate for bone age
  - Family history of delayed menarche or secondary sexual characteristics
  - Onset of adrenarche is delayed along with gonadarche
  - The combination of genetic short stature and constitutional delay lead to more profound short stature
  - Healthy child with no signs or symptoms of hypothalamic or pituitary lesion
  - Final height is often less than predicted
- **Management:**
  - Reassurance: Treatment is sometimes indicated in patient who have difficulty coping with their short stature or anxious/highly concerned
  - For boys 14 years or older:
    - Inj. Testosterone enanthate 50 mg IM every 28 days for 3 months. Higher dose may cause priapism
    - Low dose oxandrolone (2.5 mg/day orally) alternate to IM testosterone. It increase growth but does not stimulate GH secretion as it is not aromatized to estrogen. Growth velocity is temporarily increased but does not affect final height
  - For girls 13 years or older: Conjugated estrogen (0.3 mg) or ethinylestradiol 5–10 µg/day orally for 3 months.

Q. How will you approach to a patient with delayed puberty?

Ans.
- **History:**
  - Family history (consanguinity, age at onset of puberty in parents, familial history of delayed menarche or delayed secondary sexual characteristics)

- Pregnancy record (growth retardation/IUGR, time of delivery—at term or not, mode of delivery, any complication or difficulty during delivery, birth weight, any congenital disease)
- Rate of growth and milestones of development
- School performance
- History of childhood infection
- Previous or current systemic disease (respiratory, cardiac, GIT, renal)
- Dietary history (less intake, malabsorption)
- History of physical or psychological stress
- Any features of raised ICP (morning headache, vomiting, blurring of vision, focal seizure)

- **Examination:**
  - Height
  - Upper segment (crown to pubis)
  - Lower segment (pubis to floor)
  - Arm span (AS)
  - Weight
  - Midparental height
  - Secondary sexual characteristics (testicular volume/TV, stretched penile length/SPL, pubic hair, breast), body hair distribution, muscle mass and fat distribution
  - Any evidence of systemic disease (heart, lung, abdomen)
  - Test of olfaction, visual acuity, visual field and fundoscopy
  - Any stigmata or dysmorphism
  - Any features of raised ICP: Bradycardia, HTN, papilledema, false localizing signs (pupillary dilatation, sixth nerve palsy, hemiparesis, bilateral planter extensor)

- **Initial test:**
  - X-ray to determine bone age
  - Plasma testosterone or estradiol
  - Plasma FSH and LH (basal, post-GnRH or GnRH agonist)
  - Pelvic USG in girl: Ovarian morphology
  - USG in boys: Intra-abdominal testes

- **Further test:**
  - Pattern of pulsatile LH secretion
  - Karyotype
  - MRI brain with contrast enhancement
  - FT4, TSH, and prolactin
  - Testosterone level before and after hCG therapy may be used to indicate functional testicular tissue in boys
  - For systemic disease: CBC, urine R/M/E, ECG, RBS, CXR, LFTs, RFTs.

Q. How will you differentiate among different causes of delayed puberty?

Ans.

	Serum gonadotropins	Serum gonadal steroids	Criteria
Constitutional delay in growth and puberty	Prepubertal (low)	Low	Patient usually has short stature but appropriate height and growth rate for bone age. Both adrenarche and gonadarche are delayed
Hypogonadotropic hypogonadism	Prepubertal (low)	Low	Patient may have anosmia (Kallmann syndrome) or other associated pituitary hormone deficiency. If gonadotropin deficiency is isolated, patient has normal height and growth rate but lack pubertal growth spurt
Hypergonadotropic hypogonadism	Elevated	Low	Patient may have abnormal karyotype and stigmata of Turner syndrome or Klinefelter syndrome

CHAPTER 42

Male Hypogonadism

Q. Define male hypogonadism. Mention etiology of male hypogonadism.

Ans. Failure of testes to produce adequate amounts of testosterone, sperm or both.

Etiology of male hypogonadism:

1. **Hypogonadotropic hypogonadism/hypothalamic pituitary disorder/secondary hypogonadism:** Low testosterone with low or low normal FSH, LH (FSH, LH low or inappropriately normal in presence of low testosterone)
   - Hypopituitarism
   - Isolated LH deficiency/fertile eunuch syndrome
   - LH and FSH deficiency:
     - With normal sense of smell
     - With hyposmia or anosmia (Kallmann syndrome)
     - With complex neurologic syndrome:
       - Prader-Willi syndrome
       - Laurence-Moon-Bardet-Biedl syndromes
       - Mobius syndrome
   - Functional gonadotropin deficiency:
     - Chronic systemic illness (respiratory, cardiac, GIT, renal)
     - Weight loss/malnutrition
     - Anorexia nervosa
     - Stress: Physical/psychological
     - Excessive physical exercise
     - Cushing syndrome
     - Primary hypothyroidism
   - Hyperprolactinemia.

2. **Hypergonadotropic hypogonadism/gonadal failure/primary hypogonadism:** Low testosterone with increased FSH and LH
   - Klinefelter syndrome
   - Androgen receptor defect: Testicular feminization/androgen insensitivity syndrome (AIS)
   - Cryptorchidism

- Noonan syndrome/male turner syndrome
- Vanishing testes syndrome/bilateral anorchia
- Myotonic dystrophy
- Testicular insult:
  - Trauma, surgery
  - Chemotherapy/radiotherapy to gonads
  - Tuberculosis
  - Mumps orchitis (in patient with postpubertal mumps, 25% risk of orchitis, >50% of patient with orchitis will be infertile)
  - Hemochromatosis.

Q. Draw normal hypothalamic pituitary testicular axis.

Ans.

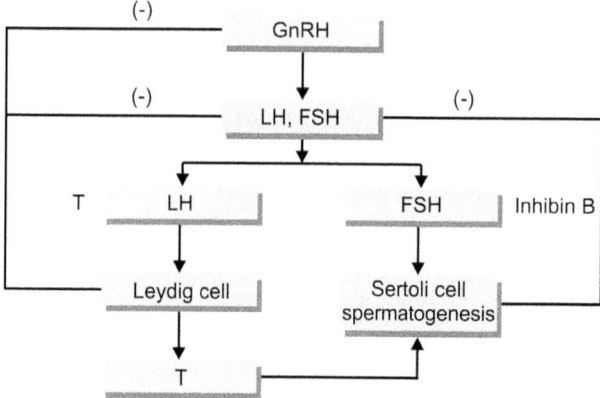

Q. Mention clinical features of androgen deficiency in male.

Ans.

1. Symptoms:

Fetal	Prepubertal	Postpubertal/adult

Ambiguous genitalia	• Delayed puberty
	• Lack of sexual interest or desire (libido)
	• Reduced morning spontaneous erections
	• Breast discomfort, gynecomastia
	• ↓ motivation and initiative
	• ↓ energy, vitality
	• No ejaculate or ejaculation (spermarche)
		• Incomplete sexual development
		• Lack of sexual interest or desire (Libido)
		• Reduced morning spontaneous erections
		• Breast discomfort, gynecomastia
		• Infertility
		• Height loss
		• Reduced shaving frequency
		• Less specific symptoms:
		  – ↓ motivation and initiative
		  – ↓ energy, vitality
		  – Feeling sad or blue, irritability
		  – Poor concentration and memory

Chapter 42: Male Hypogonadism

2. Signs:

Fetal	Prepubertal	Postpubertal/adult

• Ambiguous genitalia
• Microphallus
• Cryptorchidism
	• Reduced body and facial hair
	• Poorly developed muscle mass
	• Central fat distribution
	• High pitched voice
	• Gynecomastia
	• Delayed bone age
	• Reduced peak bone mass
	• Osteopenia or osteoporosis
	• Lack of male hair pattern growth
	• Aspermia (lack of ejaculate)
	• Severe oligozoospermia or azoospermia
	• Eunuchoidism:
	  – AS 5 cm ≥Ht (normally AS <Ht)
	  – LS >US (normally US >LS)
	  (In modified eunuchoidism, any 1 present)
	• Genitalia:
	  – TV <5 mL
	  – SPL <5 cm
	  – Lack of scrotal pigmentation and rugae
		• Loss of axillary and pubic hair
		• Gynecomastia
		• Central fat distribution/↑ body fat
		• Bone age normal, normal skeletal proportions
		• Height loss
		• Low trauma or vertebral compression fracture
		• Low BMD (osteopenia or osteoporosis)
		• Aspermia, severe oligozoospermia or azoospermia
		• Unexplained reduction of prostate size
		• Mild normocytic normochromic anemia
		• Depressed mood
		• Reduced muscle bulk and strength
		• Sparse beard, pale skin, fine facial skin wrinkles (lateral to orbits and mouth) (classic hypogonadal facies)
		• Genitalia:
		  – TV <15 mL and soft
		  – Normal SPL

AS: arm span; US: upper segment (crown to pubis); LS: lower segment (pubis to floor); TV: testicular volume; SPL: stretched penile length.

Q. How will you evaluate a male hypogonadism?

Ans.

1. **History:**
   - Age of patient
   - Birth history: Any congenital abnormality of genitalia (e.g., hypospadias, cryptorchidism, midline defects)
   - Developmental history: H/o delayed puberty or incomplete sexual development, school performance or learning disability, H/o childhood infection
   - Family history: Familial H/o delayed puberty or reproductive disorder (e.g., Young syndrome, cystic fibrosis, Kallmann syndrome)
   - Occupational history: Exposure to excessive heat or radiation
   - Medical history:
     - Hyposmia or anosmia
     - Chronic systemic illness (respiratory, cardiac, GIT, renal)
     - DM, Cushing syndrome, thyroid disorder
     - Other endocrine deficiency, for example, hypothyroidism, adrenal insufficiency

- Headache, visual field disturbance, seizure (pituitary tumor)
- Testicular insult: Trauma, surgery, chemotherapy/radiotherapy to gonads, tuberculosis, mumps orchitis, hemochromatosis, STDs
- Dietary history: Malnutrition/weight loss, anorexia nervosa
- Sexual history: Sexual interest/desire (libido), ED, difficulty in achieving orgasm/anorgasmia, anejaculation, frequency of intercourse
- Drug history: H/o chemotherapy (cytotoxic, radiation exposure, herbal preparation)
- Personal history: Smoking or alcoholism, exposure to toxin, stress (physical or psychological), excessive physical exercise, recreational drug use
- Symptoms of androgen deficiency: Reduced sharing frequency, ↓ energy, vitality.

2. **Examination:**
   - Typical hypogonadal facies: Sparse beard, pale skin, fine facial skin wrinkles (lateral to orbits and mouth)
   - Amount and distribution of body hair (e.g., pubic and axillary hair)
   - Muscle mass and fat distribution
   - Gynecomastia
   - General examination:
     - Look for evidence of systemic disease
     - Sense of smell and visual field
     - Heart/lungs/abdomen
   - Eunuchoidism: AS 5 cm ≥height, LS >US
   - Genitalia examination:
     - Penis:
       - Look for hypospadias, epispadias or chordee
       - Stretched penile length/SPL: Fully stretched dorsal penile length in flaccid state from pubopenile skin junction to tip of glans
       - In postpubertal or adult hypogonadism, SPL is normal
       - Normally, in prepuberty (SPL: 4-8 cm, width: <2 cm), In adult (SPL: 10-17 cm, width: >3 cm in flaccid state)
     - Size and consistency of testes:
       - Volume estimated with Prader orchidometer
       - Volume: $0.52 \times \text{length} \times \text{width}^2$
       - Normal volume: Prepubertal (1-4 mL), peripubertal (4-15 mL), adult (15-30 mL)
       - Consistency of testis: Normally firm. Prepubertal testicular atrophy (small and firm), postpubertal testicular atrophy (small and soft), Klinefelter syndrome (small and firm)

Chapter 42: Male Hypogonadism

- Examination of scrotum:
  - Any masses
  - Epididymis and vas deferens should be examined
  - Look for varicocele (incompetence of internal testicular vein). Patient should be examined in standing position while performing Valsalva maneuvre. Palpate the spermatic cord above the testes. A varicocele felt as impulse along the posterior portion of cord. 85% varicocele located on left side and 15% bilateral.

3. **Investigations:**
   - Serum testosterone level:
     – In normal individual frequent, rapid pulsatile changes with early morning peak at 8 AM
     – At least three blood samples taken at 20–40 min interval at morning. Testosterone may be measured in each of the samples or single-pooled sample
     – Normal serum total testosterone in male: 3.4–14 ng/mL
     – If the initial total serum testosterone is low, the measurement should be repeated 1–3 days apart to confirm
     – Testosterone deficiency should not be diagnosed during an acute or subacute illness
   - Sex hormone bonding globulin (SHBG):
     – Circulatory testosterone bound tightly to SHBG (30%), loosely to albumin (68%) or free. Bioavailable testosterone mean free testosterone and testosterone bound loosely to albumin
     – ↑ or ↓ SHBG ↑ or ↓ total testosterone, respectively, without affecting free or bioavailable testosterone
     – ↓ SHBG: Obesity, type 2 DM, hypothyroidism, acromegaly
     – ↑ SHBG: Hyperthyroidism, liver disease, estrogens
     – SHBG or free/bioavailable testosterone should be measured if clinical findings indicate hypogonadism but total testosterone level normal or borderline low and in whom alteration of SHBG is suspected
     – In primary testicular disorder (e.g., Klinefelter syndrome low testosterone and ↑ estradiol stimulate SHBG production by liver resulting in higher circulating total testosterone but low circulating free testosterone)
   - Gonadotropin/serum FSH, LH: LH and to lesser extent FSH released in pulsatile fashion, so measured in same way as testosterone (at least three blood samples or single-pooled specimen).

- Serum prolactin: Single sample is sufficient as serum PRL level is generally stable throughout the day, but patients should abstain from eating 3 h before test as protein meal stimulates PRL secretion.
- Dynamic tests:
  - hCG stimulation test:
    - Human chorionic gonadotropin (hCG) has biologic actions similar to LH
    - Diagnostic test to evaluate Leydig cell function
    - 4,000 IU IM daily for 4 days
    - Normal response: Doubling of testosterone level following last injection
    - In primary gonadal disease: Diminished response
    - In patient with Leydig cell failure secondary to pituitary or hypothalamic disease: Normal response
  - Clomiphene stimulation test:
    - Used to assess integrity of hypothalamic-pituitary axis
    - Clomiphene 100 mg daily for 7–10 days
    - Doubling of LH and 20%–50% increase in FSH indicates intact H-P axis
- Semen analysis
- Bone densitometry: As hypogonadism results in low bone mass
- Pituitary imaging/MRI: In evaluation of hypogonadotropic hypogonadism
- Karyotyping: In hypergonadotropic hypogonadism to exclude Klinefelter syndrome
- Testicular USG: Assessment of seminal vesicles and ejaculatory ducts, diagnosis of chronic epididymitis, also scrotal or testicular mass.
- Testicular biopsy: Indicated in azoospermia with normal FSH, LH, testosterone and normal testes size to distinguish between spermatogenic failure and ductal obstruction, biopsy is also used to harvest sperm for ICSI.
- Special tests:
  - Sperm cervical mucus contact test (Huner's test)
  - Sperm penetration assay
  - Acrosome reaction
  - Zona pellucida binding test
  - Motility evaluation on a postcoital test
  - DNA analysis of sperm, ovum and zygote.

Q. Draw a flowchart to evaluate androgen deficiency.

Ans.

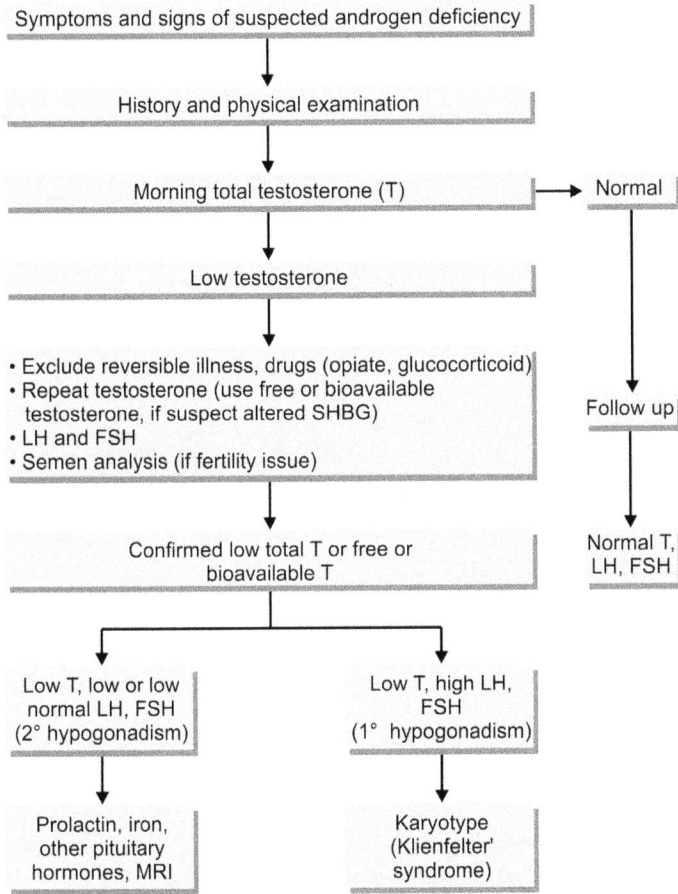

Q. Discuss about semen analysis.

Ans.

- Seminal fluid fructose (1.5-6.5 mg/mL of semen) is nutrition for sperm, derived 60% from seminal vesicle and 30% from prostate
- Normal semen analysis excludes gonadal, endocrine dysfunction and outflow obstruction
- Semen collected by masturbation after 2-7 days of sexual abstinence and examined within 1 h of collection
- A single abnormal semen analysis is not sufficient for diagnosis of testicular dysfunction. At least three samples examined over 2-3-month interval are necessary

- Fever, trauma, drug, radiation, heat exposure temporarily damages spermatogenesis
- Normal spermatogenesis: 74 ± 4 days, sperm transport: 12–21 days
- WHO criteria of normal semen analysis:

Parameter	Normal range	Abnormal values
Volume	2 mL or more	Aspermia (no ejaculate)
Total sperm count	≥40 million per ejaculate	Azoospermia (no sperm in ejaculate)
Sperm concentration	≥20 million/mL	Oligozoospermia (sperm conc. <20 million/mL of semen) Severe oligozoospermia (sperm conc. <5 million/mL of semen)
Motility	≥50% progressive motility	Asthenozoospermia (<50% motility)
Morphology	≥30% normal morphology	Teratozoospermia (<30% normal morphology)
Leukocyte	<1 million/mL	Leukocytospermia/pyospermia (leukocyte >1 million/mL)
Live sperm	>75%	Necrospermia (>25% sperm dead)
pH	7.2–7.8	
Liquefaction time	30 min	

Q. Discuss about testosterone replacement therapy.

Ans.

- **Treatment goals:**
    - Improve libido and sexual function
    - Improve energy, vitality, mood and wellbeing
    - ↑ Muscle mass and strength
    - ↑ BMD and prevent osteoporosis
    - To restore male hair growth
- Testosterone replacement does not stimulate spermatogenesis, not restore fertility in secondary hypogonadism who desire fertility (should be treated with gonadotropins, GnRH). Testosterone in these patients rather suppresses spermatogenesis by inhibiting remaining gonadotropin secretion by negative feedback mechanism
- Male with primary hypogonadism will not respond to gonadotropin or GnRH therapy
- **Indications of testosterone-replacement therapy:** Male patient with established 1 or 2°hypogonadism who is not interested in fertility or not able to achieve fertility

Chapter 42: Male Hypogonadism

- **Testosterone preparations:**

Formulation	Dose	Information
Testosterone enanthate or cypionate	150–200 mg IM every 2 weeks or 75–100 mg IM weekly	Adverse effects: • Painful IM injection • Fluctuation in mood or libido (variation in serum T level) • Cough after injection (oil vehicle microembolism)
Testosterone undecanoate	1,000 mg IM initially and at 6 weeks, then 1,000 mg IM every 10–14 weeks	
Oral testosterone undecanoate	40–80 mg with meal two or three times daily	• Poor bioavailability due to first pass hepatic metabolism • Hepatotoxicity
Testosterone gel (1%)	5–10 g gel (deliver 5–10 mg T) over shoulder or trunk	• Adverse effect: Contact transfer to others • Advice: Cover application site with shirt and washed off after 4–6 h
Transdermal testosterone patch		Adverse effect: Skin reaction
Buccal bioadhesive T tablets	Tablet applied between cheek and gum	Adverse effects: • Gum irritation and inflammation • Altered or bitter taste
Subcutaneous T pellets	2–6 pellets implanted SC every 3–6 months	Adverse effect: Bleeding, infection

- **Monitoring during testosterone treatment:** At baseline, after 3-6 months and then yearly

Parameter	Further management
Symptoms and sign of androgen deficiency	• Continue treatment in men with clinical improvement and no adverse effects • Consider discontinuing treatment in men if no clinical improvement • Men at high risk of fracture, BMD before treatment, for men with osteoporosis or low trauma fracture BMD after 1–2 years • Institute appropriate treatment for men with osteoporosis including calcium and Vitamin D
Serum testosterone	• Check serum T level to adjust dose or dosing interval to achieve serum T level in midnormal range • Testosterone ester injection: After 3–6 months, measure midway between injections or just before the next injection • Oral T undecanoate: After 1 week, at 3–5 h after oral dose • T gel: After 2 weeks, at any time after application

(Contd...)

(Contd...)

Parameter	Further management
Hematocrit	• If hematocrit >50% (risk of hypercoagulability): Stop or reduce dosage of T until hematocrit declines to normal and reinitiate T at lower dosage • Investigate for hypoxic condition, e.g., obstructive sleep apnea, chronic lung disease
DRE, PSA level and IPSS in men >40 years (IPSS: International prostate symptom score)	Urologic evaluation if any of the following: • Palpable abnormality (nodule or induration) on DRE • PSA >4 ng/mL (>3 ng/mL in men with first degree relative of prostate cancer) • PSA ↑ >1.4 ng/mL within 12-month period • Severe LUTS with BPH as indicated by IPSS score >19
Obstructive sleep apnea	A sleep study should be done if symptoms are present
Fasting lipid profile	Slight decrease in HDL cholesterol
Formulation specific adverse effects	

- **Adverse effects of testosterone replacement therapy:**
    - Erythrocytosis/polycythemia
    - Prostate growth/BPH: It is unlikely that T ↑ risk of developing prostate cancer but promote growth of existing cancer
    - Induction or worsening of obstructive sleep apnea
    - Reduced sperm production and fertility
    - Acne and oily skin
    - Male pattern balding
    - Gynecomastia
    - Growth of breast cancer
    - Cardiovascular disease: ↓ HDL
    - Hepatotoxicity: With oral testosterone
    - Fluid retention: In patient with CCF or liver cirrhosis
    - Formulation specific adverse effects
- **Contraindication of T replacement:**
    - **Absolute:**
        - Prostate cancer
        - Breast cancer
    - **Relative:**
        - BPH
        - Polycythemia
        - Obstructive sleep apnea
        - Uncontrolled CCF.

CHAPTER 43

Male Infertility

Q. Define infertility.

Ans. Inability of sexually active couple to conceive despite 1 year of unprotected intercourse (at least twice weekly).
- **Sterility:** Intrinsic inability to achieve pregnancy, whereas infertility implies a decrease in the ability to conceive and is synonymous with subfertility
- **Pituitary infertility:** The couple who have never conceived
- **Secondary infertility:** The couple who have conceived at least once in the past
- **Fecundity:** Probability of achieving a live birth in 1 menstrual cycle
- **Fecundability:** Likelihood of conception per month of exposure.

Q. Enumerate the causes of male infertility.

Ans. 15% of couple in reproductive age group is infertile. Among all causes of infertility, male factor 30%, female factor 45%, couple factor 25%, unexplained 15–20%.

1. **Hypogonadism:**
   - **Hypergonadotropic hypogonadism:**
     – Klinefelter syndrome
     – Cryptorchidism
     – Testicular insult:
       • Trauma
       • Surgery
       • Chemotherapy/radiotherapy to gonads
       • Tuberculosis
       • Mumps orchitis
       • Hemochromatosis
   - **Hypogonadotropic hypogonadism:**
     – Hypothalamic pituitary disorder/hypopituitarism
     – Kallmann syndrome
     – Hyperprolactinemia.

2. **Genital tract abnormalities:**
   - Congenital bilateral absence of vas deferens
   - Ductal obstruction: Congenital, postinfectious fibrosis (gonorrhea, chlamydia)
   - Varicocele
   - Prostatic disease
   - Anatomic defects of penis
   - Immotile cilia/Kartagener syndrome
   - Cystic fibrosis
   - Young syndrome.

3. **Systemic illness:**
   - **Endocrine:**
     - Hypothalamic pituitary disorder
     - Hyperprolactinemia
     - Hyperthyroidism
     - Hypothyroidism
     - Adrenal insufficiency
     - Congenital adrenal hyperplasia
   - **Chronic debilitating disease.**

4. **Sexual dysfunction:**
   - Erectile dysfunction
   - Retrograde ejaculation (autonomic neuropathy, prostatectomy, bladder neck surgery)
   - Decreased libido
   - Poor coital technique.

5. **Drugs:** Antimetabolites, corticosteroid, marijuana, sulfasalazine.

6. **Idiopathic.**

Q. **How will you evaluate male infertility?**

Ans.

1. **History:**
   - Age of the patient
   - Birth history: Any congenital abnormalities of genitalia, for example, hypospadias, cryptorchidism, midline defects
   - Development history: H/o delayed puberty or incomplete sexual development, H/o childhood infection
   - Occupational history: Exposure to excessive heat, radiation, toxic chemicals, for example, pesticides

- Fertility history:
  - History of previous marriage and proven fertility
  - Previous investigations or treatment for infertility
- Medical history:
  - Hyposmia or anosmia (Kallmann syndrome)
  - Chronic systemic illness (respiratory, cardiac, GIT, renal)
  - DM, adrenal disorder, thyroid disorder
  - Testicular insult: Trauma, surgery, TB, mumps orchitis
  - STD or genitourinary tract infection, for example, prostatitis
  - Surgical procedure involving inguinal and scrotal areas, for example, vasectomy, herniorrhaphy
  - Autonomic neuropathy, for example, complication of DM
  - Spinal cord injury or disease
- Sexual history:
  - Sexual interest or desire (libido)
  - Erectile dysfunction
  - Relation of sex with time of cycle
  - Details regarding coitus including erection, penetration, orgasm at right time, ejaculation, any partner experience discomfort or lack of satisfaction, use of lubricants
- Drug history:
  - H/o chemotherapy/cytotoxic drug
  - Radiation exposure
  - Herbal preparation
  - Drugs that causes hyperprolactinemia
- Personal history: Smoking and alcoholism, exposure to toxin, recreational drug use
- Symptoms of androgen deficiency: Reduced sharing frequency, ↓ energy, vitality.

2. **Examination:**
   - Typical hypogonadal facies: Sparse beard, pale skin, fine facial skin wrinkles (lateral to orbits and mouth)
   - Amount and distribution of body hair (e.g., pubic and axillary hair)
   - Muscle mass and fat distribution
   - Gynecomastia
   - General examination:
     - Look for evidence of systemic disease
     - Sense of smell and visual field
     - Heart/lungs/abdomen
   - Eunuchoidism: AS 5 cm ≥height, LS >US

- Genitalia examination:
  - Penis:
    - Look for hypospadias, epispadias or chordee
    - Stretched penile length/SPL: Fully stretched dorsal penile length in flaccid state from pubopenile skin junction to tip of glans
    - In postpubertal or adult hypogonadism, SPL is normal
    - Normally, in prepuberty (SPL: 4–8 cm, width: <2 cm), in adult (SPL: 10–17 cm, width: >3 cm in flaccid state)
  - Size and consistency of testes:
    - Volume estimated with Prader orchidometer
    - Volume: $0.52 \times \text{length} \times \text{width}^2$
    - Normal volume: Prepubertal (1–4 mL), peripubertal (4–15 mL), adult (15–30 mL)
    - Consistency of testis: Normally firm. Prepubertal testicular atrophy (small and firm), postpubertal testicular atrophy (small and soft), Klinefelter syndrome (small and firm)
  - Examination of scrotum:
    - Any masses
    - Epididymis and vas deferens should be examined
    - Look for varicocele (incompetence of internal testicular vein). Patient should be examined in standing position while performing Valsalva maneuvre. Palpate the spermatic cord above the testes. A varicocele felt as impulse along the posterior portion of cord. 85% varicocele located on left side and 15% bilateral.

3. **Investigations:**
   - Serum testosterone level
   - Sex hormone bonding globulin (SHBG)
   - Gonadotropin/serum FSH, LH
   - Serum prolactin
   - Dynamic tests:
     - hCG stimulation test
     - Clomiphene stimulation test
   - Semen analysis
   - Pituitary imaging/MRI
   - Karyotyping
   - Testicular USG
   - Testicular biopsy

- Special tests:
  - Sperm cervical mucus contact test (Huner's test)
  - Sperm penetration assay
  - Acrosome reaction
  - Zona pellucida binding test
  - Motility evaluation on a post coital test
  - DNA analysis of sperm, ovum and zygote.

4. **Treatment:**

- **Endocrine disorder:** Treatment of hyperthyroidism, hypothyroidism, adrenal insufficiency and CAH generally restores fertility
- **Hypogonadotropic hypogonadism:**
  - Human chorionic gonadotropin (hCG) 2,000-IU IM three times per week to maintain serum T within normal range for 6–12 months
  - If sperm do not appear in ejaculate, add FSH 75-IU IM three times per week for additional 6–12 months or longer
  - Sperm count following such therapy usually does not exceed 10 million/ml but still allow impregnation
  - GnRH administered in pulses every 2 h by programmable infusion pump for 6–12 months, no benefit over exogenous gonadotropin. So now not available in USA
- **Ductal obstruction:** Localized obstruction of vas deferens treated with vasovasostomy result in successful pregnancy in 40%–50% cases within 2 years
- **Genital tract infections:**
  - Acute prostatitis: Daily sitz bath, prostatic massage, antibiotic (doxycycline, ciprofloxacin for 14 days)
  - Chronic prostatitis: Ciprofloxacin 500 mg twice daily for 4 weeks
  - Acute epididymitis: Injection of local anesthetic into spermatic cord just above the testicle plus antibiotic therapy
  - Leukospermia: 14 days course of antibiotic
- **Varicocele:** Varicocele with oligospermia is indication for treatment. Surgical ligation of incompetent spermatic vein or radiographic embolization of veins with 50% success rate
- **Retrograde ejaculation:** Phenyl-propanolamine 15 mg orally twice daily. Sperm recovered from bladder following masturbation for IUI
- **Antibodies to sperm:** Prednisolone 40–60 mg/day for several months. IUI with washed spermatozoa can be done also.

Q. Draw a flowchart to evaluate male infertility.
Ans.

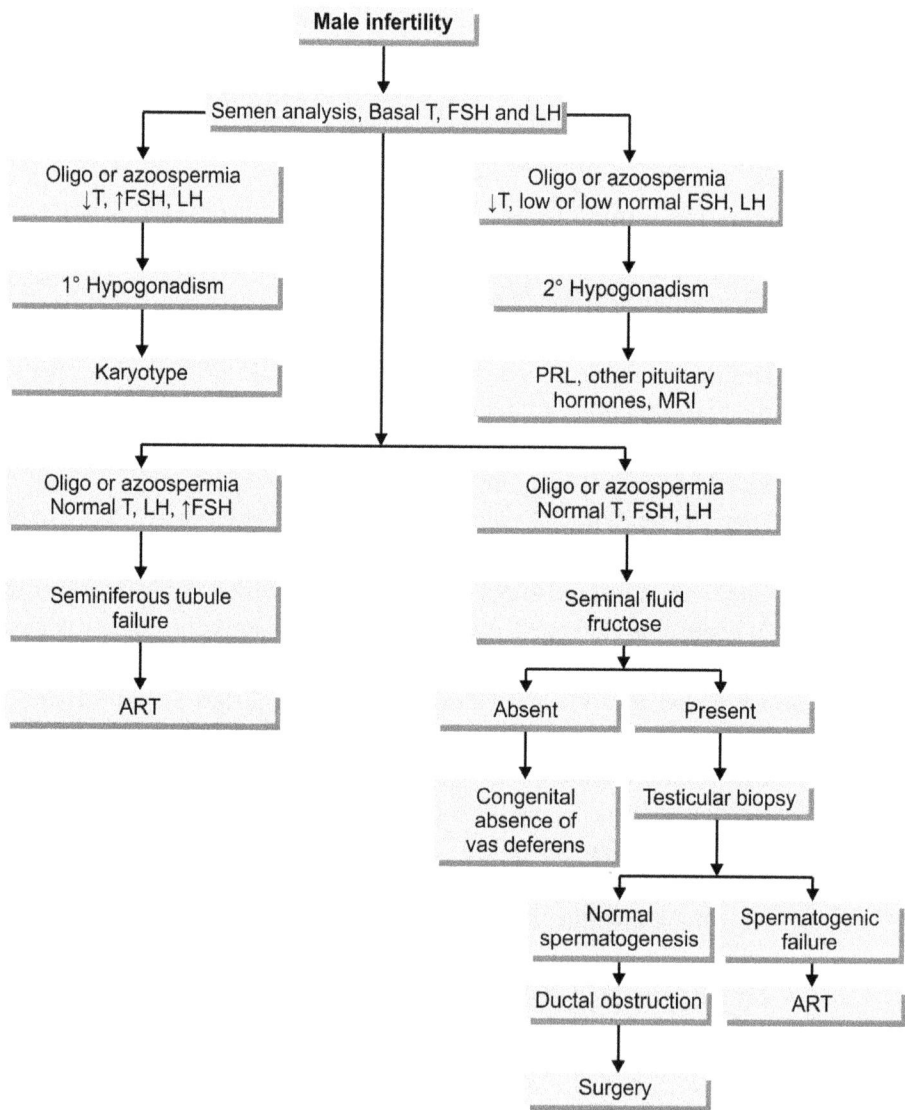

Q. Discuss about Klinefelter syndrome/seminiferous tubule dysgenesis/47, XXY.

Ans.
- Most common genetic cause of male hypogonadism occurring 1 in 600 male births
- **Pathophysiology:**
    - A male with an extra X chromosome
    - The individual is phenotypically male but chromosomal pattern is 47, XXY (90%)
    - Remaining 10% are mosaic (47, XXY/46, XY)
    - The chromosomal defect is expressed mainly during puberty. As the gonadotropins increase, the seminiferous tubule do not enlarge rather undergo fibrosis and hyalinization which results in small firm testes. Obliteration of seminiferous tubule results in azoospermia
    - Only 25% individual with Klinefelter syndrome diagnosed during life and <10% in childhood
- **Clinical features:** Klinefelter syndrome usually not diagnosed before puberty
    - Gynecomastia (>50%)
    - Signs of androgen deficiency, for example, diminished facial and body hair, poor muscular development, decreased libido, impotence
    - Small, firm testes (<4 mL)
    - Azoospermia, infertility
    - Learning disabilities, personality and behavioral disorder
    - Tall stature (androgen deficiency → lack of epiphyseal closure)
    - Disproportionate growth of legs. LS >US but AS <Ht (modified eunuchoidism)
    - Osteoporosis
    - Associated medical disorder: Chronic pulmonary disease (emphysema, chronic bronchitis), glucose intolerance/type 2 DM, primary hypothyroidism, Hodgkin lymphoma, mitral valve prolapse, 20-fold increased risk of breast cancer
- **Investigations:**
    - Serum T level: Low normal to low
    - Serum FSH and LH: Elevated
    - Elevated estradiol and SHBG
    - Semen analysis: Azoospermia
    - Buccal smear: Barr body present
    - Karyotyping of peripheral blood lymphocyte: 47, XXY karyotype. Occasionally performed of skin fibroblast or testis tissue if mosaicism is suspected
    - Testicular biopsy: Hyalinization and fibrosis of seminiferous tubule, absent or severely deficient spermatogenesis and pseudoadenomatous clumping of Leydig cell. Biopsy is also used to harvest sperm for ICSI
    - Bone densiometry: Osteoporosis
- **Treatment:**
    - Androgen deficiency should be treated with T replacement
    - If gynecomastia does not resolve with T, surgical reduction of gynecomastia

- Fertility: ICSI with sperm retrieved surgically from testes (TESE) used with some success (20–30%). Couple should be counseled about increased risk of chromosomal abnormality in offspring
- Psychological counseling
- **Prognosis:** Life expectancy is reduced by about 2.1 years.

Q. **Discuss about Noonan syndrome/male Turner syndrome.**

Ans. Autosomal dominant disorder characterized by phenotypic and genotypic males with many of the physical stigmas of classic Turner syndrome.
- **Pathology:** Reduced seminiferous tubular size with or without sclerosis, diminished or absent germ cells with Leydig cell hyperplasia
- **Clinical features:**
  - Short stature
  - Webbed neck, hypertelorism, cubitus valgus
  - Congenital cardiac abnormalities involving right side of heart in contrast to patient with Turner syndrome
  - Cryptorchidism is frequently present. Although some affected individuals are fertile with normal testes, most have small testes and mild-to-moderate hypogonadism
- **Investigations:**
  - Serum T: Low or low normal
  - Serum gonadotropins: High
  - Karyotype: Normal (46, XY)
- **Treatment:** If the patient is hypogonadal, androgen replacement therapy is indicated.

Q. **Discuss about Kallmann syndrome.**

Ans. It is the most common genetic form of isolated gonadotropin deficiency/idiopathic hypogonadotropic hypogonadism (IHH). Male:Female = 4–5:1.
- **Pathology:**
  - Hypoplasia or aplasia of olfactory lobes and bulb
  - Failed migration of GnRH containing neurons from olfactory placode to medial basal hypothalamus
- **Inheritance:**
  - Sporadic or familial cases
  - X linked recessive: Mutation of KAL_1 gene which codes for anosmin
  - Autosomal dominant: Mutation of $FGFR_1$ gene (fibroblast growth factor receptor 1)
  - Autosomal recessive
- **Clinical features:**
  - Hyposmia or anosmia. Patient may not notice that he has no sense of smell, although olfactory testing reveals the finding
  - Absent or delayed puberty
  - In infancy: Micropenis, cryptorchidism
  - Incomplete sexual maturation, androgen deficiency with eunuchoidism

- Associated disorder: Cleft lip or palate, sensorineural defect, renal agenesis, mirror hand movements
- **Diagnosis:**
  - Low T, FSH, LH level, rest of pituitary hormones normal
  - MRI: Aplasia or hypoplasia of olfactory bulbs
  - Ability of exogenous pulsatile GnRH treatment to restore normal gonadotropin secretion and testis function
- **Treatment:**
  - T replacement therapy
  - Fertility: Pulsatile GnRH treatment.

Q. Discuss about Prader–Willi syndrome.

Ans. Autosomal dominant disorder due to deletion or translocation of chromosomal 15 derived from father (genomic imprinting). If the abnormality in this area derives from mother, Angelman syndrome result.
- **Clinical features:**
  - Hypotonia
  - Small hands and feet (acromicria)
  - Developmental delay
  - Short stature
  - Poor feeding in infancy but insatiable hunger later leading to remarkable obesity, characteristics facies with almond-shaped eyes
  - Delayed puberty
  - Hypogonadotropic hypogonadism
  - Glucose intolerance
  - Learning disability
- **Treatment:**
  - Behavioral modification
  - GH therapy improves body composition and muscle strength.

Q. Discuss about Laurence–Moon–Bardet–Biedl syndrome.

Ans. Autosomal recessive disorder. Bardet–Biedl syndrome is linked to defect in basal body of ciliated cells.
- **Clinical features:**
  - Obesity
  - Short stature
  - Mental retardation
  - Polydactyly
  - Delayed puberty
  - Spastic paraplegia
  - Renal dysplasia
  - Retinitis pigmentosa
  - Hypogonadotropic hypogonadism.

CHAPTER 44

Gynecomastia

Q. Define gynecomastia.

Ans. Enlargement of male breast caused by proliferation of glandular breast tissue.

Q. Mention the causes of gynecomastia.

Ans.
- **Physiological:**
  - Neonatal: Occur in 60–90% of neonatal boys due to exposure to maternal estrogen in utero, resolves within several weeks after delivery
  - Pubertal: 70% of pubertal males due to transient increase in estrogen to androgen concentration
  - Senile obesity: Increased peripheral aromatase activity
- **Drugs:** Spironolactone, digoxin, cimetidine, isoniazid, estrogen therapy for carcinoma prostate, alcohol (possible mechanism: Estrogen-containing drugs, reduced androgen production, androgen receptor blocker)
- **Hypogonadism:**
  - Hypergonadotropic hypogonadism:
    - Klinefelter syndrome
    - Cryptorchidism
    - Testicular insult: Trauma, surgery, chemotherapy/radiotherapy to gonads, tuberculosis, mumps orchitis, hemochromatosis
  - Hypogonadotropic hypogonadism:
    - Hypothalamic pituitary disorder/hypopituitarism
    - Kallmann syndrome
    - Hyperprolactinemia
- **Endocrine:** Thyrotoxicosis, acromegaly, Cushing syndrome
- **Tumors:**
  - Estrogen secreting tumor: Adrenal carcinoma, testicular malignancy
  - hCG secreting tumor: Germ cell tumor, bronchogenic carcinoma, HCC
- **Systemic illness:** CLD, CKD, recovery from malnourishment (refeeding gynecomastia)
- **Idiopathic (25% of all cases).**

Chapter 44: Gynecomastia

Q. Mention the causes of painful gynecomastia.

Ans.
- Puberty
- Drugs (e.g. spironolactone, cimetidine, digoxin).

Q. How will you evaluate and treat a patient of gynecomastia?

Ans.

1. **History:**
   - Age of patient
   - Unilateral or bilateral
   - Duration and progression of gynecomastia
   - Associated breast pain, tenderness or galactorrhea
   - Drug history: Prescription and Over-the-counter (OTC) medicines, substance abuse or recreational drugs, herbal drugs, alcohol
   - Symptoms of hypogonadism: ↓ libido, ED, reduced shaving frequency
   - Symptoms of systemic illness: CLD, CKD
   - Symptoms of malignancy or endocrine disorder, for example, thyroid, GH, cortisol excess
   - H/o recovery from malnourishment.

2. **Examination:**
   - Breasts:
     - Unilateral or bilateral
     - Palpate the glandular tissue first with palm, then with thumb and index finger. Feeling of firm, rubbery and freely mobile disc under nipple and areola in gynecomastia but not in obesity (lipomastia in obese)
     - Tender or nontender
     - Any discharge from nipple
   - Testicular palpation: Measure TV and consistency, exclude tumor
   - 2° sex characteristics
   - Look for evidence of systemic illness: CLD, CKD, endocrine disorder.

3. **Investigations:** After exclusion of pubertal and drug induced gynecomastia
   - Serum testosterone
   - Estradiol
   - FSH, LH, Prolactin, hCG
   - LFTS, RFTS
   - Additional investigations:
     - If testicular tumor suspected: Testicular USG
     - If breast malignancy suspected: Mammography, FNAC/tissue biopsy
     - If bronchial carcinoma suspected: CXR, CT guided FNAC
     - Other investigation according to clinical suspicion, for example, karyotype in Klinefelter syndrome.

4. **Treatment:**
   - Pubertal gynecomastia usually regress spontaneously in 1-2 years
   - Treat underlying cause, stop offending drug
   - Reassurance in majority of idiopathic cases, often resolves spontaneously
   - Medical treatment: Antiestrogen or selective estrogen receptor modulator, for example, tamoxifen or raloxifene
   - Surgical treatment: Reduction mammoplasty for cosmetic reason in patient with long standing gynecomastia
   - Radiologic treatment: Prophylactic low dose breast irradiation for prostate cancer before initiation of antiandrogen.

Q. Draw a flowchart to evaluate gynecomastia.

Ans.

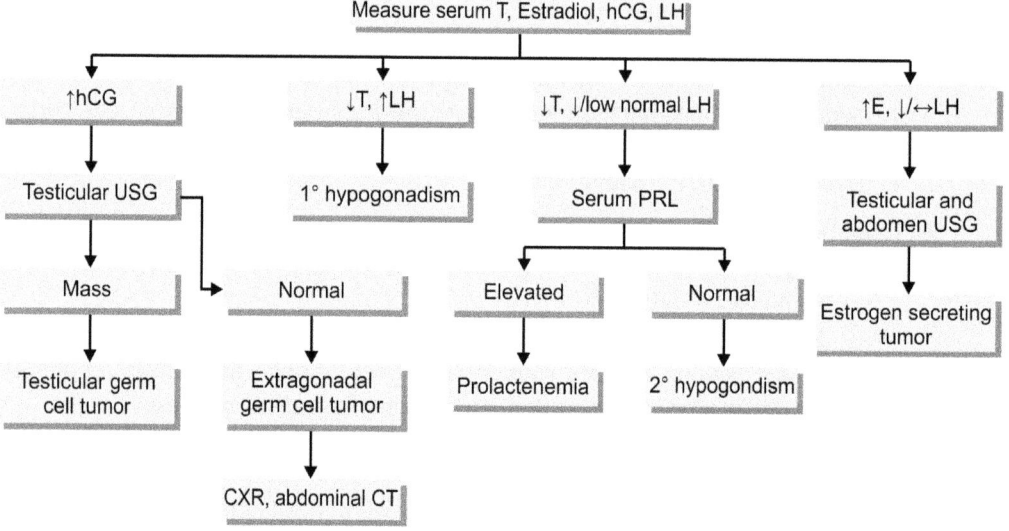

CHAPTER 45

Erectile Dysfunction

Q. Define erectile dysfunction and sexual dysfunction.

Ans.
- **Erectile dysfunction/impotence:** Inability to achieve or maintain an erection of sufficient duration and firmness for satisfactory sexual intercourse in >25% of attempts
- **Sexual dysfunction:** More general term that includes disturbances of libido, orgasm or ejaculation in addition to impotence.

Q. Discuss physiology of erectile function.

Ans.
- Erectile dysfunction (ED) affects approximately 10% of males and ↑ with age but some degree of ED is present in about 50% of men between ages 40 and 70 years.
- ED in diabetic men is about 35–50% overall.
- Erectile response is result of coordinate interaction of nerves, smooth muscle of penile erectile tissue (corpora cavernosa and spongiosum), pelvic muscles and blood vessels.
- It is initiated by psychogenic, visual or sensory stimuli that are modulated in limbic system and transmitted down the spinal cord to autonomic nervous system outflow of penile tissue.
- Penile erectile tissues consist of paired corpora cavernosa on the dorsum of penis and corpus spongiosum. These are surrounded by fibrous tissue known as tunica albuginea.
- Erection is a parasympathetic response that occurs when blood flow to penile erectile tissue increases due to cavernosal arterial vasodilation. As the corporeal sinuses fill with blood, the draining venules are compressed against tunica albuginea, so venous outflow is impaired. This results in distension, engorgement and rigidity of penis that constitute erection.
- Corporeal vasodilatation is mediated by NO, produced both in parasympathetic nerve terminal and vascular endothelium. NO activate guanylate cylase, thereby ↑ cGMP that cause smooth muscle relaxation.
- Detumescence occurs after inactivation of cGMP by phosphodiesterase 5, resulting in smooth muscle contraction and vasoconstriction.
- Ejaculation is mediated by sympathetic nervous system.

Q. Mention pathophysiological basis of erectile dysfunction.

Ans. Erectile dysfunction occurs due to
- Neurological damage
- Arterial insufficiency
- Venous incompetence
- Androgen deficiency
- Penile abnormalities.

Q. Mention etiology of erectile dysfunction.

Ans.
- **Psychological (20%):**
  - Anxiety about sexual performance
  - Depression
  - Psychiatric illness
- **Drugs (25%):**
  - Alcohol (It provokes the desire but takes away the performance!)
  - Antihypertensive: Thiazide diuretics, beta-blocker, methyldopa
  - Antidepressants: TCA, monoamine oxidase inhibitor (MAOI)
  - Antipsychotic: Phenothiazine, haloperidol
  - Drugs of abuse: Marijuana, heroin
  - Hormones: Estrogen, antiandrogen
- **Endocrine (20%):**
  - Hypogonadism
  - Hyperprolactinemia
  - DM
  - Thyroid dysfunction
- **Vascular:** PVD, pelvic trauma
- **Neurological:** Spinal cord disorder, autonomic neuropathy, multiple sclerosis
- **Systemic illness:** Cardiac disease, renal failure, liver disease
- **Penile abnormalities:** For example, Pyronie disease (idiopathic fibrosis of covering sheath of corpus cavernosum).

Q. How to differentiate psychogenic from organic erectile dysfunction?

Ans.

Phychogenic erectile dysfunction	*Organic erectile dysfunction*
Occasional ED but H/o repeated normal erection at other times	More gradual or persistent disorder
H/o nocturnal or early morning erection	No
Sudden onset of ED following a significant event, e.g., loss of job	No
Normal erection with other sexual partner, H/o extramarital relation, masturbation, watches porn movie	No
↓libido: Depression Intact libido: Anxiety/stress	↓ libido: Hypogonadism, systemic disease Intact libido: Vascular, DM, drugs

Chapter 45: Erectile Dysfunction

Q. Mention etiology of erectile dysfunction in diabetes.

Ans.
- ↓ tactile input from genitalia (somatic neuropathy)
- Disorder of parasympathetic outflow need for erection (autonomic neuropathy)
- ↓ arterial inflow to penile erectile tissue (atherosclerosis/PVD)
- Endothelial dysfunction
- Associated HTN and intensive antihypertensive medications
- Tendency to anxiety or depression (including that about diabetes)
- Low testosterone in DM patients
- Other primary penile problem, for example, balanitis, Pyronie disease associated with DM.

Q. How will you evaluate a patient of erectile dysfunction?

Ans.
1. **History:**
   - **Sexual history:**
     - Nature of sexual dysfunction: Whether the primary problem is decreased libido, ED, difficulty in achieving orgasm, premature or delayed ejaculation
     - Onset of symptoms, extent of dysfunction, its duration and progression
     - Occasional or progressive and persistent ED
     - Nocturnal or early morning erection
     - Pain with coitus/structural abnormalities of penis
     - Libido/sexual drive
   - **Symptoms of hypogonadism:** Reduced libido, ↓ energy, vitality
   - **Full medical history:**
     - For example, DM, hypertension, coronary artery disease, liver disease, renal disease, peripheral vascular disease, neurological or endocrine disease
     - Intermittent claudication suggests a vascular cause
     - History of genitourinary trauma, prostate or pelvic surgery
   - **Drug history:** Onset of ED in relation to commencing a new medication
   - **Personal history:**
     - Relationship history
     - Anxiety about sexual performance
     - Smoking history
     - Recreational drugs use including alcohol
   - **Treatment history:**
     - Coexisting CAD, use of nitrate
     - Use of vasodilator for HTN or CCF

2. **Examination:**
   - **Evidence of hypogonadism:**
     - Loss of secondary sexual characteristics
     - Eunuchoid proportions

- Small testicular volume
- Gynecomastia
- **Neurological examination:**
  - Genital and perineal sensation (spinal cord lesion or peripheral neuropathy)
  - Measure BP with posture change (autonomic neuropathy)
  - Bulbocavernosus reflex: Asses S2-4 nerves. Insert a finger into patient's rectum while squeezing his glans penis. Contraction of anal musculature represents a normal response
- **Vascular assessment:** Femoral and pedal pulses and evidences of lower extremity ischemia
- **Evidence of endocrine disorder:**
  - Hyperprolactinemia
  - Thyroid dysfunction
  - Look for other complications of DM
- **Evidence of systemic disease:** Cardiac disease, CLD, CRF
- **Genital examination:** To exclude Pyronie disease and other structural abnormalities of penis

3. **Investigations:**
   - **Baseline investigations:**
     - Serum testosterone
     - Prolactin, FSH, LH—if serum testosterone low
     - OGTT
     - Thyroid function tests: FT4, FT3, TSH
     - Liver function tests
     - Renal function tests
     - Fasting lipid profile
   - **Additional investigations:** Rarely required
     - Nocturnal tumescence monitoring: Using a plethysmograph placed around the shaft of penis overnight (healthy men and those with psychogenic ED have 3-5 erections a night associated with REM sleep. Absence or reduced frequency of nocturnal tumescence indicates organic lesion)
     - RigiScan: Ambulatory monitor to asses penile rigidity as well as tumescence
     - Vascular testing:
       - Intracavernosal injection of papaverine or PG E_1
       - Penile Doppler USG
       - Internal pudendal artery angiography
     - Psychological test: Minnesota multiphasic personality inventory.

Q. **How to manage a patient of erectile dysfunction?**

Ans.

Principle:
- Treatment of underlying disorder or withdrawal of offending drug

- Avoid smoking, alcohol or recreational drug use
- Treatment of hypogonadism with androgen and hyperprolactinemia with dopamine agonist

Stepwise approach to treatment of ED:
- All patients and their sexual partners should receive psychosexual counseling
- **First-line therapy:** Oral selective phosphodiesterase inhibitor
- **Second-line therapy:** Intracavernosal injection of alprostadil, intraurethral alprostadil, external vacuum devices
- **Third-line therapy:** Penile prosthesis, vascular surgery

1. **Psychosexual therapy:**
   - Reduce performance anxiety
   - Identify relationship problems and improve partner communication and intimacy
   - Modify sexual attitudes and belief
   - Improve couple's sexual skills.

2. **Oral selective phosphodiesterase five inhibitors (sildenafil, vardenafil, tadalafil):**
   - **Mechanism of action:** Increase cGMP activity in erectile tissue by blocking PDE-5, thereby amplifying the vasodilator action of NO. Success rate is 50–80%
   - **Contraindications:**
     - Patient taking nitrate
     - History of MI/stroke in last 6 months
     - Unstable angina
     - Hypotension (BP <90/50 mm Hg)
     - Severe CCF
     - Severe hepatic impairment
   - **Adverse effects:**
     - Headache
     - Facial flushing
     - Dyspepsia
     - Nasal congestion
     - Visual disturbance
     - Priapism
   - **ACC/AHA (American College of Cardiology/American Heart Association) guidelines for use of selective phosphodiesterase inhibitors:**
     - Do not administer selective PDE5 inhibitors to men taking long- or short-acting nitrate drugs on a regular basis
     - If the patient has stable CAD and is not taking long-acting nitrate and uses short-acting nitrates only infrequently, use of selective PDE5 inhibitor should be guided by careful consideration of risks
     - In men with preexisting CAD, assess the risk of inducing cardiac ischemia during sexual activity before prescribing selecting PDE5 inhibitors. This assessment may include a stress test

- Do not administer selective PDE5 inhibitors within 24 h of the ingestion of any form of nitrate
- Advise men about the risks of interaction between selective PDE5 inhibitors and nitrates, nitrate donors and alpha-blockers. Concurrent use of such agents could result in hypotension
- In men taking vasodilators and diuretics for the treatment of HTN or CCF, consider the potential risk of inducing hypotension with PDE5 inhibitors.

3. **Intracavernosal injection of alprostadil:**
   - **Adverse effects:**
     - Penile pain
     - Hematoma
     - Penile fibrosis
     - Priapism (unwanted prolonged painful erection of penis)
   - **Contraindication:** Predisposition to priapism (e.g. sickle cell anemia, multiple myeloma or leukemia).

4. **Intraurethral alprostail:** Given through applicator. Adverse effects: Penile pain, dizziness.

5. **External vacuum devices:** The flaccid penis is put into the device and air is withdrawn, creating a vacuum that allows blood to flow into penis. A constriction band is then placed on the base of penis, so erection is maintained. This should be removed within 30 min. Adverse effects: Penile pain, hematoma.

6. **Penile prosthesis:** Surgically implanted penile prosthesis that may be semirigid or inflatable, but the device must be replaced every 5–10 years. Adverse effects: infection, mechanical failure.

7. **Vascular surgery:** Repair of venous leaks, microsurgical revascularization of arterial lesions.

Q. How to manage priapism?

Ans.
- Do not delay treatment beyond 6 h
- Using aseptic technique, aspirate 20–25 mL blood from corpus cavernosum (19- or 21-ga butterfly needle)
- Repeat aspiration on the opposite side of penis if detumescence does not occur
- If still unsuccessful, Inj. Phenylephrine every 5–10 min into corpus cavernosum
- If still unsuccessful, refer to urgent surgical treatment, for example, shunt procedure.

CHAPTER 46

Hirsutism

Q. Define hirsutism.

Ans. Excessive growth of thick terminal hair in a male distribution pattern in a woman that affect quality of life sufficiently to prompt her to seek medical advice.

- **Etiology:**
  - Ovarian: PCOS, androgen secreting tumor
  - Adrenal: Cushing syndrome, late onset CAH, androgen secreting tumor
  - Drugs: Danazol, testosterone, anabolic steroids
  - Idiopathic hirsutism.

Q. Define hypertrichosis.

Ans. Generalized excessive growth of vellus hair in any sex which is nonandrogenic in origin.

- **Etiology:**
  - Drugs: Glucocorticoid, phenytoin, minoxidil, ciclosporin
  - Anorexia nervosa
  - Hypothyroidism
  - Familial.

Q. What is Ferriman–Gallwey scale?

Ans.
- Hair growth is rated from 0 (no growth of terminal hair) to 4 (complete and heavy cover) in 9 locations giving a maximum score of 36
- Nine locations are: Upper lip, chin, chest, upper abdomen, lower abdomen, thighs, upper arm, upper back, lower back
- Scores ≥8: Androgen excess.

Q. How will you evaluate hirsutism?

Ans.

1. **History:**
   - Onset, duration and progression of hirsutism: Slowly progressive hirsutism following puberty suggest a benign cause, whereas recent onset, rapidly progressive hirsutism with virilization require further investigation to rule out androgen secreting tumor

- Menstrual history: Menstrual irregularity or infertility
- Other features of hyperandrogenism: Acne, bitemporal hair recession
- Drug history: Some progestin used in OCP may be androgenic, for example, norethisterone
- Weight change: Weight gain in PCOS and Cushing syndrome

2. **Examination:**
   - Distinguish between androgen dependent and androgen independent hair growth
   - Extent and severity of hirsutism by Ferriman–Gallwey scale
   - Features of virilization: Clitoromegaly, male pattern/frontal balding, deepening of voice, breast atrophy, severe hirsutism, masculine habitus
   - Height, weight, BMI
   - Acanthosis nigricans: Represent insulin resistance in PCOS
   - Features of Cushing syndrome
   - Abdomen: Striae, mass (ovarian/adrenal tumor)

3. **Investigations:**
   - Serum testosterone, FSH, LH
   - 24-h UFC, overnight 1 mg DST: Suspected Cushing syndrome
   - Serum 17 OHP: Suspected late onset CAH
   - Serum DHEAS, pelvic ultrasound, CT abdomen: Androgen secreting tumor
   - Serum prolactin, TSH.

Q. Draw a flowchart to evaluate hirsutism.

Ans.

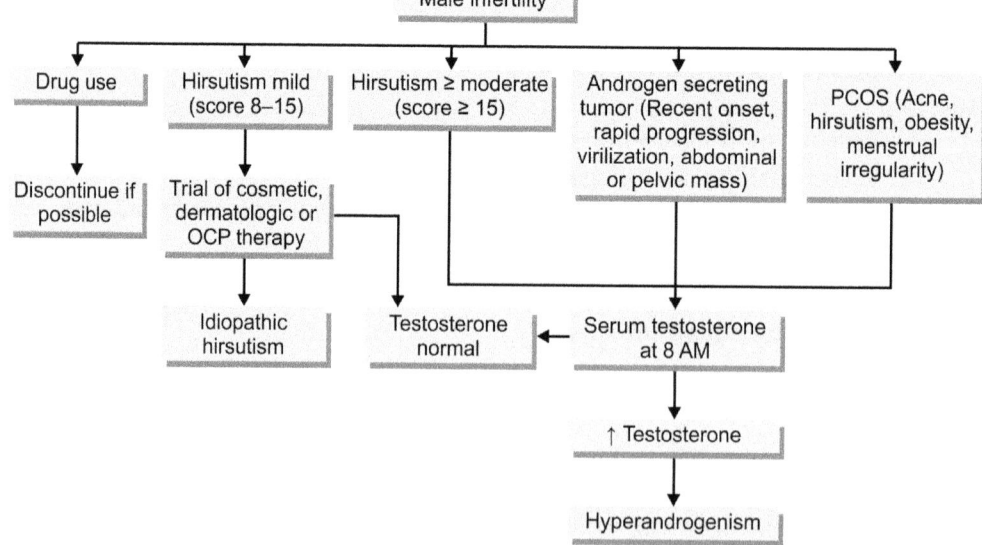

CHAPTER 47

Polycystic Ovarian Syndrome

Q. Define polycystic ovarian syndrome (PCOS)/Stein–Leventhal syndrome.

Ans.
- A heterogeneous clinical syndrome characterized by ovulatory dysfunction, hyperandrogenism and hyperinsulinemia in which other causes of androgen excess have been excluded (PCOS is a diagnosis of exclusion).
- Prevalence is 5–10% of reproductive age women.
- Accounts for 30% causes of amenorrhea, 25% of female infertility and 75% of all cases of anovulation.

Q. Mention diagnostic criteria of PCOS.

Ans.
1. **NIH (National Institute of Health) criteria (1990):** Both 1 and 2
   - Chronic anovulation
   - Clinical and/or biochemical signs of hyperandrogenism and exclusion of other etiologies.
2. **Rotterdam criteria (2003):** Any two of the following three:
   - Oligo or anovulation
   - Clinical and/or biochemical signs of hyperandrogenism
   - Polycystic ovaries and exclusion of other etiologies.
3. **AES (Androgen Excess Society) Criteria (2006):** All of the following:
   - Ovarian dysfunction: Oligo or anovulation and/or polycystic ovaries
   - Clinical and/or biochemical signs of hyperandrogenism
   - Exclusion of other etiologies (hyperprolactinemia, hypothyroidism, nonclassic CAH, androgen-secreting tumor, Cushing syndrome, drug-induced androgen excess, for example, danazol, testosterone, anabolic steroid).

Q. Discuss pathogenesis of PCOS.

Ans. The fundamental pathophysiological defect is unknown but both genetic and environmental factors are thought to play a role.

- **Genetic:**
  - Familial aggregation of PCOS in 50% cases
  - PCOS is a polygenic disorder
  - Several candidate genes have been investigated including genes involved in steroidogenesis and carbohydrate metabolism
- **Anovulation:**
  - In PCOS, functional derangement of LH secretion and frequency, amplitude. Mean level of LH is increased due to increased hypothalamic GnRH activity
  - There is chronically elevated LH without any LH surge which is essential for ovulation, so there is anovulation
  - Women with PCOS have higher mean conc. of LH but low or low-normal FSH
  - LH:FSH ratio is increased (>2.5:1), common in thin women. LH level may not be increased and the ratio is within normal range in 50% of obese with PCOS
- **Hyperandrogenism:**
  - Stimulation of theca cell to produce androgen by high LH
  - Insulin reduce hepatic synthesis of sex hormone binding globulin (SHBG), resulting elevated free testosterone and estradiol
  - The main source of hyperandrogenism is ovary but also adrenal androgen hypersecretion in 25% cases
- **Hyperinsulinemia:**
  - 50–60% of women with PCOS are insulin resistant and the defect lies in post-receptor signaling pathway
  - Hyperinsulinemia is amplified in presence of obesity but insulin resistance also observed in some thin PCOS patient also.

Q. How can you measure insulin resistance?

Ans.
- Acanthosis nigricans: Dark, thick, velvety plaque in flexural areas, particularly axilla, neck, inguinal region, inframammary region
- Frequently sampled intravenous glucose tolerance test: ADA gold standard
- Insulin tolerance test
- Euglycemic insulin clamp: ADA gold standard
- Fasting insulin level
- Glucose/insulin ratio
- Insulin resistance index = glucose × insulin/25.

Q. What are the clinical features of PCOS?

Ans.
- Onset of symptoms around puberty after weight gain or after stopping OCP but can present at any time
- Due to oligo or anovulation (≤9 times/year): Oligomenorrhea, amenorrhea, irregular cycle. These females are usually well estrogenized, so there is little risk of osteoporosis unlike other causes of amenorrhea

- **Due to hyperandrogenism:**
  - Hirsutism (70%), also suffer from acne or frontal baldness
  - Virilization is not a feature of PCOS
  - Infertility: PCOS account for 75% of all cases of anovulation
  - Risk of spontaneous miscarriage is also higher than general population
- **Obesity:**
  - 50% of PCOS are obese
  - Symptoms worsen with obesity as it is associated with increased testosterone conc. as a result of associated hyperinsulinemia
  - Acanthosis nigricans found in insulin resistant female with PCOS
- **HAIR-AN syndrome:** Combination of hyperandrogenism, insulin resistance and acanthosis nigricans.

Q. What are the risks associated with PCOS?

Ans.
- Type 2 DM: Type 2 DM is two to four times more common in PCOS (diabetes of bearded women). IGT and GDM is also more prevalent
- Dyslipidemia
- Cardiovascular disease common in PCOS due to HTN, dyslipidemia, DM
- Endometrial hyperplasia and carcinoma: In anovulatory female, endometrial stimulation by unopposed estrogen results in endometrial hyperplasia and two- to fourfold increased risk of endometrial carcinoma. Risk of breast and ovarian cancer also increased.

Q. How to rule out androgen-secreting tumor?

Ans.
- Evidence of virilization
- Testosterone >3 times × ULN (>2 ng/mL or DHEAS >8 µg/mL)
- Rapidly progressive hirsutism
- MRI of adrenals and ovaries will detect adrenal and ovarian tumors
- Selective venous sampling:
  - Occasionally necessary to locate virilizing tumor undetected by imaging
  - Blood sample taken from both adrenal and ovarian veins and from peripheral circulation
  - A virilizing tumor is likely if androgen conc. gradient is detected.

Q. Mention criteria of polycystic ovaries.

Ans.
- 10 or more cystic follicles 2–8 mm in diameter, arranged along the subcapsular edge of the ovary in string-of-pearls fashion (the increased ovarian volume and displacement of follicles toward periphery is due to hyperplastic stroma containing theca cells capable of androgen synthesis)
- Ovarian volume ≥10 cm³
- More than 20% of normal women have similar ovarian morphologic feature
- Polycystic ovaries are not unique to PCOS, also seen in late onset CAH, HIV, epilepsy.

Q. How will you investigate a patient of PCOS?

Ans.

1. **To confirm diagnosis:**
   - Total testosterone: Elevated but normal androgen level in a patient of hirsutism (40%) does not exclude PCOS
   - Serum LH FSH:
     - LH elevated with low or low-normal FSH
     - LH:FSH ratio is increased (>2.5:1, normal 1:2-3), common in thin women
     - LH level may not be increased and the ratio is within normal range in 50% of obese with PCOS
     - Higher the LH level, increased risk of anovulation and infertility
   - Fasting insulin level: Elevated
   - Ultrasound: Sensitivity 75%, better to do TVS
     - Polycystic ovaries
     - Endometrial thickness: >10 mm is diagnostic of endometrial hyperplasia in presence of anovulation.

2. **Exclusion of differential diagnosis:**
   - Serum prolactin: Mild hyperprolactinemia is present in up to 30% of PCOS and dopamine agonist treatment is necessary, if pregnancy is desired
   - Serum TSH: To exclude hypothyroidism
   - 17-OHP (8 AM): Used to exclude late onset CAH
   - DHEAS (dehydroepiandrosterone) and androstenedione: Moderately raises in PCOS. DHEAS is a useful adrenal marker of hyperandrogenism. In case of PCOS, DHEAS is usually up to 8 µg/mL
   - If Cushing syndrome suspected: 24-h urinary free cortisol, overnight 1 mg DST.

3. **To screen for complications:**
   - Fasting lipid profile, OGTT: Dyslipidemia, DM
   - Endometrial biopsy: If long history of irregular cycle (>1 year), endometrial hyperplasia.

Q. Discuss about treatment of PCOS.

Ans. Depends on presenting symptoms and according to need of the patient.

1. **Weight loss:** Diet with 500 kcal/day deficit and exercise 30–60 min/day. Weight loss improves insulin sensitivity and reduces hyperandrogenism with improvement in hirsutism, restoration of menstrual regularity and fertility.

2. **Metformin:** Metformin reduce insulin resistance and reduction in serum androgen. Use of metformin is not recommended unless there is metabolic derangements that is not fixed with diet and exercise alone. Clomiphene is superior to metformin in achieving ovulation but ovulatory response to clomiphene is increased in obese women with PCOS with addition of metformin.

3. **Hirsutism:**
   - Pharmacological treatment of hirsutism is directed at slowing the growth of new hair but has little impact on established hair
   - It should be combined with mechanical methods of hair removal (shaving, bleaching, waxing, plucking, chemical depilation and permanent method like electrolysis, laser treatment)
   - Hair cycle length is 4 months, so response should not be expected before 6 months of treatment
   - Facial hair is slow to respond, treatment is prolonged and symptoms may recur after discontinuation of drugs
   - Adequate contraception is mandatory during pharmacological treatment of hirsutism because of possible teratogenicity
   - **Pharmacological treatment of hirsutism:**
     - Ovarian androgen suppression: OCP containing ethinylestradiol and cyproterone
     - Androgen receptor antagonist: Spironolactone, cyproterone acetate, flutamide
     - 5α-reductase inhibitor: Finasteride
     - Insulin sensitizers: Metformin
     - Topical inhibitor of hair follicle growth: Eflornithine
   - **OCP:**
     - OCP containing 30-35 µg ethinylestradiol increase SHBG leading to reduce free androgen conc., progestogen inhibits LH secretion and thus ovarian androgen production
     - Preparation containing ethinylestradiol (35 µg) and cyproterone acetate (2 mg) commonly used
   - **Spironolactone:** 100-400 mg/day. Start at low dose. Adverse effect is diuresis in first few days. K^+ level should be monitored and other K^+ sparing drugs should be avoided
   - **Cyproterone acetate:** Adverse effect is hepatotoxicity. 50-100 mg/day at D1-10 of the pill cycle in combination with OCP
   - **Eflornithine cream:** Irreversibly block enzyme ornithine decarboxylase which is involved in growth of hair follicles. Used for facial hirsutism, discontinue if no improvement after 4 months. It is not a depilatory cream, so must be combined with mechanical method of hair removal. Adverse effect is skin irritation with burning, acne.

4. **Amenorrhea:** A minimum of withdrawal bleed every 3 months minimizes risk of endometrial hyperplasia with OCP.

5. **Infertility:** Ovulation induction regimen is indicated:
   - Clomiphene citrate
   - Letrozole
   - Low dose gonadotropin: FSH used
   - Laparoscopic ovarian drilling
   - Wedge resection
   - In vitro fertilization (IVF).

CHAPTER 48

Female Infertility

Q. Enumerate the causes of female infertility.

Ans.

- Ovulatory disorder (25%):
  - PCOS
  - Hypothalamic/pituitary disease
  - Hyperprolactinemia
  - Late onset CAH
  - Cushing syndrome
  - Androgen secreting tumor
  - Thyroid disorders
  - Adrenal insufficiency
  - DM
  - Obesity
  - Chronic systemic illness
  - Ovarian failure: Turner syndrome, Premature ovarian failure (POF)
- **Tubal disorder:** PID (chlamydia, gonorrhea), endometriosis, previous pelvic or abdominal surgery
- **Uterine factors:** Congenital abnormalities, fibroids, Asherman syndrome
- **Cervical factors:** Congenital abnormalities, trauma to cervix (including surgery)
- **Unexplained/idiopathic.**

Q. How will you evaluate a case of female infertility?

Ans.

1. **History:**
   - Age of patient (Fertility declines after the age of 35)
   - Duration of infertility and results of previous evaluation and treatment
   - Infertility being primary or secondary
   - H/o previous marriage with proven fertility
   - In secondary infertility: Details of previous pregnancy including abortion (spontaneous and therapeutic), ectopic pregnancy

Chapter 48: Female Infertility

- Menstrual history:
  - Age at menarche
  - Length of menstrual cycle and its regularity, for example, oligo/amenorrhea
  - Intermenstrual spotting (Regular cycles are usually associated with regular ovulation)
  - Premenstrual molimina (Breast tenderness, spasmodic dysmenorrhea, fluid retention, mood change suggestive of ovulation)
  - Midcycle pain or bleeding (indicate ovulation). Ovulation pain is called mittelschmerz
- Sexual history: Frequency of intercourse, sexual dysfunction, use of lubricants
- Medical history:
  - Headache, visual disturbance (hypothalamic/pituitary disease)
  - Galactorrhea (hyperprolactinemia)
  - Acne, hirsutism, obesity, menstrual irregularities: PCOS
  - Rapid onset virilization: Androgen secreting tumor
  - Thyroid disorder, Cushing syndrome
  - PID, TB, DM, pelvic surgery
  - Fibroid, endometriosis
  - Chronic systemic illness
- Drug history:
  - Drugs that cause hyperprolactinemia
  - OCP
  - Cytotoxic chemotherapy/radiotherapy
- Family history of POF, PCOS, endometriosis
- Personal and lifestyle history: Occupation, exercise, stress, dieting/weight changes, smoking, alcohol.

2. **Examinations:**
   - Height, weight, BMI
   - Secondary sexual characteristics: If absent look for evidence of Turner syndrome
   - Breast: Atrophied, galactorrhea
   - Evidence of hyperandrogenism or virilization
   - Evidence of thyroid disorders, Cushing syndrome
   - Abdomen: Striae, mass in abdomen
   - Vulvovaginal examination.

3. **Investigations:**
   - CBC with ESR
   - Chest X-ray P/A view: to exclude TB
   - OGTT: To exclude DM
   - To see evidence of ovulation:
     - Basal body temperature: After ovulation, temperature rises .5-1F

- Cervical mucus test: Cervical mucus is thin, acellular and show fern pattern during follicular phase. During ovulation, it becomes thin, watery and copious and during luteal phase, it becomes thick, cellular and loss of fern pattern
- Midluteal progesterone level: On D21 of menstrual cycle/7 days before expected onset of menses, progesterone level ≥3 µg/L (9.5 nmol/L) consistent with ovulation
- Serial estimation of LH level: Ovulation occurs 24–36 h after onset of LH surge and 10–12 h after peak LH surge
- Endometrial biopsy: Done at D18–22 of the cycle to see the secretory phase which is a progestational effect. It also excludes TB endometritis
- Serial ultrasound to follow the development and ultimately disappearance of follicle. Mature follicle is 18–24 mm in diameter by D14
- Laparoscopic visualization of corpus luteum

- Patient with irregular cycle or who are not ovulating: FT4, TSH, PRL
- Assessment of ovarian reserve: Early follicular cycle (D2–4) FSH, LH, estradiol
  - FSH <10 mIU/mL: Adequate ovarian reserve
  - FSH >10 mIU/mL: ↓ Ovarian reserve
  - FSH >40 mIU/mL: Ovarian failure
- Serum T, DHEAS, 17 OHP, 24 h UFC, CT abdomen: If clinical evidence of hyperandrogenism or virilization
- Karyotype: If Turner syndrome suspected
- MRI of pituitary region: If hyperprolactinemia and hypogonadotropic hypogonadism
- TVS: To assess uterine and ovarian anatomy
- To see uterine pathology: Hysteroscopy
- To see tubal pathology:
  - Hysterosalpingography
  - Laparoscopic dye test
  - Tubal insufflation test
- Exclude cervical infection, send vaginal discharge for culture and do Chlamydia serology
- Special tests:
  - Sperm cervical mucus contact test (Huner's test)
  - Sperm penetration assay
  - Acrosome reaction
  - Zona pellucida binding test
  - Motility evaluation on a postcoital test
  - DNA analysis of sperm, ovum and zygote.

Q. Classify ovulatory disorders (WHO).

Ans.
- Class I: Hypogonadotropic hypogonadal anovulation
- Class II: Normogonadotropic normoestrogenic anovulation, for example, PCOS
- Class III: Hypergonadotropic hypoestrogenic anovulation.

Q. Discuss about ovulation induction.

Ans.
- **Indications:**
  - Chronic anovulation. Normal ovarian reserve and absence of other endocrine abnormalities (e.g. hyperprolactinemia, hypothyroidism)
    - PCOS
    - Hypogonadotropic hypogonadism
  - Controlled ovarian hyperstimulation for ART
- **Pretreatment assessment:**
  - Exclude thyroid dysfunction and hyperprolactinemia
  - Confirm normal semen analysis
  - Confirm tubal patency prior to gonadotropin use and/or after failed clomiphene use
  - Baseline pelvic USG to exclude ovarian mass and uterine abnormalities prior to treatment
- **Methods of induction of ovulation:**

1. **General:**
   - **Assurance:** Psychotherapy to improve emotional status
   - **Body weight:** Optimize lifestyle, maintain ideal BMI, moderate exercise, stop smoking and alcohol intake
   - **Metformin:** Given in obese patient of PCOS with glucose intolerance. Metformin inhibits hepatic glucose production and thereby ↓ insulin secretion. Metformin ameliorates hyperandrogenism and abnormalities of gonadotropin secretion in women with PCOS and can restore menstruation cyclically and fertility.

2. **Medical:**
   - **Clomiphene citrate:**
     - Indicated in patient with adequate level of estrogen with normal level of FSH, for example, PCOS
     - Mechanism of action: Synthetic nonsteroidal compound with estrogen agonist-antagonist action, bind to estrogen receptor at hypothalamus and block normal negative feedback by circulating estrogen, thereby ↑ gonadotropin release to stimulate follicular recruitment and ovulation

- Dose: 50 mg/day for 5 days starting at D2-6 of spontaneous or induced menstrual period. Ovulation should be documented in each treatment cycle. If ovulation does not occur, dose to be increased 50 mg/day increment per cycle. Maximum dose is 150 mg/day
- Advice to patient: Couples are advised to have intercourse every other day for 1 week beginning 5 days after last day of medication
- Result: Ovulation expected to occur in 80% and pregnancy in 35%–40% in first 6 ovulatory cycles
- Clomiphene citrate should not be continued for >6-9 cycles
- **Adverse effects:**
  - Hot flushes
  - Mood swing
  - Abdominal pain
  - Multiple pregnancy (7-10%)
  - Ovarian enlargement (5%)
  - Ovarian hyperstimulation syndrome (1%): Abdominal pain, vomiting, hypovolemia, ascites
  - Ovarian cancer: In patient receiving >12 cycles clomiphene
- **Letrozole:** Aromatase inhibitor. Dose is 2.5 mg/day for 5 days starting at D2-6 of menstrual period, maximum dose is 7.5 mg/day.
- **Gonadotropins:** Indicated in hypogonadotropic hypogonadism.
- **GnRH:** Indicated in hypogonadotropic hypogonadism with normal pituitary function.

3. **Surgery:**
   - Laparoscopic ovarian drilling: By diathermy or laser. Four punctures to a depth of 4 mm made in each ovary
   - Wedge resection: Bilateral wedge resection of one third of ovarian mass of each side.

Q. What is assisted reproductive technology (ART)?

Ans. Procedure for infertile couple in which there is oocyte or embryo manipulation.
- **Methods:**
  - Intrauterine insemination (IUI)
  - In vitro fertilization (IVF)
  - IVF with micromanipulation: ICSI (intracytoplasmic sperm injection)
  - Other methods:
    - Gamete intrafallopian transfer (GIFT)
    - Zygote intrafallopian transfer (ZIFT)
    - Embryo intrafallopian transfer (EIFT).

Q. Discuss about intrauterine insemination (IUI).

Ans. Procedure in which processed and concentrated motile sperm are placed directly into uterine cavity.

- **Indication of IUI:**
  - **Male factor infertility:**
    - Abnormal sperm quality (oligo-, astheno-, teratozoospermia)
    - Hypospadias
    - Impotence, for example, spinal cord injury or other neurological problems
    - Retrograde ejaculation
  - **Severe vaginismus**
  - **Cervical factor infertility:** Scanty, thick or absent cervical mucus
  - **Unexplained infertility**
- **Procedure of IUI:**
  - **Semen preparation:**
    - Semen is collected by masturbation
    - Semen is centrifuged, sperm collected at the bottom of tube that is mixed with culture media (Ham's 10 media)
    - The mixture is incubated. Actively motile spermatozoa swim up at the top of tube forming a cloud that is taken for IUI (swim-up technique)
  - **Timing of insemination:**
    - IUI should be done at the time of ovulation that may be natural or controlled ovarian hyperstimulation
    - Insemination should be done twice on the day of LH surge and within next 24 h
  - **Procedure of insemination:** .3 mL of prepared semen is placed directly into uterine cavity by various types of catheter
  - **Result:** Pregnancy rate is 10–30% with IUI. 3–5 cycles attempt is needed for success
  - **Complication:** Mild to severe uterine bleeding, pelvic infection.

Q. Discuss about in vitro fertilization (IVF).

Ans. Procedure in which sperm and egg are fertilized in vitro, then fertilized egg is transferred into uterine cavity. First performed in 1978 (Louise Brown/test tube baby).
- **Indication:**
  - Severely damaged or occluded fallopian tubes
  - Male factor infertility
  - Cervical hostility
  - Diminished ovarian reserve
  - Unexplained infertility
- **Procedure of IVF:**
  - Controlled ovarian hyperstimulation
  - Oocyte retrieval: By ultrasound-guided transvaginal puncture
  - Fertilization in vitro: Collected oocytes are mixed with spermatozoa in a small volume of culture medium
  - Embryo transfer: Carried out 48–50 h after oocyte recovery at 4–8 cell cleavage stage or blastocyst stage

- Luteal phase support: By progesterone supplement
- Complication: Complication of procedure, multiple gestation, ectopic pregnancy.

Q. Discuss about ICSI (intracytoplasmic sperm injection).

Ans. Procedure in which a single sperm is injected directly into cytoplasm of a mature oocyte.
- **Indication:**
  - Severe deficit in semen quality
  - Failed routine IVF
  - Obstructive azoospermia
- **Procedure:**
  - Oocyte retrieval
  - After incubation, those oocytes which have extruded the first polar body (oocyte at metaphase II) are candidate for ICSI
  - Sperm sources include fresh and frozen specimen from collected by masturbation, microepididymal sperm aspiration or testicular biopsy specimen
  - A single sperm is injected directly into cytoplasm of mature oocyte using special microinjection pipette
  - Embryo transfer
  - Luteal phase support
  - Result: Success rate 24–30%.

Q. Discuss about premature ovarian failure (POF).

Ans. Ovarian failure manifested by amenorrhea, estrogen deficiency and hypergonadotropic hypogonadism (FSH >40 IU/L) before the age of 40 years.
- **Etiology:**
  - Genetic origin: Turner syndrome, Fragile X syndrome
  - Autoimmune ovarian dysfunction (concomitant autoimmune disease in 20% patients with POF)
  - Iatrogenic: Ovarian insult resulting from trauma, surgery, chemotherapy/radiotherapy to gonads
  - Idiopathic (>50% of patient with POF)
- **Investigations:**
  - Serum FSH, LH, estradiol
  - Karyotype
  - Screening for autoimmune disease: Evaluate for APS (autoimmune polyglandular syndrome), screen for thyroid and adrenal insufficiency
  - Fragile X testing
  - TVS: Ovarian volume and blood flow
  - DEXA
- **Treatment:** HRT.

Q. Discuss about Turner syndrome/45, XO/gonadal dysgenesis.

Ans. Chromosomal disorder in which the individual is phenotypically female but the chromosome pattern is 45, XO. Here a female who has lost an X chromosome.

- **Chromosomal abnormality:**
  - 45, XO (57%)
  - Structural abnormalities of X chromosome (19%)
  - Mosaics 45, XO/46, XX (29%)
- **Clinical features:**
  - Sexual infantilism:
    - Primary amenorrhea (menopause occur before menarche)
    - Failure to develop the breasts
    - Widely spaced nipples
    - Broad shield like chest
    - Scanty pubic hair
    - Infantile external genitalia
    - Ovaries are severely atrophic and contain only fibrous stroma arranged in whorls, devoid of ova and follicles (streak gonads)
    - Gonadoblastoma in mosaic
  - Short stature: Mean final height is 143 cm (133–153 cm)
  - Micrognathia, epicanthal fold, low set ear, low posthairline
  - Fish like mouth, high arched palate
  - Conductive/sensorineural hearing loss (due to recurrent otitis media)
  - Webbing of neck/pterygium colli (40%): In infancy, swelling of the nape of neck due to lymph stasis (cystic hygroma). Later, the swelling subside but often leave bilateral neck webbing and persistent looseness of skin on the back of neck
  - Lymphedema of hands and feet
  - Learning disabilities with impaired visuospatial processing, usually normal intelligence
  - Short fourth metacarpals and metatarsals
  - Madelung deformity of wrist (bilateral bowing of wrist with dorsal subluxation of distal ulna)
  - Wide carrying angle of elbows (cubitus valgus)
  - Cardiovascular anomalies of left side of heart: Coarctation of aorta, bicuspid aortic valve, aortic aneurysm
  - 10% patient may undergo spontaneous puberty, menarche and even pregnancy
  - Associated conditions:
    - Obesity, HTN, type 2 DM, IHD, stroke, osteoporosis
    - Horseshoe kidney
    - Pigmented nevi, tendency to keloid formation
    - Autoimmune thyroid disease

- IBD, intestinal telangiectasia with bleeding
- Abnormal liver enzymes
- **Diagnosis:** Phenotypic females with the following features should have a karyotype analysis:
  - Short stature (>2.5 SD below the mean for age) with or without somatic anomalies associated with syndrome of gonadal dysgenesis
  - Delayed puberty with ↑ FSH
  - Patient with clinical features of Turner syndrome, for example, lymphedema of hands or feet, left-sided cardiac anomalies, characteristic facies, short fourth metacarpals or metatarsals
- **Investigations:**
  - Lymphocyte karyotype as well as FISH of 200 cells to rule out mosaicism: 45, XO
  - Barr bodies (buccal smear, PMN): Absent
  - Serum estrogen: ↓, FSH: ↑
  - AMH (Anti-Müllerian hormone): Provide an estimate of number of antral follicles. Low AMH herald ovarian failure
  - Inhibin B: To determine status of gonad. Measurable level indicate presence of functional follicles and possibility of spontaneous puberty
  - Echocardiography/MRI: To evaluate cardiac anomalies, aortic size
  - Renal ultrasound: Renal or urinary tract anomalies
  - Periodic evaluation of
    - Thyroid function test
    - CBG, LFTs, lipid profile
    - Echocardiography
    - Renal USG
    - DEXA
    - Hearing evaluation
    - Orthodontics
    - Psychosocial and school performance
- **Treatment:**
  - **Treatment goal:**
    - Maximizing growth
    - Hormone replacement at puberty for orderly progressive development of secondary sexual characteristics
  - High dose of GH 45-67 µg/kg/day or 1.3-2 mg/m²/day subcutaneous daily start earlier in childhood (as soon as growth failure is evident) with or without Oxandrolone (.0625 mg/kg/day by mouth). Height increase 7-10 cm after 3-7 years of therapy. Dose adjustment to maintain IGF-1 to high normal range
  - Estrogen replacement therapy initiated at 11-13 years of age. Conjugated estrogen (0.3 mg) or ethinylestradiol (3-5 µg) given orally for first 21 days of calendar month. Dose of estrogen increased gradually to 1.25 mg conjugated estrogen or

10 μg ethinylestradiol daily over next several years. The minimal dose of estrogen necessary to initiate and maximize uterine development, secondary sexual characteristics should be administered. After 18–24 months of estrogen therapy, MPA (5 mg) given on D12–21 of the month to ensure menses and ↓ risk of endometrial carcinoma due to unopposed estrogen
- Patient should be reassured about sexual function and potential for maternity with donor eggs and IVF. The success rate of ovum donation is 40% per treatment cycle but only 50% pregnancy achieve live birth due to high miscarriage rate
- Complete cardiac evaluation prior to egg implantation with close monitoring if pregnancy ensues. Caesarean section to avoid ↑ stress to CVS is recommended.

CHAPTER 49

Amenorrhea

Q. Define amenorrhea and different types of amenorrhea.

Ans.
- **Amenorrhea:** Absence of menstruation
- **Primary amenorrhea:**
  - Absence of menarche by age 16 in presence of normal secondary sexual characteristics or by age 14 if secondary sexual characteristics have not developed
  - Mean age of menarche is 12.8 years
- **Secondary amenorrhea:** Absence of menstruation for >3 cycles interval or 6 consecutive months in a previously menstruating woman during reproductive phase
- **False amenorrhea/cryptomenorrhea/hidden menstruation:** Menstruation is taking place but menstrual blood fails to come out from genital tract due to obstruction in the passage
- **Oligomenorrhea:** Reduction in the frequency of menstruation to <9 periods a year.

Q. What are the causes of primary amenorrhea?

Ans.
- Constitutional delayed puberty
- Developmental abnormality of genital tract: Imperforate hymen and vaginal agenesis
- Hypothalamic etiology: Hyperprolactinemia and hypopituitarism
- Ovarian etiology:
  - Turner syndrome
  - Other causes of ovarian failure: Trauma, surgery and chemotherapy/radiotherapy to gonads
- Hyperandrogenic state:
  - PCOS
  - Nonclassic CAH
  - Cushing syndrome
  - Androgen secreting tumor
- Other endocrine disorder: Thyroid disorder, DM and adrenal insufficiency

- Uterine cause: TB endometritis
- Systemic disease: TB, respiratory, cardiac, GIT and renal.

Q. **What are the causes of secondary amenorrhea?**

Ans.
- **Physiological:** Pregnancy and lactation
- **Hypothalamic etiology:** 15%
  - Hypothalamic dysfunction: Injury and Infiltration
  - Functional hypothalamic amenorrhea:
    - Stress: Physical/psychological
    - Excessive physical exercise/athlete
      (athlete triad: disordered eating, amenorrhea and osteoporosis)
    - Anorexia nervosa
    - Weight loss/malnutrition
    - Chronic systemic illness
- **Pituitary etiology:** 5%
  - Hyperprolactinemia
  - Hypopituitarism
- **Ovarian etiology:** 70%
  - PCOS
  - Premature ovarian failure:
    - Genetic
    - Autoimmune ovarian destruction
    - Iatrogenic: Surgery and chemotherapy/radiotherapy to gonads
- **Hyperandrogenic state:**
  - PCOS
  - Nonclassic CAH
  - Cushing syndrome
  - Androgen secreting tumor
- **Other endocrine tumor:** Thyroid disorders, DM and adrenal insufficiency
- **Uterine cause:**
  - TB endometritis
  - Asherman syndrome (endometrial adhesion after D&C, infection).

Q. **How will you evaluate a case of amenorrhea?**

Ans.
1. **History:**
   - Age of patient
   - Duration of amenorrhea
   - Mode of onset (sudden or following oligomenorrhea, following PPH with absence of postpartum lactation-Sheehan syndrome)

- Pregnancy symptoms
- Stress: Physical/psychological
- Excessive physical exercise/athlete and chronic systemic illness (functional hypothalamic amenorrhea)
- Weight changes:
    - Weight loss: Anorexia nervosa, TB and malabsorption
    - Weight gain: Hypothyroidism, Cushing syndrome and hypothalamic lesion
- Features of hyperandrogenism: Acne, hirsutism, obesity and menstrual irregularity (PCOS)
- Features of hyperandrogenism with rapid onset virilization, progressive symptoms: Androgen secreting tumor (adrenal and ovary)
- Headache, visual disturbance: Hypothalamic and pituitary lesion
- Any symptom of estrogen deficiency: Hot flushes, decreased libido and vaginal dryness
- Drug history: Drugs that cause hyperprolactinemia, contraceptive, chemotherapy/radiation and recreational drug use
- Galactorrhea: Hyperprolactinemia
- Obstetric history:
    - Recent delivery, abortion and MR
    - Breast feeding
    - Severe PPH
    - Postpartum or postabortal D&C
    - Hysterectomy
- Medical history:
    - H/o TB or contact
    - Chronic systemic illness
    - Pituitary/thyroid/adrenal disorder
- Family H/o POF and autoimmune disorder

2. **Examination:**
    - Height, weight and BMI
    - Features of Turner syndrome or other dysmorphic features (primary amenorrhea)
    - Secondary sexual characteristics
    - Breast: Atrophied and galactorrhea
    - Evidence of hyperandrogenism or virilization
    - Abdomen: Striae, mass in abdomen

- Evidence of thyroid disorder
- Visual field defect
- Vulvovaginal examination: Clitoromegaly and vaginal dryness.

3. **Investigations:**
   - Urine for pregnancy test/serum hCG: To exclude pregnancy
   - Serum FSH, LH, estradiol, prolactin, FT4 and TSH
     - Normally LH/FSH = 1:2–3
     - In PCOS-LH/FSH = >2.5:1 (LH elevated with low or low normal FSH, E normal >50 pg/mL)
     - In functional hypothalamic amenorrhea—FSH/LH >1, estrogen <50 pg/mL
   - Clinical evidence of hyperandrogenism: Serum T, 17 OHP, DHEAS and 24-h UFC
   - CBC with ESR, CXR and MT: If TB suspected
   - MRI of sella turcica: If FSH low or hyperprolactinemia
   - Karyotype: If Turner syndrome suspected
   - Transvaginal USG:
     - Ovarian and uterine abnormalities: Exclude anatomical abnormalities, PCOS and Turner syndrome
     - Endometrial thickness: To assess estrogen status
   - Assessment of estrogen status:
     - Progesterone challenge test
     - Endometrial thickness on TVS
     - Serum estradiol
- **Progesterone challenge test:**

  Medroxyprogesterone acetate (MPA) 10 mg orally daily for 10 days. If withdrawal bleeding occurs, it indicates sufficient circulating estrogen produced by ovary that has "primed" the endometrium and the diagnosis is normoestrogenic anovulation, for example, PCOS.

  If withdrawal bleeding does not occur, combined estrogen and progesterone challenge done. Oral conjugated estrogen .625 mg/day from D1 to D21 with medroxyprogesterone 10 mg daily from D12 to D21 (last 10 days).

  If withdrawal bleeding occurs, it indicates hypoestrogenic amenorrhea. FSH and LH should be done to differentiate ovarian failure from hypothalamic-pituitary etiology. If withdrawal bleeding does not occur, it indicate outflow problem. Hysteroscopy should be done to exclude Asherman syndrome.

Q. Draw a flowchart to evaluate secondary amenorrhea.
Ans.

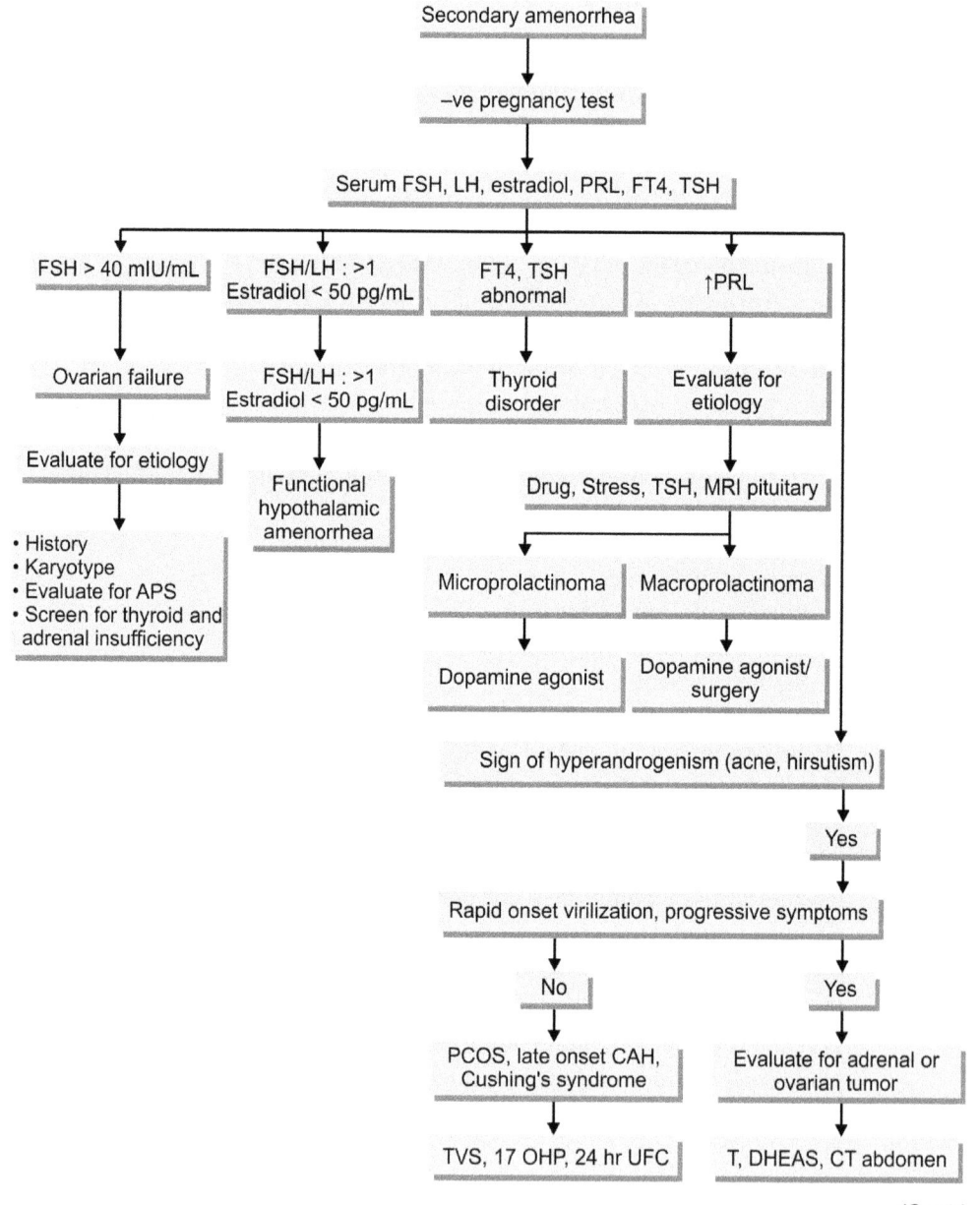

(Contd...)

(Contd...)

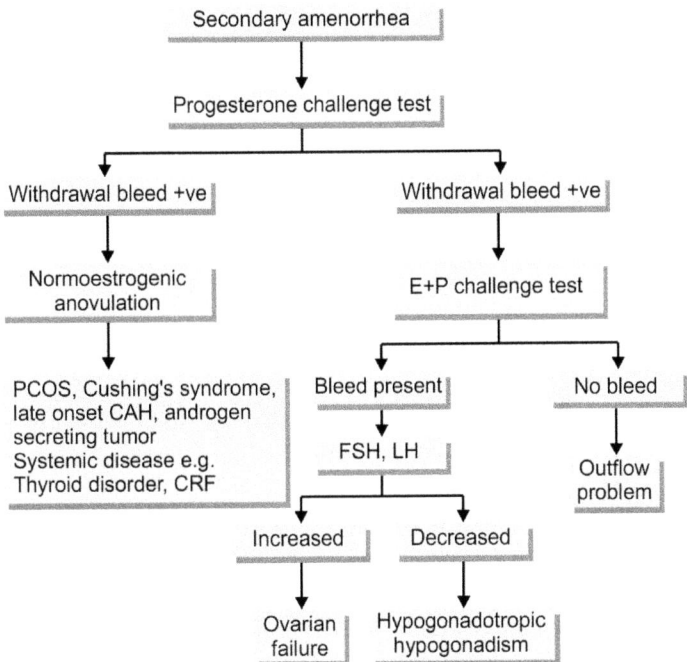

CHAPTER 50

Menopause

Q. Define menopause and different types of menopause.

Ans.

- **Menopause:** Counterpart of menarche and refers to permanent cessation of menstruation for at least 1 year at the end of reproductive life. Globally, it is observed at 46–55 years (mean 51.2 years)
- **Climacteric/perimenopause/menopausal transition:** Counterpart of puberty and is transitional phase lasting for 1–3 years during which a woman passes from reproductive to nonreproductive stage due to waning of ovarian activity
- **Early postmenopause:** First 5 years following the final menstrual period
- **Late postmenopause:** Begin 5 years after final menstrual period and continue until death
- **Premature menopause:** Menopause before the age of 40 years. Etiology is the same as POF
- **Early menopause:** Menopause before the age of 46 years
- **Late menopause:** When menstruation continues beyond 55 years. May be constitutional, DM, uterine fibroid, estrogenic tumor of ovary
- **Artificial/induced menopause:** Due to bilateral surgical removal of ovaries (surgical menopause), chemotherapy, pelvic radiation
- **Senescence:** After the age of 60 years.

Q. What are the symptoms of menopause?

Ans.

1. **Vasomotor symptoms/hot flushes:** Episodic subjective sensation of intense warmth of upper body, last for 30 s–5 min and may occur as frequently as every hour or several times per week. Hot flushes occur in 70% women undergoing natural menopause and in almost all women who have undergone surgical menopause. 80% of women have symptoms lasting for at least 1 year. Only 25% women are still symptomatic at 5 years after final menstruation period. The episode usually ends in profuse sweating and cold sensation.
    - **Mechanism:** Defect in central thermoregulatory function related to fluctuation in estrogen concentration

- **Differential diagnosis:**
  - Thyrotoxicosis
  - Pheochromocytoma
  - Carcinoid tumor
  - Panic disorder
  - Diabetes
- **Treatment:**
  - Estrogen
  - Life-style modification: Avoiding of smoking, spicy food, hot bath, coffee, use fan, air conditioning, light cotton clothing, relaxation therapy, exercise
  - SSRIs, for example, Fluoxetine 20 mg orally daily
  - Centrally acting alpha-blocker: Clonidine .1 mg orally daily. Adverse effects: Dry mouth, postural hypotension
  - High-dose progestins
  - Gabapentin 300–900 mg daily in divided doses
  - Vitamin E 400 IU orally twice daily
  - Phytoestrogens/bioidentical hormone.

2. **Genitourinary:**
   - Pruritus vulvae, vaginal dryness, dyspareunia, loss of libido, urgency, recurrent UTI
   - Cellular glycogen diminishes, leading to ↓ in lactobacilli and lactic acid production with concomitant rise in vaginal P^H that favors vaginal colonization with fecal flora
   - Treatment/prevention of recurrent UTI: Vaginal estrogenic preparation for at least 1–3 months

3. **Skeletal:** Osteoporosis, bone pain, fracture.

4. **Psychological:** Anxiety, irritability, emotional lability, depression, insomnia.

5. **Cardiovascular:** ↑ risk of CAD, CVA (estrogen is cardioprotective).

6. **Connective tissue:** Skin changes are
   - ↓ in elasticity
   - ↓ sweat and sebaceous gland, so skin becomes dry
   - loss of subcutaneous adipose tissue →↓ thermal insulating capacity.

Q. Discuss management for menopause or workup before HRT.

Ans.

1. **History:**
   - Time of menopause
   - Presence of vasomotor, genitourinary and psychological symptoms
   - Sexual life
   - Any gynecological problem
   - Obstetrical history

- Smoking habit
- Dietary habit
- Work pattern
- Social and economic status
- Assessment of mental buildup of patient
- Family history of osteoporosis, DM, HTN, dyslipidemia
- H/o thromboembolism or use of OCP
- Assessment of risk factors of osteoporosis and coronary artery disease.

2. **Examination:**
   - Weight
   - BP
   - Examination of breasts
   - Examination of abdomen and pelvis to exclude any gynecological abnormality.

3. **Investigation:**
   - OGTT
   - Baseline mammogram
   - ECG
   - Fasting lipid profile
   - LFTs, RFTs
   - DEXA
   - Pelvic USG:
     - Endometrial thickness: Normal up to 5 mm. >5 mm needs endometrial biopsy
     - Ovarian volume: Normal volume 3–4 cm^3. If more than normal volume, screen for ovarian carcinoma
     - Any fibroid
   - Endometrial biopsy:
     - Perimenopausal women with irregular/heavy bleeding
     - Postmenopausal bleeding
     - Endometrial thickness >5 mm
   - Progesterone challenge test: MPA 10 mg/day for 10 days
     - Withdrawal bleeding: Endometrial biopsy to be done as risk of endometrial carcinoma
     - No bleeding: Atrophic endometrium (normal).

Q. What are the indications of hormone replacement therapy (HRT)?

Ans.
- In male: Testosterone replacement in hypogonadism
- In patient desiring fertility: Gonadotropin (FSH, LH), GnRH
- In female: Estrogen, progesterone, combined E + P in postmenopausal state
- Tibolone: Synthetic steroid with tissue-specific estrogenic, progestogenic and androgenic effect. 10% patient experience irregular bleeding.

Q. Discuss about hormone replacement therapy (HRT) in postmenopausal state.

Ans.
- **Hormone used in HRT:** Estrogen, progesterone, combined E + P
- **Indications of HRT:**
    - Moderate-to-severe vasomotor symptoms associated with menopause
    - Moderate-to-severe symptoms of vulvar and vaginal atrophy associated with menopause
    - Prevention of postmenopausal osteoporosis
- **Contraindications of HRT:**
    - Current, past or suspected breast cancer
    - Uncontrolled HTN
    - Undiagnosed vaginal bleeding
    - Active liver disease
    - Active or recent thromboembolic disease
    - Endometrial hyperplasia
    - Porphyria cutanea tarda
- **Benefit of HRT:**
    - Vasomotor symptoms
    - Genitourinary symptoms
    - Osteoporosis
- **Risks of HRT:**
    - Endometrial carcinoma, breast carcinoma, ovarian cancer
    - HTN, CAD, CVD
    - Thromboembolism
    - Change in liver function
    - Gall stones
    - Migraine
- **Estrogen preparation:**
    - Conjugated equine estrogen (CEE): .3–1.25 mg/day
    - Ethinylestradiol
    - Transdermal estradiol
    - Micronized 17 β estradiol
    - Topically applied estradiol emulsion, gel and spray
    - Vaginal estrogenic preparation including CEE vaginal cream
- **Disadvantages of oral route:**
    - Due to first pass hepatic metabolism, plasma estrogen level variable and symptoms not always respond
    - May be associated with nausea and exacerbate liver disease
    - Adverse lipid changes and increased venous thromboembolism risk in comparison with transdermal route
- **Transdermal route:** Preferred in patient with liver disease and ↑ TG. Viewed as endometrial protective agents

- **Progesterone preparation:**
  - Medroxyprogesterone acetate (MPA), 5 mg/day (least androgenic)
  - Norethisterone, 5 mg/day (most androgenic)
  - Micronized progesterone
  - Drospirenone, 3 mg/day (antimineralocorticoid progesterone)
  - Levonorgestrel, .075 mg/day.
- **Adverse effects of progesterone:**
  - Premenstrual tension like symptoms, for example, mood swing, fluid retention, sleep disturbance
  - Adverse effect on lipid profile
  - Breast cancer
- **Common regimen of HRT:**
  - Women who have hysterectomy: Estrogen alone
- **Types of HRT:**

Regimen	Estrogen	Progesterone	Withdrawal bleeding
Cyclic sequential	D_1-D_{21}	$D_{12}-D_{21}$ (10–12 day/month)	Each month
Continuous sequential	Everyday	$D_{12}-D_{21}$ (10–12 day/month)	Each month
Continuous	Everyday	Everyday	No withdrawal bleeding but breakthrough bleeding (20%), ↑ breast cancer risk
Seasonal	Everyday	Last 10–12 day/every 3rd month	Every 3 month

  - Women who have uterus: Combined estrogen and progesterone as unopposed estrogen ↑ risk of endometrial hyperplasia and carcinoma
- **Duration of HRT:**
  - Still a matter of debate
  - HRT should be given in lowest dosage possible for shortest period for symptom relief only
  - For 2–3 years but rarely >5 years
  - In patient with gonadal dysgenesis, surgical menopause, premature menopause: Low dose OCP until age 45 years, then CEE .625 mg ± P
- **Factors to be considered before selection of HRT regimen:**
  - Presence or absence of uterus
  - Willing to experience bleeding or not
  - Presence of risk factors, for example, osteoporosis, CVD.

CHAPTER 51

Precocious Puberty

Q. Define precocious puberty. Classify precocious puberty with etiology.

Ans.

- **Definition:** Appearance of secondary sexual characteristics before the age of 9 years in boys or 8 years in girls
- **Types of precocious puberty:**
    - **Central/complete/true precocious puberty:** Premature activation of hypothalamic-pituitary axis and it is gonadotropin dependent
    - **Incomplete precocious puberty:** If ectopic gonadotropin secretion occurs in boys or autonomous sex steroid secretion occurs in either sex and it is gonadotropin independent
    - **Isosexual precocity:** If feminization occurs in girls and virilization occurs in boys
    - **Contrasexual precocity:** If feminization occurs in boys and virilization occurs in girls
- **Etiology of precocious puberty:**
    - **Central precocious puberty:**
        - Constitutional
        - Idiopathic
        - CNS disorders (congenital defects, tumors, infection, trauma)
    - **Incomplete isosexual precocious puberty:**
        - Males: Gonadotropin secreting tumor, androgen secreting testicular/adrenal tumor, and virilizing CAH
        - Females: Estrogen secreting tumors, severe hypothyroidism
        - Both sex: McCune-Albright syndrome
    - **Incomplete contrasexual precocious puberty:**
        - Males: Estrogen secreting tumor
        - Females: Androgen secreting tumor, virilizing CAH.

Q. Write down the management of precocious puberty.

Ans.

- **Clinical features:**
    - Secondary sexual characteristics: Take H/o age when first noted and order
    - ↑ in growth velocity but short final height (early epiphyseal fusion)

- Tendency toward obesity
- Epilepsy or other CNS abnormality
- Abdominal discomfort
- Family H/o early puberty

■ **Investigations:**
- Bone age
- FSH and LH (↑ in central type and ↓ in peripheral type)
- Sex hormones (testosterone, estradiol, androstenedione, and DHEAS)
- FT4, TSH
- CT scan or MRI of brain
- 17 OH progesterone (↑ in CAH)
- USG or CT of abdomen (adrenals and ovaries)
- Tumor markers (α-fetoprotein and β-hCG)

■ **Treatment:**
- Central: GnRH analogs down regulate GnRH receptors of pituitary gonadotroph and reduce response to endogenous GnRH (medical gonadectomy). Triptorelin acetate subcutaneous or deep IM every 28 days given
- Incomplete:
  • Girls: Medroxyprogesterone acetate (MPA) and aromatase inhibitor (letrozole)
  • Boys: Ketoconazole, flutamide, and MPA
- Counseling and support
- Treatment of underlying cause.

Q. How will you differentiate central from peripheral precocious puberty?

Ans.

Point	Central	Peripheral
Cause	CNS pathology	Adrenal, gonadal tumor, CAH
2° sex characteristics	Appear in normal pubertal order	Appear in isolation
Testes enlargement	First sign and significant	Not enlarged unless tumor
Virilization	Not usual	Can occur
CNS features	May be present	Absent
FSH, LH	↑	↓
GnRH stimulation	Responsive	Not responsive
Imaging	Brain	Abdomen
Gonadotropin	Dependent	Independent
Treatment	GnRH analogs	MPA

CHAPTER 52

Miscellaneous Endocrine Disorders

RECURRENT ABORTION

Q. Define recurrent abortion. Write down its etiology.

Ans. Occurrence of three or more consecutive spontaneous pregnancy losses before the age of viability. Repeated pregnancy loss may be primary (woman without any previous live-born infant) or secondary (woman with at least one prior live-born infant).
- **Etiology of recurrent abortion:**
  - Chromosomal abnormality (numerical or structural)
  - Anatomical abnormalities: Cervical incompetence, fibroids
  - Endocrine disease: Hypo- or hyperthyroidism, uncontrolled DM, PCOS
  - Immunological: Antiphospholipid antibody syndrome, SLE
  - Infection: Toxoplasmosis, rubella, untreated syphilis, HIV, genital tract infection
  - Environmental: Smoking, tobacco, alcohol, radiation, drugs, for example, quinine.

RENAL STONE

Q. Write down types of renal stone and predisposing factors.

Ans.
- **Types of renal stone:**
  - Mixed calcium oxalate and calcium phosphate
  - Calcium oxalate
  - Calcium phosphate
  - Struvite/magnesium ammonium phosphate—staghorn calculi (associated with infection)
  - Cystine stone
  - Uric acid stone, xanthine stone (radiolucent, not seen in X-ray)
- **Predisposing factors for renal stone:**
  - **Environmental and dietary:**
    - Low urine volume: High temperature, low fluid intake
    - Diet: High protein, high Na^+, low Ca^{2+}
    - High Na^+, oxalate, urate excretion
    - Low citrate excretion
  - **Acquired:**
    - Hypercalcemia due to any cause

- Ileal disease or resection (oxalate stone)
- RTA type I (Distal)
  - **Congenital and inherited:**
    - Medullary sponge kidney
    - Familial hypercalciuria
    - Primary hyperoxaluria
    - Cystinuria
  - **Drugs:** Indinavir, ephedrine.

Q. What are the measures to prevent calcium renal stone?

Ans.
- **Diet:**
  - Fluid intake 3–4 L/day (At least 2 L output/day)
  - ↓ Na^+ intake
  - Moderate protein intake, not high
  - Maintain good Ca^{2+} intake in diet, avoid supplement away from meals
  - ↓ oxalate intake, for example, spinach
- **Drugs:**
  - Thiazide: ↓ Ca^{2+} excretion
  - Allopurinol: If urate excretion is high
  - Avoid vitamin D supplement
  - Avoid vitamin C supplementation (more oxalate stone).

Q. What are the indications for intervention of renal stone?

Ans.
- Obstructive anuria or severe infection (pyonephrosis)
- Severe pain or solitary kidney
- Pain and failure of stone to move.

Q. How will you evaluate recurrent stone formers?

Ans.
- **Indications of evaluation:**
  - Recurrent stone >1/3 years
  - ↑ in number or size of stones (metabolically active stones)
  - All children
  - All noncalcium stone formers
  - Positive family history
- **Basic evaluation:**
  - **History:**
    - Stone history
    - Medical history
    - Family history
    - Medications
    - Occupation and lifestyle
    - Diet and fluid intake

- **Physical examination:** To find any etiology that may cause hypercalcemia
- **Investigations:**
  - Urine R/M/E and culture
  - Blood urea, creatinine, electrolytes
  - Urinary pH
  - Serum Ca^{2+}, PO_4, ALP, PTH
  - Serum uric acid
  - Biochemical analysis of passed stones
  - 24-h urinary screen to determine volume and levels of Na^+, Ca^{2+}, PO_4, oxalate, urate, citrate
  - Blood pH (ABG) and acid/NH_4Cl challenge test: If RTA suspected
  - Imaging: Plain X-ray KUB, IVU, unenhanced CT scan.

Q. Discuss about nephrocalcinosis.

Ans.
- **Definition:** Deposition of calcium in renal parenchyma, usually in medulla, rarely cortex
- **Etiology:**
  - RTA—Type I/distal
  - Hypercalcemia due to any cause, for example, hyperparathyroidism, vitamin D intoxication
  - Medullary sponge kidney
  - Chronic pyelonephritis
  - Healed renal TB
- **Clinical features:**
  - Asymptomatic
  - Recurrent renal colic or loin pain
  - Recurrent UTI
  - Hematuria
  - Polyuria
- **Investigations:**
  - Urine R/M/E
  - RFTs (urea, creatinine, electrolyte)
  - USG of KUB
  - IVU
  - Serum Ca^{2+}
  - Other investigations according to suspicion of causes.

MULTIPLE ENDOCRINE NEOPLASIA

Q. Define multiple endocrine neoplasia (MEN).

Ans. Autosomal dominant disorder with hyperplasia and formation of benign or malignant tumors in multiple glands.

- **MEN 1 (Wermer syndrome):**
  - Tumors: Primary hyperparathyroidism, pancreatic neuroendocrine tumors (gastrinoma, insulinoma), pituitary tumors
  - Genetics: Mutation of *MEN1* gene on long arm of chromosome 11
  - Screening in asymptomatic mutation carrier:
    - Annual serum Ca^{++}, PO_4, albumin, ALP, PTH, fasting gastrin, insulin, glucose, prolactin, IGF-1
    - Imaging studies: MRI of pituitary, CT abdomen at presentation and 3 yearly
- **MEN 2:**
  - MEN 2A (Sipple syndrome): Tumors: Medullary carcinoma of thyroid, pheochromocytoma, primary hyperparathyroidism
  - MEN 2B: Tumors: Medullary carcinoma of thyroid, pheochromocytoma, somatic manifestations, for example, marfanoid habitus. Primary hyperparathyroidism is typically absent
  - Genetics: Mutation of RET protooncogene on long arm of chromosome 10
  - Screening in asymptomatic mutation carrier: Annual calcitonin ± pentagastrin stimulation test, plasma or urine catecholamines or metabolites, Ca^{++}, PTH, CT/MRI adrenals.

CARCINOID SYNDROME

Q. Define carcinoid tumor.

Ans. Tumor derived from enterochromaffin cells and is common in appendix and rectum. Spread locally, also metastasis to liver.

Q. Discuss about carcinoid syndrome.

Ans.
- **Carcinoid syndrome:** Systemic symptoms produced when secretory products of neoplastic enterochromaffin cells reach systemic circulation. When produced by primary tumor, they are usually metabolized in liver and do not reach systemic circulation. Carcinoid syndrome only seen when 5-HT/serotonin, bradykinin, and other peptide hormones are released by hepatic metastases
- **Clinical feature:**
  - Small bowel obstruction due to tumor mass
  - Intestinal ischemia (due to mesenteric infiltration or vasospasm)
  - Hepatic metastasis causing pain, hepatomegaly, and jaundice
  - Flushing and wheezing
  - Diarrhea
  - Cardiac involvement (TR, PS) leading to HF
  - Facial telangiectasia
- **Investigation:** 24-h urinary 5-HIAA (5-hydroxyindoleacetic acid, a 5-HT metabolite)
- **Management:**
  - Surgical resection of tumor
  - Hepatic metastasis: Excision to reduce tumor mass, hepatic artery embolization, octreotide
- **Prognosis:** Even with hepatic metastasis, prolonged survival is common.

SECTION 3

METABOLISM

53. Spontaneous Hypoglycemia
54. Homocystinuria
55. Phenylketonuria
56. Obesity
57. Alkaptonuria
58. Glycogen Storage Disease
59. Lysosomal Storage Disease
60. Galactosemia
61. Wilson Disease
62. Hemochromatosis
63. Acute Intermittent Porphyria
64. Renal Tubular Acidosis
65. Hypomagnesemia
66. Nonalcoholic Fatty Liver Disease
67. Gout

CHAPTER 53

Spontaneous Hypoglycemia

Q. Define spontaneous hypoglycemia. How will you evaluate spontaneous hypoglycemia?

Ans.
- **Definition:** Spontaneous hypoglycemia mean hypoglycemia develop in non-diabetic person
- **Evaluation:**

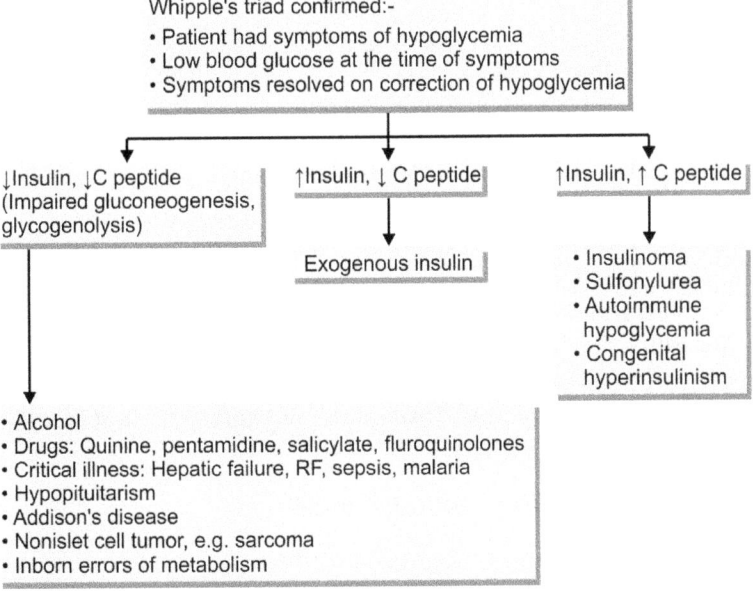

Q. Discuss about insulinoma.

Ans.
- **Insulinoma:**
    - Insulin secreting tumor of islets of Langerhans
    - 90% of insulinomas are benign, 10% are malignant. 80%—solitary and remainder—multiple

- May be familial and associated with MEN 1 in 10% cases
- 99% located in pancreas with equal frequency throughout head, body and tail of pancreas and 1% in ectopic pancreatic tissue (one published report at cervix)
- Any age but common in fourth to sixth decades
- No gender predilection but slight predominance in women

- **Clinical features:**
  - Symptoms of hypoglycemia at fasting or during exercise, relieved by eating
  - Weight gain occurs in 30% patients
  - Sign and symptoms are chiefly those of subacute or chronic neuroglycopenia rather than adrenergic discharge

- **Investigations:**
  - Blood glucose level during symptoms (glucometer and laboratory-based glucose measurement)
  - Plasma insulin, C peptide, alcohol, sulfonylurea level
  - 72 h supervised fasting in hospital
  - Tumor localization studies: CT scan, MRI, endoscopic USG, intraoperative USG, selective calcium stimulated angiography

- **Treatment:**
  - Surgical resection of tumor
  - Small, frequent complex carbohydrate diet
  - Medical treatment:
    - Diazoxide (adverse effects: Edema, hirsutism)
    - Verapamil (orally, 80 mg three times daily)
    - Somatostatin analog, for example, octreotide
  - Malignant insulinoma:
    - Streptozocin, radiolabeled somatostatin analog
    - Resection/embolization of hepatic metastasis

- **Prognosis:**
  - Following removal of solitary insulinoma, life expectancy is restored to normal
  - Average 5 years survival 35%.

Q. Discuss about 72 h supervised fasting in hospital.

Ans.

- **Procedure:**
  - Obtain baseline serum glucose, insulin, proinsulin and C peptide at onset of fast and place intravenous cannula
  - Calculate the onset of fast from the time of last food intake, discontinue all non-essential medications
  - Permit only calorie free and caffeine free fluids and encourage supervised activity, for example, walking
  - Measure urine for ketones at the beginning and every 12 h
  - Obtain capillary glucose with reflectance meter 4 hourly until values <60 mg/dL (3.3 mmol/L), then check hourly

- If symptoms of hypoglycemia occur or if blood glucose <45 mg/dL (2.5 mmol/L) or 72 h elapsed, conclude the fast with sample send for plasma glucose, insulin, pro insulin, C peptide, β-hydroxybutyrate and sulfonylurea
- Give oral fast acting carbohydrate followed by meal. If patient is confused, give 50 mL 25% glucose IV over 3–5 min
- **Diagnostic criteria for insulinoma after 72 h fast:**
  - Plasma glucose: <45 mg/dL
  - Plasma insulin (RIA): ≥6 μU/mL
  - Plasma C peptide: ≥200 pmol/L
  - Beta hydroxybutyrate: ≤2.7 nmol/L (hyperinsulinemia suppress ketogenesis)
  - Sulfonylurea screen: Negative.

Q. Discuss about alimentary hypoglycemia.

Ans.
- Alimentary/reactive/postprandial hypoglycemia mean hypoglycemia in postprandial state
- Common following gastric surgery (including Roux-en-Y gastric bypass), also known as late dumping syndrome
- Patients develop hypoglycemia 1–3 h after a meal especially after consumption of large meal with rapidly absorbable carbohydrate. Rapid delivery of carbohydrate load in small intestine cause sharp rise of plasma glucose which cause increased insulin secretion followed by hypoglycemia
- Mixed meal test used to precipitate the symptoms or patient is requested to consume a meal that leads to symptoms during everyday life. Prolonged (5 h) OGTT not recommended due to false-positive result in some healthy subjects
- **Management:**
  - Small frequent complex carbohydrate diet, avoid large meal with high carbohydrate content
  - Alpha glucosidase inhibitors (acarbose, miglitol)
  - Octreotide prior to each meal.

Q. Discuss about late hypoglycemia of occult diabetes.

Ans. This condition is characterized by initial exaggeration of hyperglycemia during OGTT leading to exaggerated delayed insulin release produces late hypoglycemia 4–5 h after ingestion of glucose. These patients are often obese, frequently have a family H/o DM and have IGT.
- **Management:**
  - Weight reduction in obese patient
  - Small frequent complex carbohydrate diet
  - Avoid refined sugar
  - Advised to have periodic medical checkup.

CHAPTER 54

Homocystinuria

Q. Discuss about homocystinuria.

Ans.
- **Definition:** Autosomal recessive disorder due to cystathionine beta synthase deficiency that convert homocysteine to cystathionine leading to ↑ urinary excretion of homocysteine and methionine
- **Clinical features:**
    - Skeletal: Phenotypes similar to Marfan syndrome (tall stature, hypermobility), osteoporosis
    - Eyes: Ectopia lentis (dislocation of lens)
    - Vascular: Thromboembolism
    - CNS: Developmental delay, mental retardation, seizure, psychiatric disturbance
    - Skin: Hypopigmentation
- **Investigations:**
    - ↑ Plasma homocysteine and methionine but low plasma cystine
    - Cyanide nitroprusside test in urine: +ve due to ↑ homocysteine in urine
    - Spectroscopic examination of urine: Homocysteine detected
- **Treatment:**
    - Dietary: Methionine restricted and cystine supplement diet
    - Large dosage of pyridoxine.

Q. Mention the difference between Marfan syndrome and homocystinuria.

Ans.

Points	Marfan syndrome	Homocystinuria
Inheritance	Autosomal dominant	Autosomal recessive
Lens	Dislocated upward	Dislocated downward
Osteoporosis, mental retardation, thromboembolism	No	Common
Cyanide nitroprusside test in urine	−ve	+ve
Pyridoxine	No	May respond

CHAPTER 55

Phenylketonuria

Q. Discuss about phenylketonuria.

Ans.
- **Definition:** Autosomal recessive disorder due to deficiency of phenylalanine hydroxylase enzyme that convert phenylalanine to tyrosine
- **Clinical features:**
  - Mental retardation
  - Seizure
  - Hypopigmentation (light skin color, fair hair and blue eyes)
  - Growth failure
  - Mousy odor of sweat (metabolites of phenylalanine)
- **Investigations:**
  - ↑ Blood level of phenylalanine (Guthrie test)
  - Urine test for phenylpyruvic acid (metabolite of phenylalanine)
- **Treatment:** Lifelong adherence to low phenylalanine diet
- **Neonatal screening:** Blood level of phenylalanine determined 48 h after infant has ingested protein (not at birth).

CHAPTER 56

Obesity

Q. Define obesity.

Ans. Excess of body fat sufficient to adversely affect health.

Q. Compare between abdominal and gluteofemoral obesity.

Ans. Central/abdominal/visceral/android/apple obesity is more associated with ↑ cardiovascular risk, metabolic syndrome, T2DM than gluteofemoral obesity (pear shaped/gynoid).

Q. What is Body mass index (BMI)?

Ans. Body mass index = weight in kg/height in m².
- <18.5: Underweight
- 18.5–24.9: Healthy weight
- 25–29.9: Overweight
- ≥30: Obese
  - 30–34.9: Class I (moderate)
  - 35–39.9: Class II (severe)
  - ≥40: Class III (very severe/morbid obesity)
  - WHO recommends for Asians: BMI >23 (overweight), >25 (obese).

Q. Discuss about metabolic syndrome.

Ans.
- **Metabolic syndrome/syndrome X/insulin resistance syndrome/Reaven syndrome:** Clustering of metabolic abnormalities that ↑ risk of cardiovascular disease and DM
- **National cholesterol education program (NCEP) adult treatment part III: (ATP III) 2001 criteria for metabolic syndrome: 3 or more out of 5 risk factors**
  - Central/abdominal obesity: Waist circumference >102 cm (male), >88 cm (female)
  - HTN ≥130/≥85 mm Hg or specific medication
  - FBS ≥6.1 mmol/L or specific medication or previously diagnosed T2DM
  - Triglyceride ≥150 mg/dL or specific medication
  - HDL cholesterol <40 mg/dL (male), <50 mg/dL (female) or specific medication
  - Other associated factors: Hyperinsulinemia, microalbuminuria, ↑ fibrinogen, ↑ plasminogen activator inhibitor-1, ↑ CRP, ↑ uric acid, PCOS, NASH.

Q. Mention complications of obesity.

Ans.
- Metabolic syndrome (T2DM, HTN, Dyslipidemia): Coronary artery disease, stroke, diabetic complications
- NASH → Liver cirrhosis
- GERD, hiatal hernia
- Restricted ventilation: Exertional dyspnea, sleep apnea, respiratory failure (Pickwickian syndrome)
- Mechanical effects of weight: Urinary incontinence, osteoarthritis, varicose veins
- ↑ Peripheral steroid interconversion in adipose tissue: Hormone-dependent cancers (breast, endometrium), PCOS (infertility, hirsutism)
- Gall stone
- Colorectal, prostate, renal cell carcinoma
- Skin infections (groin and submammary candidiasis)
- Psychological (low self-esteem, depression).

Q. Mention etiology of progressive weight gain.

Ans.
- Primary/simple obesity
- Endocrine: Cushing syndrome, hypothyroidism, PCOS, acromegaly, insulinoma, pseudohypoparathyroidism
- Drugs: OCP, corticosteroids, insulin, sulfonylurea, TCA, Na valproate, cyproheptadine
- Hypothalamic tumors or injury
- Depression (over eating)
- Nephrotic syndrome
- Prader-Willi syndrome, Laurence-Moon-Bardet-Biedl syndrome.

Q. Discuss about management of obesity

Ans.

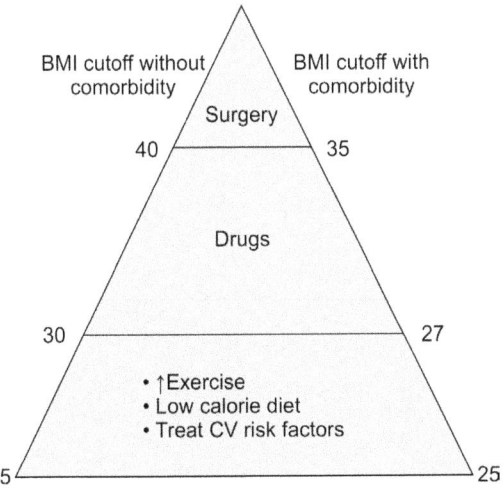

1. **Diet:** Reduce calorie intake 600 kcal below current intake. Goal is to lose .5 kg/week. Ensure minimum 50 g protein/day (M) or 40 g/day (F) to minimize muscle degradation
2. **Exercise:** 60 min/day
3. **Target:** Weight loss ≥10% of initial body weight and maintaining the loss ≥1 year
4. **Drugs:** Orlistat → Inhibit pancreatic and gastric lipase →↓ hydrolysis of digested TG →↓ fat absorption (30%). Dose is 60–120 mg with three main meals. Adverse effects are loose stool, oily spotting, fecal urgency, flatulence, malabsorption of fat soluble vitamins
5. **Bariatric surgery:**
    - **Indication:**
        - Obese patients with BMI ≥40 (without comorbidity) or ≥35 (with at least one comorbid disease, e.g. T2DM, HTN, dyslipidemia, cardiovascular disease, sleep apnea) in motivated patient in whom extensive dietary and drug therapy fails
        - No other reversible endocrine disorders causing obesity
        - No current substance abuse
        - No severe psychiatric illness
    - **Types of bariatric surgery:**
        - Gastric banding
        - Sleeve gastrectomy
        - Roux-en-Y gastric bypass: Stapling the upper stomach into a small 30 mL pouch and attaching it to jejunum bypassing the lower stomach and duodenum
        - Duodenal switch
    - **Mechanism of weight loss:**
        - ↓ Quantity of food ingested at any one time
        - Malabsorptive procedure cause wasting of fat calories
        - ↓ Hunger and ↑ satiety by disrupting release of ghrelin from stomach or other peptides from small bowel
    - **Complication of bariatric surgery:**
        - Operative complications
        - Dumping syndrome:
            - Early dumping: Rapid gastric emptying leads to abdominal discomfort and diarrhea after eating
            - Late dumping (reactive hypoglycemia)
        - Persistent vomiting
        - Micronutrient deficiency: Iron, Vitamin B_{12}, folate
        - Gastric cancer
        - Metabolic bone disease/osteoporosis.

CHAPTER 57

Alkaptonuria

Q. Discuss about alkaptonuria/ochronosis.

Ans.
- **Definition:** Autosomal recessive disorder due to deficiency of enzyme homogentisic acid oxidase that convert homogentisic acid to methylacetoacetic acid in tyrosine degradation pathway
- **Clinical features:**
  - Homogentisic acid binds to collagen of connective tissue, tendon and cartilage leading to
    - Blue-black pigmentation of ear, nose and cheeks (ochronosis)
    - Arthritis later in life (30 years)
  - Black color of urine if allowed to stand (oxidation of homogentisic acid)
- **Treatment:** Alkaptonuria is benign.

CHAPTER **58**

Glycogen Storage Disease

Q. **Discuss about glycogen storage disease/glycogenoses.**
Ans.
- **Definition:** Autosomal recessive disorder due to deficiency of one of the enzymes involved in synthesis or breakdown of glycogen
- **Types:** 11 major types:
    - Type I: Von Gierke
    - Type II: Pompe
    - Type III: Cori
    - Type IV: Andersen
    - Type V: McArdle
    - Type VI: Hers
    - Type VII: Tarui
    - Type VIII
    - Type IX
    - Type 0

    (Easy way to remember: Vice president Cori Andersen makes her trip)
- **Clinical features:**
    - **Hepatic form (all types except 2, 5, 8):** Primarily affects the liver, manifested as hypoglycemia, hepatomegaly, liver failure
    - **Myopathic form (type 2, 5, 8):** Primarily affects the muscle, manifested as muscle weakness, muscle cramp after exercise. Lactate level in blood fails to rise after exercise due to block in glycolysis
- **Diagnosis:** Muscle or liver biopsy to confirm enzyme defect
- **Treatment:** Avoid hypoglycemia (frequent feeding, avoid profound fasting), enzyme replacement, liver transplantation.

CHAPTER **59**

Lysosomal Storage Disease

Q. **Discuss about lysosomal storage disease.**

Ans.
- **Definition:** Autosomal recessive disorder due to deficiency of functional lysosomal enzymes leading to accumulation of partially degraded insoluble metabolite within lysosomes
- **Type:**
    - Gangliosidosis: Tay-Sachs disease, manifested as progressive neurological disorder
    - Sulfatidosis:
        - Fabry disease
        - Gaucher disease
        - Niemann-Pick disease
    - Mucopolysaccharidosis: Hurler syndrome, manifested as short limb and short spine
- **Treatment:** Enzyme replacement.

CHAPTER 60

Galactosemia

Q. Discuss about galactosemia.

Ans.
- **Definition:** Autosomal recessive disorder due to deficiency of galactose-1 phosphate uridyltransferase (GALT) enzyme
- **Clinical features:**
  - Neonate is unable to metabolize galactose, one of the hexose sugars contained in lactose
  - Vomiting or diarrhea usually begins within a few days of ingestion of milk
  - Neonate may become jaundiced
  - Failure to thrive
  - Hepatomegaly, cataract, mental retardation, fulminant infection with *Escherichia coli*
- **Treatment:** Lifelong avoidance of galactose and lactose containing foods.

CHAPTER 61

Wilson Disease

Q. Discuss about Wilson disease/hepatolenticular degeneration.

Ans.
- **Definition:** Autosomal recessive disorder due to failure of synthesis of ceruloplasmin leading to increased total body copper with excess copper deposited in and causing damage to several organs
- **Clinical features:**
  - Age: 5–45 years. Hepatic disease occurs predominantly in childhood, but neurological disease occurs in later adolescence
  - **Liver disease:** Acute hepatitis, recurrent acute hepatitis, fulminant liver failure, chronic hepatitis, cirrhosis of liver
  - **Neurological disease:** Tremor, choreoathetosis, dystonia, Parkinsonism, dementia
  - **Kayser Fleischer rings:** Greenish-brown discoloration at the junction of cornea and sclera. Sometimes seen only by slit lamp examination. Seen in 60% adults with Wilson disease, less often in children but almost always in neurological Wilson disease. Disappear with treatment
- **Investigations:**
  - Serum ceruloplasmin: low
  - Serum free copper level: ↑
  - 24 h urinary copper excretion: ↑
  - 24 h urinary copper excretion while giving D-penicillamine: Confirmatory
  - Liver biopsy: High hepatic copper content
- **Management:**
  - Penicillamine, 1–4 g/day (copper binding agent)
  - Zinc acetate
  - Trientine dihydrochloride
- **Prognosis:** Good, provided treatment started before there is irreversible damage
- **Family screening:** Siblings and children of patients must be investigated and treatment must be given to affected individuals, even asymptomatic.

CHAPTER 62

Hemochromatosis

Q. Discuss about hemochromatosis.

Ans.

- **Definition:** Hemochromatosis is a condition in which total body iron is increased to 20–60 g (normal 4 g) with excess iron deposited in and causing damage to several organs
- **Causes:**
  - Hereditary hemochromatosis
  - Secondary iron overload:
    - Repeated blood transfusion (>50 L)
    - Chronic hemolytic disorder: Thalassemia, sideroblastic anemia
    - Alcoholic liver disease
    - Porphyria cutanea tarda
- **Hereditary hemochromatosis:** Autosomal recessive disorder caused by increased absorption of dietary iron. 90% in male (iron loss in menstruation primarily protect female)
- **Clinical features:**
  - Features of liver disease (with hepatomegaly)
  - DM
  - Heart failure or cardiac arrhythmia
  - Leaden-gray skin pigmentation (due to excess melanin) in exposed parts like axilla, groin, genitalia (bronzed diabetes)
  - Arthropathy
- **Investigations:**
  - Iron profile:
    - ↑ serum iron
    - ↑ serum ferritin: >1,000 µg/L (iron overload)
    - Transferrin saturation: >45% (iron overload)
    - TIBC: Saturated
  - Liver biopsy: Assessment of fibrosis. Hepatocyte iron is characteristic (Perls stain)
- **Management:**
  - Weekly venesection of 500 mL blood (250 mg iron) until serum ferritin <50 µg/L
  - Family screening.

CHAPTER 63

Acute Intermittent Porphyria

Q. Discuss about acute intermittent porphyria (AIP).

Ans.
- **Definition:** Autosomal dominant disorder due to partial enzyme deficiency of Heme biosynthetic pathway
- **Precipitating factors:** Alcohol, fasting, drug (anticonvulsant, sulfonamide, OCP)
- **Clinical features:**
  - Photosensitive skin manifestations: Pain, erythema, blistering, pigmentation on sun exposed area
  - Acute relapsing and remitting neurological syndrome:
    - Acute abdominal pain with autonomic dysfunction (tachycardia, HTN, constipation)
    - Neuropsychiatric manifestation
    - Hyponatremia (SIADH)
    - Acute neuropathy (motor)
  - Urine turns dark on standing in light and air
  - Triad of acute intermittent porphyria: Recurrent episode of peritonism, neuropsychiatric manifestations, hyponatremia
- **Investigations:**
  - Measurement of porphyrins and porphyrin precursor in blood, urine, feces
  - Measurement of enzyme: Porphobilinogen (PBG) deaminase activity in RBC
- **Treatment:**
  - Avoid drug that precipitate porphyria
  - IV glucose (5,000 kJ/day)
  - Administration of heme
  - Cyclical acute attack in women: GnRH analog (suppress menstruation)

- Photosensitive skin manifestation:
  - Avoid sun exposure and skin trauma
  - Barrier sun cream: Zinc cream
  - Beta carotene
- **Porphyria cutanea tarda:**
  - Precipitated by alcohol, Fe overload, HCV, HIV, estrogen
  - ↑ Skin fragility and blistering on light exposed area, for example, back of fingers
- **Treatment:** A course of venesection, avoid precipitant, prolonged course of chloroquine.

CHAPTER 64

Renal Tubular Acidosis

Q. Discuss about renal tubular acidosis (RTA).

Ans.
- **Definition:** Systemic acidosis caused by impairment of the ability of renal tubules to maintain acid–base balance
- **Suspected in:** Hyperchloremic (normal Cl^-: 95–107 mmol/L) with normal anion gap acidosis with no evidence of gastrointestinal disturbance and urinary pH inappropriately high (>5.5) in presence of systemic acidosis (Plasma HCO_3^- <21 mmol/L)
- Normal anion gap is 12 ± 4 mmol/L. Anion gap: $(Na^+ + K^+) - (Cl^- + HCO_3^-)$
- **Types of RTA and difference:**

Points	Type 1/classical distal	Type 2/proximal RTA	Type 4/hyperkalemic distal RTA/hyporeninemic hypoaldosteronism
Renal defect	Distal H^+ secretion	Proximal HCO_3^- reabsorption	Distal Na^+ reabsorption with secondary ↓ secretion of K^+ and H^+
Serum K^+	↓	↓	↑
Renal stone, nephrocalcinosis, osteomalacia	Yes	No	No
Cause	• Congenital • SLE • Lithium • Amphotericin	• Congenital (Fanconi syndrome, Wilson disease) • Multiple myeloma • Hyperparathyroidism • Amyloidosis	• Hypoaldosteronism (primary or secondary) • Obstructive nephropathy • Amiloride • Spironolactone
Treatment		• Treatment of underlying cause • $NaHCO_3$ or $KHCO_3$ • Target: Plasma HCO_3^- >18 mmol/L with normal K^+	• Loop or thiazide diuretics • Fludrocortisone

- **Investigations of RTA:**
  - Blood pH (ABG)
  - Urine pH
  - Serum electrolytes

- Plain X-ray KUB
- Confirmatory test: Acid load test/NH_4Cl challenge test: Measurement of urinary pH after oral $NH_4Cl \rightarrow$ Urine pH >5.5 despite plasma HCO_3^- <21 mmol/L $\rightarrow$ RTA. (failure to acidify urine despite giving acid load).

Q. How renal stone formed in type 1 RTA?

Ans. In type 1 RTA, Acidosis $\rightarrow Ca^{++}$ mobilization from bone $\rightarrow$ Hypercalciuria, renal stone, nephrocalcinosis, osteomalacia.

CHAPTER 65

Hypomagnesemia

Q. Discuss about hypomagnesemia.

Ans.
- **Definition:** Plasma magnesium below the reference range (0.7–1.0 mmol/L). Mg^{++} is an important element required for neuromuscular and neurological function
- **Etiology:**
    - Inadequate intake: Starvation, malnutrition (esp. alcoholism), TPN
    - Excessive losses:
        - GIT: Prolonged vomiting, chronic diarrhea, malabsorption
        - Renal: Diuretics (loop and thiazide), DKA, transport defect (Bartter, Gitelman syndrome)
    - Others: Acute pancreatitis, hungry bone syndrome, DM
- **Clinical features:**
    - Hypomagnesemia is frequently associated with hypocalcemia
    - Tetany, cardiac arrhythmia, CNS excitation, seizure
    - Magnesium depletion also associated with $\downarrow$ Na and $\downarrow$ K^+
- **Investigations:**
    - Serum Mg^{++}
    - Serum Ca^{++}
    - Serum electrolytes
    - ECG
- **Treatment:**
    - Treatment of cause (stop alcohol, diuretic)
    - Oral Mg salts: Poor absorption and may cause diarrhea
    - If symptomatic: IV Mg. Serum Mg level monitored daily and dose repeated daily till Mg level normal. K^+ and Ca^{++} replacement may be added also
    - Tendon reflex checked as $\downarrow$ reflex in hypermagnesemia
    - Mg rich food: Tomato, tea, nuts, beans.

CHAPTER 66

Nonalcoholic Fatty Liver Disease

Q. Discuss about nonalcoholic fatty liver disease (NAFLD).

Ans.
- **Definition:** NAFLD represents spectrum of liver disease with
  - Evidence of hepatic steatosis either by imaging or by histology
  - No cause for secondary hepatic fat accumulation such as significant alcohol consumption, hereditary disorders or use of steatogenic medications, for example, amiodarone, MTX, tamoxifen, corticosteroid
- **Classification of NAFLD:** NAFLD is histologically classified into
  - **Nonalcoholic fatty liver (NAFL):** Presence of hepatic steatosis with no evidence of hepatocellular injury or fibrosis. The risk of progression to cirrhosis and liver failure is minimal
  - **Nonalcoholic steatohepatitis (NASH):** Presence of hepatic steatosis and inflammation with hepatocyte injury (ballooning) with or without fibrosis. This can progress to cirrhosis, liver failure and rarely hepatocellular carcinoma (HCC)
- **Risk factors associated with NAFLD:**
  - Obesity
  - T2DM
  - Dyslipidemia
  - Metabolic syndrome
  - PCOS
  - Hypothyroidism
  - Hypogonadism
- **Clinical features:**
  - Asymptomatic, abnormal LFTs (↑ transaminases or isolated ↑ GGT)
  - Jaundice occurs when cirrhosis established
  - Complication of cirrhosis, for example, variceal hemorrhage or HCC
  - Presence of risk factors, for example, obesity, DM, metabolic syndrome
- **Investigation:**
  - LFTs: ↑ transaminases (SGPT > SGOT), ↑ ALP (30%)
  - USG: Bright liver

- Liver biopsy: Indicated in individuals with SGPT >2XULN with features of metabolic syndrome. Findings are
    - Macrovesicular fat deposition
    - Mallory bodies
    - Neutrophil infiltration and pericellular fibrosis
- **Management:**
    - Weight loss (at least 3–5%): Hypocaloric diet, ↑ exercise
    - Metformin: Improve LFTs in T2DM with NASH, also pioglitazones
    - Vitamin E (α-tocopherol): 800 IU/day improve liver histology in nondiabetic adult
    - Statin: For coexisting dyslipidemia
    - Bariatric surgery: In morbid obese patient with NAFLD
- **Prognosis:** Once cirrhosis develops, 5-year survival rate (90%) and 10-year survival rate (84%).

CHAPTER 67

Gout

Q. Define gout.

Ans.
- Crystal deposition disease and is pathological reaction of the joint and periarticular tissue to the presence of monosodium urate monohydrate (MSU) crystals
- Male:Female = 5:1.

Q. Discuss metabolism of uric acid.

Ans.

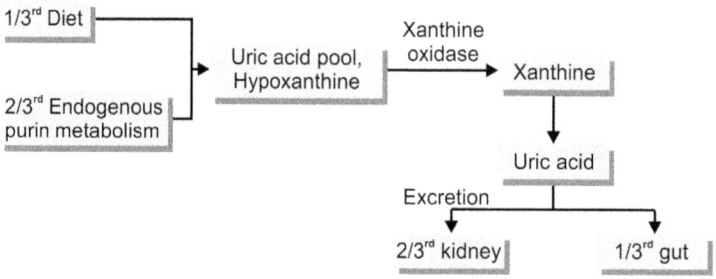

- Normal serum uric acid: male: 3.4–7 mg/dL, female: 2.4–5.7 mg/dL.

Q. Mention etiology of hyperuricemia (serum uric acid >6.8 or 7 mg/dL).

Ans.
- Primary gout (inherited renal tubular defect)
- Renal failure
- Chronic drug therapy: Thiazide and loop diuretics, low dose aspirin, ciclosporine, pyrazinamide
- Lead toxicity
- Lactic acidosis (alcohol)
- Chronic myeloproliferative or lymphoproliferative disorder, for example, PRV, CLL
- Psoriasis, hypothyroidism, hyperparathyroidism (hyperuricemia is present in 5% population, but 95% of hyperuricemic patients never develop gout).

Q. Mention clinical features and investigations of gout.

Ans.
- **Acute gout:**
  - First MTP joint affected/podagra (>50%)
  - Also ankle, midfoot, knee, small joints of hand, wrist and elbow
  - Very rapid onset, maximum in 2–6 h, worst pain ever with extreme tenderness
  - Marked swelling with overlying red shiny skin
  - Self limiting over 5–14 days with complete return to normal
  - Differential diagnosis: Septic arthritis, cellulitis
- **Chronic tophaceous gout:** Large MSU crystal deposit produce white irregular firm nodule (tophi) at extensor surface of finger, hand, forearm, elbow, Achilles tendon and helix of ear
- **Uric acid calculi (10%)**
- **Progressive renal impairment**
- **Investigations:**
  - Serum uric acid: ↑ Uric acid does not confirm gout. Uric acid may be normal in acute attack as it falls as a part of acute phase response
  - Synovial fluid study: ↑ Turbidity in acute attack (due to PMN). Polarized microscopy reveal MSU crystal that is needle shaped, bright birefringence (also found in tophus aspirate)
  - Renal function tests (urine R/M/E, urea, creatinine)
  - OGTT, fasting lipid profile
  - X-ray of involved joint.

Q. Discuss about management of gout.

Ans.
- **General management:** Weight loss for obese patient. Stop smoking, alcohol. Exercise, stay well hydrated and avoid high protein diet (red meat, sea food, liver, kidney)
- **Acute attack:**
  - NSAID with local ice pack
  - Colchicine (Neutrophil microtubular assembly inhibitor): .5 mg 6, 8 or 12 hourly. Adverse effect includes vomiting and severe diarrhea
  - Joint aspiration with intra-articular steroid
  - Severe polyarticular attack: Parenteral corticosteroid
- **Indication of urate lowering drug:**
  - Recurrent attacks of acute gout (≥2/year)
  - Tophi
  - Evidence of bone or joint damage
  - Associated renal disease and/or nephrolithiasis
  - Gout with greatly elevated serum uric acid

- **Target uric acid:** Serum uric acid <6 or <5 mg/dL if needed to improve gout sign and symptoms
- **Drugs:**
  - Allopurinol 100 mg/day or febuxostat 80 mg/day. Xanthine oxidase inhibitor → may trigger acute attack, continue it. So start colchicine for initial 6 months
  - Uricosuric drug: Probenecid, sulfinpyrazone
  - Biological agent: Pegloticase
  - Thiazide diuretics should be stopped if possible and replaced with ACEI, as it has uricosuric effects.

Bibliography

1. ABM Abdullah. Long Cases in Clinical Medicine. Jaypee Brothers Medical Publishers, 2013
2. David G Gardner, Dolores Shoback (Eds). Greenspan's Basic and Clinical Endocrinology, 10th Edition.
3. Denise Ferrier. Lippincott Illustrated Reviews: Biochemistry, 6th Edition (2017)
4. Endocrine Secrets, 7th Edition
5. Guidelines by American Thyroid Association, American Diabetic Association, American Association of Clinical Endocrinologists
6. Harrison's Principles of Internal Medicine, 20th Edition
7. J Alastair Innes, Anna Dover, Karen Fairhurst (Eds). Macleod's Clinical Examination, 14th edition (2018)
8. John E. Hall. Guyton and Hall Textbook of Medical Physiology, 13th Edition (2016)
9. Kim E Barrett, Susan M Barman, Scott Boitano, Heddwen Brooks. Ganong's Review of Medical Physiology, 25th Edition (2015)
10. Kumar and Clark's Clinical Medicine, 9th Edition
11. Maxine A. Papadakis, Stephen J. McPhee, Michael W. Rabow (Eds). Current Medical Diagnosis and Treatment, 2018
12. Michael Glynn, William M Drake (Eds). Hutchison's Clinical Methods: An Integrated Approach to Clinical Practice, 24th Edition.
13. Oxford Handbook of Endocrinology and Diabetes, 4th Edition (2014)
14. Richard IG Holt, Allan Flyvbjerg, Barry J Goldstein (Eds). Textbook of Diabetes, 5th Edition, 2017.
15. Shlomo Melmed, Kenneth S Polonsky, P Reed Larsen, Henry M Kronenberg (Eds). Williams Textbook of Endocrinology, 13th Edition (2016).
16. Stuart Ralston Ian Penman Mark Strachan Richard Hobson (Eds). Davidson's Principles and Practice of Medicine, 23rd Edition
17. Various books and leaflets by Diabetic Association of Bangladesh, in Bangla Bangladesh Diabetic Somiti (BADAS).
18. Victor Rodwell, P Anthony Weil, David Bender, Kathleen M Botham, Peter J Kennelly. Harper's Illustrated Biochemistry, 30th Edition (2015)
19. Vinay Kumar, Abul K Abbas, Jon C Aster. Robbins Basic Pathology, 10th Edition (2018).

Index

A

Abdominal obesity 348
Abdominal pain 21-23
Abortion, etiology of recurrent 337
Acanthosis nigricans 115
Acarbose 32
Acromegaloidism 133
Acromegaly
   causes of 134
      death in 136
   clinical features of 135
   pathophysiology of 134
   patients, treatment of 140
Acrosome reaction 284
Acute intermittent porphyria
   clinical features 357
   investigations 357
   treatment 357, 358
Addison disease 237
   clinical features of 238
   triad of 238
Adrenal androgen insufficiency 238
Adrenal carcinoma 235
Adrenal crisis, acute 242
Adrenal dependent 250
Adrenal hemorrhage 238
   acute 239
Adrenal incidentaloma 221, 222, 232
   differential diagnosis of 221
   evaluate 221
   treat 222
Adrenal insufficiency 199
Adrenal malignancy, extra 222
Adrenal mass
   incidental 221
   types of 263
Adrenal tumor, primary 225
Adrenal venous sampling 254
Adrenalectomy, bilateral 233
Adrenarche 272
Adrenocortical insufficiency 236, 239, 243
   causes of 237
   etiology of 237, 239
   pathophysiology of 236

   primary 241, 243
   secondary 239, 241
Adrenocorticotropic hormone
   dependent 223
   independent 223
   stimulation test 240
Aerobic exercise 25
   benefits of 25
Agranulocytosis 167
Alanine transaminase 33
Albright hereditary
   osteodystrophy 207
Alcoholic liver disease 356
Aldose reductase inhibitor 67, 83
Aldosterone 251
Aldosterone-renin ratio 253
Aldosteronism
   clinical features of primary 252
   detect primary 252
   primary 251
   testing for primary 252
   treat primary 255
Alendronate 218
Alimentary hypoglycemia 345
Alkali syndrome, milk 199
Alkaptonuria 351
Allergic reactions, minor 167
Alpha glucosidase inhibitors 36
Alprostadil, intracavernosal
   injection of 306
Aluminum toxicity 76
Amenorrhea 313, 324, 325
   causes of
      primary 324
      secondary 325
   false 324
   primary 324
   secondary 324, 328
   types of 324
American Diabetic Association 20
Amino acids 39
Ampicillin 89
Anaerobic exercise 25
   benefits of 26
Analog insulin 45
   safety of 103

ANCA positive vasculitis 168
Androgen 220
   deficiency 285
      in male, clinical features of 280
      sign of 287
      symptoms of 287
   Excess Society criteria 309
Androgen-secreting tumor,
   rule out 311
Anemia
   causes of 74
   in hypothyroidism, types of 180
   treatment modalities of 75
Angiography 244
Anovulation 310
Antidepressants, tricyclic 83
Antidiabetic
   agent, selection of 31
   drugs, types of 31
   medication 100, 103, 112
   treatment 115
Antidiuretic hormone 122
Antioxidant 21, 84
Antithyroid drugs 165, 166, 168
   contraindication of 169
   dose of 166
Aplasia cutis of scalp 168
Appetite, normal or increased 162
Aptonuria 351
Argon laser phototherapy 66
Arteria dorsalis pedis 88
Arterial ulcer 91
Arthritis 351
   and lupus like syndrome 168
Assisted reproductive
   technology 318
Atonic bladder 84
Atorvastatin 95
Attack, acute 365
Autoantibodies 14
Autoimmune
   adrenalitis 237
   hypothyroidism 164
Autonomic neuropathy 82
   clinical features of 82

B

Bacterial infection 114, 160
Ballet sign 162
Bariatric surgery 350
   complication of 350
   types of 350
Basal bolus
   insulin regimen 47, 110
   regimen 49
Basal fasting growth hormone
   level 138
Basal plus regimen 46
Baseline investigations 304
Beta-blocker 168
Beta-cell function, genetic
   defects of 3
Betamethasone 247
Biguanides 34
Bile acid sequestrants 95
Biosynthesis of catecholamine,
   steps of 256
Bisphosphonate 217
   adverse effect of 217
   contraindications of 218
   swallowing of 217
   use of 217
Block and replace therapy 167
Blood
   glucose monitoring 110
   loss, chronic 76
   pressure regulation, abnormal 82
   sugar 22
   transfusion 356
Body mass index 348
Body weight 317
Bone
   and mineral disorders 198
   biopsy 210
   densitometry 213, 214
      indications of 214
   turnover, biochemical
      markers of 213
Brain, magnetic resonance
   imaging of 138
Breast 274
Brittle diabetes 10
Bruns-Garland syndrome 81
Buccal bioadhesive T tablets 287

C

C peptide estimation 23
Calciphylaxis 79
Calcitonin 219
Calcium
   concentration in body fluid 198
   deficiency 209
   deposition of 205, 339
   in body, role of 198
   renal stone, prevent 338
Calcium-creatinine clearance
   ratio 198
Canagliflozin 32
Candida infection of mouth 114
Carbimazole 166
Carbohydrate
   intake 72
   metabolism 41
Carcinoid syndrome 340
Carcinoid tumor 340
Cardiac autonomic
   neuropathy 83, 105
Cardiac risk 105
Cardiovascular disease,
   screening for 100
Cardiovascular risk factors 92
Carney syndrome 225
Carpal tunnel syndrome 137
Cataract 67
Catecholamine metabolism, steps
   of 256
Cell of origin 192
Cells of islets 40
Central nervous system
   disorders 275
   effects 200
Central precocious puberty 335
Central puberty 335
Cerebral circulation 18
Cerebrospinal fluid 123
Cervical factor 314
   infertility scanty 319
Cervical mucus 319
Charcot joints 84
   clinical features 85
   etiology 84
   indication of surgery 85
   investigations 85
   management 85
   pathogenesis 85
Chemosis 162
Chemotherapy 145
Chest 164
Cholecystographic agents 168
Cholestatic jaundice 168
Cholesterol absorption inhibitors 95
Cholestyramine 95, 168
Chvostek sign 206
Ciprofloxacin 89
Climacteric transition 330
Clindamycin 89
Clomiphene citrate 317
Clonidine suppression test 261
Cold and sweaty hand 136
Cold nodule 165
Colesevelam 95
Colestipol 95, 168
Combination therapy 97
Complete puberty 335
Computed tomography scan 21
Congenital adrenal hyperplasia 266
   classify 267
   diagnose 268
   enzyme deficiency in 266
   in pregnancy, case of 270
   late onset 268
   management of 269
   simple virilizing 267
   types of 267, 268
Congenital malformations 103
Conjunctival edema 162
Constipation 84
Contrasexual precocious puberty,
   incomplete 335
Contrasexual precocity 335
Conventional irradiation 128
Coronary circulation 18
Cortical adenoma 263
Cortical carcinoma 263
Hormone stimulation test,
   corticotropin-releasing
   229
Cranial diabetes insipidus 148, 150
Creatinine clearance rate 71
Cretinism 178
Cryptomenorrhea 324
Cryptorchidism 289
Cushing's disease 224
   treatment of 233
Cushing's syndrome 223, 227, 231,
   232, 234
   causes of 223, 229
   classify 223
   clinical features of 226
   cyclic 232
   endogenous 224
   food-dependent 225
   prognosis of 234
Cutaneous infections 114

Index

Cutaneous metabolic
　　manifestations 114
Cyanide nitroprusside test 346
Cypionate 287
Cyproterone acetate 313
Cytologic diagnosis 190

D

Dapagliflozin 32
Debilitating disease, chronic 290
Deep breaths 83
Dehydration 251
Dehydroepiandrosterone
　　replacement 243
Delayed puberty 274, 276
　　causes of 275, 278
Denosumab 219
Dermopathy 161
Dexamethasone 168, 247
　　suppression test 228
Diabetes 21, 23
　　medical evaluation 11
　　microvascular complication of 19
　　ocular complication of 67
　　of young 1, subtypes of 15
　　syndrome 14
　　testing for 116
Diabetes insipidus 148-150
　　clinical features of 148
　　from primary polydipsia 150
Diabetes management 104
　　during surgery, strategies of 107
Diabetes mellitus 3, 20, 30, 92
　　acute complications of 57
　　amelioration of 122
　　and Ramadan 108
　　and surgery 105
　　chronic complications of 18
　　classification of 3
　　diagnosis of 3, 5
　　disease spectrum, natural
　　　　history of type 2 18
　　during Ramadan 108
　　exercise in 25
　　malnutrition-related 20
　　manage during 108
　　microvascular
　　　　complications of 69
　　pathogenesis of 13
　　　　type 1 13
　　prevention of 116
　　primary prevention 116
　　risk of surgery in 105

　　secondary prevention 117
　　skin manifestation of 114
　　tertiary prevention 117
　　treatment of 7, 106
　　type 1 3, 69, 107, 113
　　type 2 3, 69, 107, 113, 115
　　well-controlled type 2 107
Diabetic amyotrophy 81
Diabetic autonomic
　　neuropathy 28, 81
Diabetic dermopathy 115
Diabetic diarrhea 84
Diabetic dyslipidemia 94
Diabetic foot 86, 89
　　avoid heat injury 90
　　cut nails 90
　　examine 87
　　footwear for 90
　　high-risk of 86
　　inspect 90
　　lesions 88
　　　　pathogenesis of 87
　　prevalence of 86
　　screening for high-risk 90
　　treatment of 89
　　ulceration, risk factors of 86
Diabetic ketoacidosis 57, 62, 108
　　causes of death of 62
　　clinical features of 59
　　complications of 62
　　pathophysiology of 57
Diabetic nephropathy 18, 28, 69,
　　　　71, 72
　　epidemiology of 69
　　natural history of 69
　　progression of 70
Diabetic neuropathy 18, 80, 81
　　diagnosis of 80
　　epidemiology 80
　　histopathology of 80
　　management of 80, 83
　　pathogenesis of 64, 80
Diabetic peripheral neuropathy 28
　　chronic sensorimotor 81
Diabetic retinopathy 18, 28, 64-67
Diarrhea 243
Diastolic blood pressure 83
Diet 23
　　and nutrition 72
Dopamine 260
　　agonist 144, 145
　　on fetus 146
　　resistance 145

Drug 212
　　choice of 165
　　treatment 144
Dual energy X-ray absorptiometry
　　advantage of 215
　　disadvantage of 215
Ductal obstruction 293
Dyslipidemia 92, 94, 96
　　clinical manifestations of 94
　　management of 94
　　primary 92
　　secondary 92

E

Early morning hyperglycemia 55
Ectopic adrenocorticotropic
　　hormone syndrome 225,
　　235
Eflornithine cream 313
Electrocardiogram 28
Electrocardiography 164
Embryo intrafallopian transfer 318
Empty Sella syndrome 125
Endocrine 290, 298
　　disorder 212, 293, 337
　　　　evidence of 304
　　hypertension 250
　　　　causes of 250
　　neoplasia, multiple 339
　　pancreatic function test 23
　　tumor 325
Endoscopic retrograde cholangio-
　　　　pancreatography 21
Endoscopy 244
Epilepsy 232
Erectile dysfunction 84, 301, 303, 304
　　etiology of 302
　　in diabetes, etiology of 303
　　pathophysiological basis of 302
Erectile function, physiology of 301
Erythropoiesis stimulating agent 75
Erythropoietin 74, 75
　　therapy, monitoring of 75
Escherichia coli 39, 354
Estimated average glucose 9
Estrogen 219, 334
　　preparation 333
　　receptor modulator,
　　　　selective 219
Euglycemic ketoacidosis 58
Excessive sweating 84
Exercise 25, 350
　　benefits of 25

contraindications of 27
during pregnancy 29
during Ramadan 29
during sick days 29
tolerance test 28
types of 25
Exocrine pancreas, disease of 3
Exocrine pancreatic function tests 23
Exophthalmos 162
Ezetimibe 95

F

Fabry disease 353
Familial/genetic short stature,
    criteria for 153
Fasting glucose, impaired 18
Fasting lipid profile 8
Fasting plasma glucose 33
Fatigue overtones 202
Fecal chymotrypsin test 23
Fecundability 289
Fecundity 289
Female infertility 314
    causes of 314
Fenofibrate 95
Ferriman-Gallwey scale 307
Fetal growth, monitoring of 103
Fetal life 272
    to puberty, endocrine changes
        from 271
Fever 243
Fibrate 96
Fibric acid derivatives 95
Fibrocalculous pancreatic
    diabetes 20
    complications of 22
    epidemiology of 20
    etiopathogenesis of 20
    heterogenecity of 22
    management of 23
Flucloxacillin 89
Fluid
    intake 113
    replacement 60
    restriction 72
Fluorodeoxyglucose 261
Fluvastatin 95
Folate deficiency 76
Folic acid supplementation 100
Follicle-stimulating hormone 121
Follicular adenoma, benign 192
Follicular carcinoma 195
Follicular cells 192
Foot deformity, severe 86
Fracture risk assessment tool 215
Friedewald equation 94
Fructosamine 9
Fuel metabolism
    in aerobic exercise 26
    in anaerobic exercise 26
Fulminant hepatic necrosis 168
Fundus fluorescein angiography 65
Fungal infections 114

G

Gadolinium enhancement 230
Galactorrhea 143
Galactosemia 354
    clinical features 354
    treatment 354
Gamete intrafallopian transfer 318
Gastroparesis 84
Gaucher disease 353
Gemfibrozil 95
Genetic susceptibility 160
Genetic testing 261
Genital examination 304
Genital tract
    abnormalities 290
    infections 293
Genitalia 274
Gestational diabetes mellitus 4, 101
    complications of 101
    manage 102
    screening for 101
Giant cell thyroiditis 185
Gigantism 133
Glaucoma 68
Glibenclamide 32
Gliclazide 32
Glimepiride 32
Glipizide 32
Glomerular filtration rate 69
Glucocorticoid 175, 240, 248
    classify 246
    induced osteoporosis 212
    insufficiency 238
    judicious use of 246, 247
    metabolic effects of 247
    properties of 247
    replacement 124, 243
    therapeutic use of 246
    treatment 247
Gluconeogenesis 58
Glucose
    metabolism 58
    suppression 137
    tolerance, impaired 5, 18
Glucotoxicity 16
Glutamic acid decarboxylase 14
Gluteofemoral obesity 348
Glyburide 32
Glycated hemoglobin 8
Glycemic control 73
    goals of 30
    good 83
Glycemic targets 99
    during pregnancy 102
Glycogen storage disease 352
Glycogenesis 58, 352
Glycogenolysis 58
Glycolysis 58
Goitrous hypothyroidism, causes
    of 178
Gonadal dysfunction 143
Gonadal dysgenesis 321
Gonadal failure 279
Gonadotropins 318
Gout 364
    acute 365
    clinical features of 365
    investigations of 365
    management of 365
Graves' disease 160, 164, 186
    drug treatment of 165
    drugs used in 167
    eye
        changes in 163
        signs of 162
    indication of surgical treatment
        of 170
    medical treatments to 168
    pathogenesis of 160
    potential risk factors for 160
    surgical treatment of 170
Graves' ophthalmopathy 174
    activity of 174
    pathogenesis of 161
    severity of 175
    treatment of 175
Growth and puberty, constitutional
    delay in 275, 278
Growth failure 155, 347
Growth hormone
    deficiency 155
        clinical features of 155
        diagnose 156

diabetogenic effect of 134
hypersecretion, causes of 134
ketogenic effect of 134
physiology of 134
replacement 124
response 158
stimulation test
    with clonidine 156
    with levodopa 156
    testing 156
    precaution about 156
therapy 157, 158
    adverse effects of 157
    monitoring of 157
Gynecomastia 298-300
    causes of 298

H

HAIR-AN syndrome 311
Hashimoto thyroiditis 178, 187
Health benefits of fasting 108
Heart rate 83
    fixed 82
    resting 83
Heat intolerance 136
Hematocrit 288
Hematological disorder 212
Hemochromatosis 356
    causes 356
    clinical features 356
    investigations 356
    management 356
Hemoglobinopathy 76
Hemolytic disorder, chronic 356
Hemorrhage 251
Hepatic disease 96
Hepatic form 352
Hepatolenticular degeneration 355
Hereditary hemochromatosis 356
Hidden menstruation 324
Hirsutism 307, 308, 313
Homocystinuria 346
Homogentisic acid, oxidation of 351
Hormonal therapy,
        monitoring of 269
Hormone 58
    in pubertal growth spurt,
        role of 272
Hormone replacement therapy 333
    benefit of 333
    common regimen of 334
    contraindications of 333
    duration of 334
    indication of 332, 333

    risks of 333
    types of 334
Hot flushes 330
Human insulin 45
Huner's test 284, 293
Hurthle cell carcinoma 192
Hydrocortisone 247
Hygiene hypothesis 13
Hyperalgesia 81
Hyperandrogenic state 325
Hyperandrogenism 310, 311
Hypercalcemia 198-200, 339
    asymptomatic 201
    causes of 199
    mild 201
    severe 201
    treatment of 201
Hypercalcemic crisis 201
Hypercholesterolemia 94
    secondary 92
Hyperfunctioning 165
Hyperglycemia 105
    intermediate 6
Hyperglycemic neuropathy 81
Hypergonadotropic hypogonadism 275, 278, 279, 289
Hyperinsulinemia 310
Hyperlipidemia 92
Hyperosmolar nonketotic coma 57, 58, 62
    clinical features of 63
Hyperparathyroid
    bone disease 77, 202
    kidney disease 202
Hyperparathyroidism 77
    primary 79, 202, 203
    secondary 77
    severe 76
    tertiary 79
Hyperprolactinemia 143, 144
    case of drug induced 146
    causes of 142
Hypertension 69
    control of 66, 73
Hypertensive retinopathy 67
Hyperthyroidism 159
    accelerated 171
    risks of subclinical 173
    subclinical 173
Hypertrichosis 307
Hypertriglyceridemia 94
    secondary 92
Hyperuricemia, etiology of 364

Hypocalcemia 205, 206, 208
    acute 208
    case of 208
    causes of 205
    chronic 208
Hypocalciuric hypercalcemia,
        familial benign 200
Hypofunctioning 165
Hypoglycemia 51, 52, 54, 55, 57
    associated autonomic failure 52
    causes of 53
    clinical features of 51
    complications of 54
    first defense against 52
    in type 1 diabetes 27
    in type 2 diabetes 28
    mild 54, 55
    relative 54
    second defense against 52
    severe 54, 55, 108
    spontaneous 343
    third defense against 52
    unawareness 52
Hypogonadal states 212
Hypogonadism 289, 298
    evidence of 303
    hypogonadotropic 275, 278, 279, 289, 293
    low testosterone, primary 279
    secondary 279
    symptoms of 303
Hypomagnesemia 361
    clinical features 361
    etiology 361
    investigations 361
    treatment 361
Hypophosphatemia 209
Hypopigmentation 347
Hypopituitarism 121, 123
    causes of 121
    clinical features of 121
    investigate 122
Hypothalamic disorder 121
Hypothalamic pituitary
    disorder 279
    testicular axis, normal 280
Hypothyroidism 177, 180-182
    causes of 177
    clinical features of 178
    in pregnancy 183
        complications of 183
        treatment of 183
    management of subclinical 185
    preclinical 184
    subclinical 184

I

Iatrogenic Cushing's syndrome 223
Ibandronate 218
Idiopathic hyperprolactinemia 142
Illness, severe 244
Impotence 301
In vitro fertilization 318, 319
 procedure of 319
Incretin 32, 36
 based therapy 36
 hormones 36
 effect of 37
Infections 4, 76, 237
Infertility 289, 313
 secondary 289
 unexplained 319
Inflammation 76
Influence puberty 271
Insemination
 procedure of 319
 timing of 319
Insulin 39, 44, 45, 103
 absorption 42
 action of 41
 genetic defects of 3
 adverse effects of 41
 analogs 49
 autoantibodies 14
 dose adjustment 110
 hyposecretion, relative 105
 induced hypoglycemia test 156
 inhaled 44
 initiation guideline 48
 injection sites 42
 metabolic effects of 41
 neuritis 81
 regimen, types of 45
 sensitizers 32, 34
 synthesis 40
 therapy, indication of 103
 tolerance test 156
 vial syringe mismatch of 43
Insulin administration
 routes of 42
 technique of 42
Insulin resistance 17, 105, 310
 in adipose tissue 17
 in liver 17
 in muscle 18
 mechanism of 17
 syndrome 348
Insulin secretion
 abnormalities of 16
 causes of abnormalities of 16
 mechanism of 40
 pattern of 40
Insulinoma 343, 345
Insulitis 14
Intercurrent illness 243
Intermittent porphyria, acute 357
Intracranial calcification, causes of 132
Intracytoplasmic sperm injection 320
Intraurethral alprostail 306
Intrauterine insemination 318
 indication of 319
Intravenous insulin infusion, indications of 48
Invasive localizing studies 203
Iodide
 excess 160
 induced hyperthyroidism 160
 transport inhibitor 168
Iodine
 agent 168
 deficiency 165
Iodine-containing agent 168
Iron 75
 deficiency 76
 overload, secondary 356
 replacement, indication of 76
 therapy 76
 targets of 76
Islands of Langerhans 39
Islet antigen 2 autoantibodies 14
Islets of Langerhans 39
Isolated gonadotropin deficiency 275
Isosexual precocious puberty, incomplete 335
Isosexual precocity 335

J

Jendrassik sign 162
Jod Basedow effect 160
Joffroy sign 162
Joints 202
Juxtaglomerular apparatus 250

K

Kallmann syndrome 296
Kayser-Fleischer rings 355
Keith-Wagener-Barker classification 67
Keratitis 162
Ketoacidosis 105
Ketogenesis 58
 hormonal regulation of 58
Ketone bodies 63
Ketosis
 causes of 63
 resistant 22
Kidney disease
 chronic 33
 stages of chronic 70
Klinefelter syndrome 289, 295

L

Lactic acidosis 57
Laser treatment, complications of 67
Laurence-Moon-Bardet-Biedl syndrome 297
Leg arteries, anatomical position of 88
Leg ulcer, causes of 91
Lens 346
Leptin 272
Letrozole 318
Levothyroxine therapy for benign nodule 191
Lid retraction 162
Light skin color 347
Linagliptin 32
Lipid
 metabolism 41
 presence of 222
 regulating drug 95, 98
Lithium 168
 therapy 200
Liver disease 355
Localized osteoporosis 212
Low turnover disease 77
Lymphocytic thyroiditis 187
Lymphoma 192
Lysosomal storage disease 353

M

Macroadenoma 146, 147
Macroglossia 137
Macroprolactinemia 141
Macroprolactinoma 143, 144
Maculopathy 66
Male factor infertility 319
Male hypogonadism 279, 281
 etiology of 279

Index

Male infertility 289, 290
  causes of 289
  evaluate 294
Male turner syndrome 296
Malnutrition 20, 76
Marfan syndrome 346
Marshall stage 274
Meal plan 112
Medullary carcinoma 192, 195
  management of 196
  treatment of 196, 197
Meglitinides 32, 33
Menopausal transition 330
Menopause 330
  artificial 330
  early 330
  induced 330
  late 330
  management for 331
  premature 330
  symptoms of 330
  types of 330
Mental retardation 346, 347
Metabolic syndrome 348
Metaiodobenzylguanidine 261
Metanephrine 260
Metastasis 263
Metastatic malignancy 238
Metformin 32, 35, 103, 109, 312, 317
  metabolic of 34
  vascular effects of 34
Methimazole 166
Methylprednisolone 247
Metronidazole 89
Microadenoma 146, 147
Microalbuminuria 70
Micronutrient deficiency 21
Microprolactinoma 143, 144
Midnight salivary cortisol 228
Midnight serum cortisol 229
Miglitol 32
Mineralocorticoid
  insufficiency 238
  replacement 243
Mobius sign 162
Mohan's diagnostic criteria 21
Multinodular goiter 164
Myocardial infarction 18
Myocardial ischemia 18
Myopathic form 352
Myxedema 178
  coma 183
    mortality rate of 184

N

National Cholesterol Education
  Program 348
National Institute of Health
  Criteria 309
Neck, ultrasonography of 164
Necrobiosis lipoidica
  dibeticorum 115
Nelson syndrome 234
Neonatal diabetes 14
Neonatal hypoglycemia 104
Nephrocalcinosis 339
Nephrogenic diabetes insipidus
  148, 150
Nephropathy, screening for 100
Neurological disease 355
Neurological examination 304
Neuromuscular manifestations 206
Neuropathic ulcer 91
Neuropathy, screening for 100
Newborn
  infants 178
  screening 178
Niacin 95, 97
Nicotinic acid 95
Niemann-Pick disease 353
Nocturnal hypoglycemia 54
Nodule in thyroid scan, types of 165
Nonalcoholic fatty liver disease 362
  classification of 362
  clinical features 362
  investigation 362
  management 363
  prognosis 363
Nonalcoholic steatohepatitis 362
Nonesterified fatty acid 26
Nonfunctioning nodule, benign 190
Nongoitrous hypothyroidism,
  causes of 178
Nonthyroidal illness 165
Noonan syndrome 296
Normetanephrine 260

O

Obesity 311, 348
  complication of 349
  management of 349
Ochronosis 351
Oligomenorrhea 324
Opioids 83
Optical coherence tomography 65
Oral antidiabetic drugs 30
  contraindication of 30
  failure 38
  indication of 30
Oral candidiasis 114
Oral glucose tolerance test 5, 22
  importance of 5
Oral iron preparations 77
Oral route, disadvantages of 333
Oral sodium loading test 253
Oral testosterone undecanoate 287
Orbital decompression 176
Organic erectile dysfunction 302
Osteitis fibrosa cystica 77
Osteomalacia 77, 209, 210, 359
  causes of 209
  clinical features of 209
Osteomyelitis 89
Osteoporosis 77, 143, 202, 211, 213,
  216, 346
  causes of secondary 212
  classification of 211
  clinical features of 213
  diagnosis of 213
  drug used for 218, 219
  nonpharmacological
    treatment of 216
  pathophysiology of 211
  primary 211
  secondary 211
    cause of 213
  treatment for 220
Osteoporotic fracture,
  surgery for 220
Osteosclerosis 77
Ovulation induction 317
Ovulatory disorders 317
Oxidative stress 21

P

Painful bones 202
Painful diabetic peripheral
  neuropathy 83
Painful gynecomastia, causes of 299
Pancreatic islets 37
Pancreatic structure, tests of 23
Pancreaticojejunostomy, role of 24
Panhypopituitarism 121
Papillary carcinoma 192, 193, 195
Para aminobenzoic acid test 23
Paraganglioma 257
Parathyroid
  dependent hypercalcemia 199
  gland
    abnormal 203
    anatomy of 201

independent hypercalcemia 199
related disorder 205
Parathyroidectomy 204
    complications of 204
Pendred syndrome 180
Penile abnormalities 302
Penile prosthesis 306
Percutaneous ethanol injection 191
Perimenopause transition 330
Periodic paralysis 171
Peripheral densitometry 215
Peripheral precocious puberty 336
Peripubertal gonadotropin
    increase 272
Petrosal sinus sampling, inferior 230
Pharmacological treatment 255
    of hirsutism 313
Phenylethanolamine
        N-methyltransferase 256
Phenylketonuria 347
Pheochromocytoma 256-259,
        261-263
    case of 260, 264
    clinical features of 258
    complications of 259
    differential diagnosis of 259
    in pregnancy, treat 265
Phosphate
    homeostasis, disorder of 209
    restriction 72
Phychogenic erectile dysfunction 302
Pioglitazone 32
Pituitary adenoma 126, 127
    causes of 126
    clinical features of 126
    types of 126
Pituitary apoplexy 124
Pituitary disorder 121, 142
Pituitary gigantism 133
Pituitary hormone deficiency 122
Pituitary incidentaloma 130
    case of 130
    differential diagnoses of 130
    surgery for 131
Pituitary infertility 289
Pituitary macroadenoma 126
Pituitary microadenoma 126
Pituitary radiotherapy 128
Pituitary stimulation insulin
        tolerance test 123
Plain X-ray abdomen 23
Plasma
    cortisol, diurnal rhythm of 229

fractionated
    catecholamines 260
    metanephrines 260
    glucose 102
Pneumonia 244
Polycystic ovarian syndrome 7,
        309, 310
    diagnostic criteria of 309
    pathogenesis of 309
    treatment of 312
Polycystic ovaries, criteria of 311
Polydipsia, primary 150
Porphyria cutanea tarda 356, 358
Postcoital test, motility evaluation
        on 284
Postexercise growth hormone
        stimulation test 156
Postmenopausal women 214
Postmenopause
    early 330
    late 330
Postpituitary surgery 129
Postural hypotension 82-84
Potassium
    replacement 61
    restriction 72
Prader-Willi syndrome 297
Pravastatin 95
Prebreak fast hyperglycemia 55
Precocious puberty 335
    etiology of 335
    incomplete 335
    management of 335
    types of 335
Prediabetes 6, 116
    categories of 6
Prednisolone 247
Pregnancy 160, 232
    on tumor size 146
Premature ovarian failure 320
Premixed insulin 45, 46
    regimen 109
Pretibial myxedema 176
Priapism 306
Progesterone 334
    adverse effects of 334
    challenge test 327
    preparation 334
Progressive weight gain,
        etiology of 349
Prolactin 141
Prolactinoma 141, 142, 144
    clinical features of 143

in pregnancy 146
select therapy for 146
treatment of 145
Proliferative diabetic retinopathy 66
    complications of 67
Prominent supraorbital ridge 137
Protein
    energy malnutrition 20
    excretion in urine, normal 70
    kinase C activation 19
    metabolism 41
    restriction 72
    sparer effect of growth
        hormone 134
Proximal myopathy
    endocrine cause of 137
    metabolic cause of 137
Pseudo-Cushing syndrome 223, 232
Pseudohypoparathyroidism 207
    resistance 207
Pseudomonas 114
Pseudopseudohypoparathyroidism
        207
Psychic moans 202
Psychological stress 14
Psychosexual therapy 305
Puberty 271
    stages of 274
Pubic hair 274
Pure red cell aplasia 76
Pyogenic thyroiditis, acute 186
Pyridoxine 346

R

Radiation, external 175
Radioactive iodine
    therapy 169
    uptake test 163
Radiology 178
Radiotherapy 139, 145
    focal forms of 128
Raloxifene 219
Rapid acting analogs 49
    advantages of 50
    disadvantage of 50
Reaven syndrome 348
Recurrent abortion 337
Recurrent stone formers 338
Renal bone disease 77, 78
    clinical features of 78
    treatment of 78
Renal defect 359
Renal disease 96

Index

Renal failure 232
Renal impairment, progressive 365
Renal osteodystrophy 77
   components of 77
Renal parenchyma 339
Renal stone 202, 337, 359
   intervention of 338
   types of 337
Renal tubular acidosis 359
   investigations of 359
   types of 359
Renin angiotensin system 251
Repaglinide 32
Reproductive endocrinology 271
Resistance exercise 25
   benefits of 26
Retinal assessment 103
Retinal detachment, fractional 66
Retinopathy, screening for 100
Retrograde ejaculation 293
Rheumatological disorder 213
Rickets 209, 210
   causes of 209
   clinical features of 209
Risedronate 218
Rosiglitazone 32
Rosuvastatin 95
Rothera's test 63
Rotterdam criteria 309

S

Saline infusion test 254
Salmon calcitonin 219
Salt restriction 72
Sarcoidosis 200
Sarcoma 192
Seizure 347
Sella and parasellar mass,
   differential diagnosis
   of 129
Semen
   analysis 285
   preparation 319
Seminiferous tubule dysgenesis 295
Senescence 330
Sensory neuropathy, acute 81
Serum
   calcium 198
   chromogranin A 260
   gonadal steroids 278
   gonadotropins 278
   testosterone 287
      level 283
   uric acid 364

Sex hormone
   bonding globulin 283
   replacement 124
Sexual dysfunction 290, 301
Sheehan syndrome 124
Short stature 152, 153, 155
   criteria of constitutional 153
   etiology of 152
   idiopathic 153
Short synacthen test 240
Sick thyroid syndrome 165
Sick-day management 112
Sideroblastic anemia 356
Sildenafil 305
Simvastatin 95
Sitagliptin 32
Sleep apnea syndrome 137
Snow flake cataract 67
Sodium
   bicarbonate 61
   glucose cotransporter 2
      inhibitors 38
Solitary thyroid nodule 188
   differential diagnosis of 188
Sperm
   antibodies to 293
   cervical mucus contact test 284
   concentration 286
   penetration assay 284
Spironolactone 313
Split mixed regimen 46
   insulin 109
Spontaneous atrophic
   hypothyroidism 178
Staphylococcus aureus 114
Statins 96
Steatorrhea 21, 23
Stein-Leventhal syndrome 309
Stellwag sign 162
Sterility 289
Steroid 249
   biosynthesis 267
   bracelet 245
   card 244
   contraindications of 246
   withdrawal protocol 249
Stimulated tests 156
Stress 160
   diabetes 6
   ketosis 58
Struma ovarii 176
Subclinical hypothyroidism,
   treatment of 185

Subcutaneous T pellets 287
Sulfonylurea 32, 33, 109
Surgery
   contraindications of 170
   preparation for 170
Sweating, endocrine causes of
   increased 162
Systemic disease, evidence of 304
Systemic disorders 142
Systemic illness 302
Systemic metastatic calcification 200

T

T replacement, contraindication
   of 288
T_4 overdose, adverse effects of 182
Tachycardia, resting 82
Tadalafil 305
Tanner stage 274
Target uric acid 366
Teratoma 192
Teriparatide 219
Testicular insult 289
Testosterone
   enanthate 287
   gel 287
   preparations 287
   replacement therapy 286, 288
      indications of 286
   treatment, monitoring
      during 287
   undecanoate 287
Tetracosactide 240
Thalassemia 356
Thiazide diuretics 199
Thiazolidinediones 35, 36, 109
Thionamides, mechanism of
   action of 166
Thromboembolism 346
Thyroglobulin 164
Thyroid
   color flow Doppler of 164
   dermopathy 176
   disorders 159
   failure, early 184
   function tests, indications of 180
   neoplasm 192
   ophthalmopathy 164
   peroxidase 164
   reserve, decreased 184
   scan 163, 165
   scintigraphy 163, 190

stimulating hormone 121
surgery, complications of 170
tumors 192
USG 189
Thyroid autoantibodies 163
  prevalence of 164
Thyroid hormone
  extrathyroidal source of 160
  peripheral resistance to 177
  replacement 124
Thyroid nodules 188
  evaluate 188
  fate of untreated 191
  features of malignant 189
  investigation of 189
Thyroid storm 171
  causes of death and mortality rate of 171
  treatment of 171
Thyroiditis 160, 185
  causes of 185
  chronic 187
Thyrotoxic crisis 171
Thyrotoxicosis 159, 163, 199
  causes of 159
  clinical features of 161
  factitia 176
  high uptake 165
  in children and elderly, features of 162
  in pregnancy 173
    treatment of 174
  low uptake 164
Thyroxine replacement 182
Tibial artery, posterior 88
Tissue, connective 331
Tongue, large 137
Tophaceous gout, chronic 365
Total sperm count 286
Toxic substances 14

Transdermal route 333
Transdermal testosterone patch 287
Transient thyroiditis 164
Trans-sphenoidal
  pituitary surgery 128
  surgery 234
Triamcinolone 247
Tropical calcific diabetes 20
True precocious puberty 335
Tubal disorder 314
Tuberculous Addison disease 237
Tumor
  effects of 136
  type 192
Turner syndrome 321

U

Unconsciousness, causes of 56
Urate lowering drug, indication of 365
Uric acid
  calculi 365
  high 73
  metabolism of 364
Urinary fractionated catecholamines 260
Urine routine microscopic examination 22
Uterine factors 314

V

Vacuum devices, external 306
Vaginismus, severe 319
Valsalva maneuver 83
Vanillylmandelic acid 260
Vardenafil 305
Varicocele 293
Vascular assessment 304

Vascular surgery 306
Vasomotor symptoms 339
Vildagliptin 32
Viral infection 13, 160
Vision
  causes of loss of 68
  sudden loss of 68
Vitamin
  B_{12} 76
  B_3 95
  D
    deficiency 205
    disorder of 205, 209
    intoxication 199
Vitrectomy 67
Vitreous hemorrhage 66
Vomiting 243
von Graefe sign 162

W

Warm and sweaty hand 136
Water deprivation test 149
Weight gain but weakness 136
Weight loss 312
  mechanism of 350
Wermer syndrome 340
Werner classification 163
Whipple's triad 51
Wilson disease 355
World Health Organization 20

Z

Zinc transporter and autoantibodies 14
Zoledronic acid 219
  precaution for 218
Zona pellucida binding test 284
Zygote intrafallopian transfer 318

EU GSPR Authorised Reprsentative
Logos Europe, 9 rue Nicolas Poussin
1700, La Rochelle, France
Phone: +33 (0) 6 67 93 73 78
E-mail: contact@logoseurope.eu

www.ingramcontent.com/pod-product-compliance
Ingram Content Group UK Ltd.
Pitfield, Milton Keynes, MK11 3LW, UK
UKHW050456150426
5217IPUK00025B/1709